Britta Rutert
Contested Properties

Culture and Social Practice

Britta Rutert, born 1974, works as a research associate at Charité Universitätsmedizin Berlin. She received her PhD from Free University Berlin in 2016. She is also an ethnographic researcher at the Open African Innovation Research (openAIR) Network.

BRITTA RUTERT

Contested Properties

Peoples, Plants and Politics in Post-Apartheid South Africa

[transcript]

Bibliographic information published by the Deutsche Nationalbibliothek
The Deutsche Nationalbibliothek lists this publication in the Deutsche Nationalbibliografie; detailed bibliographic data are available in the Internet at http://dnb.d-nb.de

Cover layout: Maria Arndt, Bielefeld

Print-ISBN 978-3-8376-4794-5
PDF-ISBN 978-3-8394-4794-9
https://doi.org/10.14361/9783839447949

Contents

Acronyms and Abbreviations

ABS	Access and benefit sharing
ACB	African Centre for Biosafety
ANT	Actor-Network Theory
BCP	Biocultural Community Protocol
CBD	Convention on Biological Diversity
CEO	Chief Executive Officer
CITES	Convention of International Trade in Endangered Species of Flora and Fauna
COP	Conference of the Parties
CSIR	Council for Scientific and Industrial Research
DAC	Department of Arts and Culture
DAFF	Department of Agriculture, Forestry and Fishery
DEAT	Department of Environmental Affairs and Tourism
DoH	Department of Health
DST	Department of Science and Technology
DTI	Department of Trade and Industry
F2P	Farmer to Pharma
GATT	General Agreement on Tariffs and Trade
GTZ	Gesellschaft für Technische Zusammenarbeit
GUCM	Guangzhou University of Chinese Medicine

HIV/AIDS	Human Immunodeficiency virus/ Acquired Immune Deficiency Syndrome
HPLC	High Performance Liquid Chromatography
IKS	Indigenous Knowledge Systems (Health) Lead Program
IP	Intellectual Property
IPR	Intellectual Property Rights
IPUF	Indigenous Plant Use Forum
K2C	Kruger to Canyon (Biosphere Region)
LC-MS	Liquid Chromatography-Mass Spectrometry
MCC	Medicines Control Council
MOU	Memorandum of Understanding
MRC	Medical Research Council
MTA	Material Transfer Agreement
NDA	Non-Disclosure Agreement
NEMBA	(South African) National Environmental Biodiversity Act
NEPAD	New Partnership for Africa's Development
NGO	Non Governmental Organization
NIKSO	National Indigenous Knowledge Systems Office
PIC	Prior Informed Consent
PTO	Permission to occupy
R& D	Research and Development
SAHGA	South African Hoodia Growers Association
SAWC	South African Wildlife College
SMME	Small, Medium and Macro Enterprise
STS	Science and Technology Studies
TB	Tuberculosis

THO	Traditional Healers Organization
THPB	Traditional Health Practitioners of Bushbuckridge
TICIPS	The International Centre for Indigenous Phytotherapy Studies
TLC	Thin Layer Chromatography
TRAMED	Traditional Medicine Database
TRIPS	Trade-Related Aspects of Intellectual Property Rights
UCT	University of Cape Town
UWC	University of the Western Cape
WIPO	World Intellectual Property Organization
WTO	World Trade Organization

Chapter I
Opening Pandora's Box: Bioprospecting in South Africa

> Writing is a question of becoming, always
> incomplete, always in the midst of being
> formed, and goes beyond the matter of any
> livable or lived experience. It is a process,
> that is, a passage of Life that traverses both
> the livable and the lived.
> Gilles Deleuze (1997: 1)

Introduction: A Plant Exchange in Thulamahashe

In November 2011, nine people of different ethnic groups and languages gathered in a small, dusky room of a guesthouse on the road between Thulamahashe and Acornhoek, two of the foremost trading towns in Bushbuckridge Municipality, Mpumalanga Province, South Africa. The group was assembled around bags and bottles filled with medicinal plants and extracts. The white tattered plastic bags typically used for maize powder were filled with green leaves, which left a soapy sensation when rubbed between the fingers. Aged, dusty Klipdrift brandy bottles held a brown oily liquid. The executive committee of the Kukula Traditional Healers Association (hereafter Kukula Healers) had brought the bags and bottles to the meeting, which had been arranged to share the plant material and selected knowledge associated with it with the local cosmetic company Godding & Godding, which specializes in cosmetic silk products with 'African additives' such as Baobab or Marula essence. The company was represented by two members of the Kruger to Canyon (K2C) Management Committee, an organization that manages activities in the Kruger to Canyon Biosphere Region.

The meeting was not the first between the Kukula Healers and the K2C committee members. Together with the non-profit organization Natural Justice, a bio-cultural community protocol (BCP) had been developed over the preceding three years to ensure the healers' custody of and stewardship over their traditional knowledge and natural resources. But it was actually the first time since this ongoing cooperation that plant material and associated knowledge were being exchanged. Indeed, such an 'official' exchange had never occurred before in the region. Prevailing segregation between black and white citizens, a vestige of colonial and Apartheid politics, still characterizes the region. Ultimately, it was global, national and regional political developments, as well as the efforts of NGOs and the government to bridge past and present inequalities by means of local community empowerment and poverty alleviation that made this meeting possible.

It was my first week in the K2C region, and the first time I was meeting the Kukula Healers. Rodney Sibuyi, the healers' tall, self-confident and determined chief executive officer (CEO), introduced himself and his fellow healers. The members of the K2C committee, Marie-Tinka Uys and Debby Thompson, two women from the neighboring Maruleng Municipality, also introduced themselves and briefly explained the purpose of the meeting. After the introductions, they sat together with the healers to write down the names of the plants, the parts used for treatment, the method of preparation and the purpose of use. As an observer who had not been involved in the preliminary meetings, I noticed a sense of wariness and politeness on the part of the K2C committee. Marie-Tinka was vigilant and diplomatic, while Debby was more direct, demanding and fact-oriented. Carefully, Marie-Tinka explained what would happen to the exchanged material and repeatedly ensured the confidential treatment of the plant material and knowledge at all times. The laboratory of the cosmetic company would receive the material and information for content analysis, and later, if a product was eventually developed and marketed, an access and benefit sharing (ABS) agreement would be negotiated between the concerned parties. Product development, however, is an interminable, unpredictable and expensive process, for which success cannot be guaranteed.

At first glance, the meeting seemed efficient and framed by mutual respect and acceptance between the two parties. I was curious, however, about the ambivalent attitude of the K2C members, somewhere between politeness, cautiousness and business engagement. Obviously, they were aware that sharing plants and knowledge is a sensitive, yet lucrative matter. The healers, in contrast, seemed confident about the value of plant material and relaxed in their interaction with the K2C members. Later, Marie-Tinka told me that it had taken three years of ongoing cooperation to build trust between the K2C committee and the healers. A non-disclosure agreement (NDA) had been negotiated between the healers and Godding & Godding that ensured the confidential treatment of the shared knowledge. Rodney, in contrast to Marie-Tinka, said that the healers had never had an issue with sharing their knowledge, as long as they came to an agreement. I also learned later that the healers generally trusted the K2C committee, but secretly had an issue with Debby, whom they alleged had given some of the shared plant material to a German cosmetic company without informing them. Although this accusation turned out to have no valid grounds, it nonetheless reveals an underlying tension between the healers and the K2C committee, and a protective and circumspect attitude of the healers towards their property.

I came to know in a later interview with the cosmetic company owner that the plant material had been analyzed but had so far (as of my last contact with her in March 2012) been found to have little marketable cosmetic value. She said: "There is a bit of sun block factor in the oily plant extract, but it is not high enough for a product. And the soapy plant unfortunately leaves a burning sensation on the scalp skin. We can't use it for our shampoo series." When I asked Rodney during a conference in Cape Town in 2013 about what had happened with the plants, he almost indignantly replied: "Ah no, they never came back to us to inform us what happened to our plants." What Rodney did not know was that Godding & Godding had encountered serious problems with the government for not having complied correctly with the bioprospecting regulations of the South African Biodiversity Act (2004). They had allegedly not conducted the necessary administrative work for the exchange of plant materials, as well as other earlier bioprospecting activities. The healers did not know about these behind-the-scenes rumors due to their lack of direct communication with the company, since all communication between the two parties was mediated by Marie-Tinka.

The plant exchange had therefore been arranged and carried out with great expectation and hope, but ended in a slew of consequences that eventually led to disappointing outcomes for both parties: no new cosmetic product for Godding & Godding, and no shared benefits for the Kukula Healers. And yet were the interactions themselves invaluable.

Situating the Field: Research Questions and Contextualization

The plant exchange in Thulamahashe is an example of bioprospecting, a process that was first defined as "chemical prospecting" (Eisner 1989, see also 1994) and was then re-defined as "biodiversity prospecting" (Reid et al. 1993, Reid 2002). Today, bioprosecting is being applied as "the exploitation and utilization of biological diversity for commercial purposes" (Soejarto et al. 2005: 16). This definition delineates the scientific exploration and utilization of biological or genetic resources for commercial purposes, either within or beyond the context of traditional knowledge (ibid.). When traditional or indigenous knowledge[1] is involved, bioprospecting comprises many questions and challenges, which come into being at a particu-

---

1   The terms 'indigenous' and 'traditional' are often used interchangeably, depending on when they are used and by whom (cf. Anderson 2009: 5ff). In this book, I will also use both terms interchangeably according to the context and user. For a detailed discussion about the con-

lar moment in the bioprospecting activity, namely *the moment of knowledge disclosure*. During the plant exchange in Thulamahashe, the Kukula Healers exchanged medicinal plants and disclosed associated knowledge via the K2C committee members to the cosmetic company Godding & Godding. The exchange illustrates how the moment of knowledge disclosure assembles different people, materials, interests, motivations, languages, cultural backgrounds and values. Each party involved in the exchange – as with any other exchange – brings with them expectations and values that meet and sometimes collide. Collision, however, has two sides of a coin. Although no product developed from the plant exchange, a working relationship had been established that did not exist before.

Accordingly, this book intends to give voices to the actors involved in the field of bioprospecting in South Africa in the years 2009 to 2012, which are traditional healers[2], scientists, NGO members, politicians, and traders, and to portray their interaction with and use of medicinal plants or muthi[3] by following the trajectory of values attached to medicinal plants and associated but changing knowledge(s) to different sites and environments, here traditional healers' communities in Eastern Cape and Mpumalanga Provinces and a biochemical laboratory in Cape Town. Depicting these changing values will help understanding the clash of these values that can occur in terms of negotiating fair and appropriate ABS agreements and the protection of (indigenous) knowledge and may provide partial resolution on how to make use of these clashes and provide future advance of ABS and knowledge protection politics.

With delineating this trajectory, this book intends to fill existing gaps in research on the bioprospecting of medicinal plants and associated (indigenous) knowledge, an underrepresented area in (South) African anthropology, by looking at the multiple human and non-human actors, which produce these different "regimes of values" (Appadurai 1986). The overall research questions are therein: What values are produced exactly in the field of bioprosecting of medicinal plants, how and by whom are these values produced and why are these values so strongly contested in post-Apartheid South Africa?

---

ceptually and analytically problematic terms 'indigenous', 'indigenous peoples', 'indigenous communities' and 'indigenous knowledge', see page 72.

2   A traditional healer in South Africa is called sangoma or inyanga, depending on the region and ethnic identity of the healer. In this book, I will either use the term traditional healer or *sangoma*, unless the interview partners used a different term.

3   *Muthi* is the South African term for traditional medicinal plants used as medicine for healing purposes or for witchcraft and spells (Ashforth 2005a, 2005b).

Situating the Research Field

To situate the complexity of this 20-month long, multi-sited, ethnographic field re-search project conducted in three different regions of South Africa, and to curtail the stream of actors, sites and situations, emotions and rationales, contexts and content, containment was and is crucial. This book will contribute to the South African bioprospecting discourse by drawing a picture of bioprospecting as a field in the process of "becoming" (Deleuze & Guattari 1987; Biehl & Locke 2010; Rutert et al. 2012), where hope for economic and political participation that biodiversi-ty politics like the Convention on Biological Diversity (CBD) enables, interchanges with rational consideration and contestation over the increasingly growing value of medicinal plants and associated knowledge and the growing global demand for natural products and for information in the global knowledge economy. Because of the breadth and constant flux of these bioprospecting assemblages (Deleuze & Guattari 1987), "complicated new configurations of global, political, technical, bio-logical, and other segments" (Biehl & Locke 2010), and the phenomenon's reach from the past of (colonial) bioprospecting to present activities and agencies and on to future hopes (Hirokazu 2004, 2006) for upcoming products, profits, political articulations and empowerment, containment of the complexity is crucial. Anne-marie Mol and John Law state that "there is complexity if things relate but don't add up, if events occur but not within the process of linear time, and if phenomena share a space but cannot be mapped in terms of a single set of three-dimensional coordinates" (Law and Mol 2002: 2). The complexity of the bioprospecting situation will be contained as depicted below:

First, this research concentrates on bioprospecting of traditional medicinal plants or *muthi*. The term *muthi* is frequently and most commonly used by tra-ditional health practitioners – but also by other South African citizens – and is bound up with indigenous knowledge. Medicinal plants, next to the technologies they are made and preceded with, i.e. the mortar of a traditional healer or the grin-ding machine in a biochemical laboratory, are the main non-human actors of this research.

Second, the many actors, who influence each other interdependently and the-refore cannot be looked at independently, constitute the field of bioprospecting. For the human (i.e. traditional healers and biochemists or pharmacologists) and non-human (i.e. different medicinal plants) actors involved in the field, actor-net-work theory (ANT) provides a methodological framework for their examination. Although it is called a theory, "ANT is not a theory or, if it is, then a theory does not necessarily offer a coherent framework, but may as well be an adaptable, open repository" (Mol 2010: 253). ANT engages with crossing the boundaries of recurring dualisms like natural versus social science (Latour & Wolgar 1986), nature versus culture/society (Latour 2005) or traditional versus modern (Latour 1991), and instead focuses on processes of *translation* between the actors and an analysis of how actors interact with and speak to each other. Translation expels fractures, frictions and failings, but at the same time offers a commonsense code of understanding that enables communication and interaction between the actors (cf. Rottenburg 2012, 2014).

Third, the choice of various research sites situates the work as a multi-sited ethnography (Marcus 1995; Hannerz 2003; Falzon 2009). In my case, multi-sited ethnography methodologically contained the three dispersed and yet geographically centered main research sites and their actors, namely: (i) the IKS Lead Program and its biochemical laboratory in Cape Town; (ii) traditional healers of Eastern Cape Province; and (iii) the Kukula Healers of Bushbuckridge Municipality in Mpumalanga Province. Additional sites emerged through cooperation, encounters and connections made at the IKS Lead Program – as well as those made independently of it – and in cooperation with the Kukula Healers and the NGO Natural Justice.

Fourth, three main analytical categories form the theoretical foundation of this book. Something as highly contested as medicinal plants and associated indigenous knowledge can be regarded as possessing highly valuable tangible and intangible *properties*, which call for thorough contextual scrutiny. Property never stands alone, however, and is always relational to people and the rights of those people to the property (cf. Hann 1989; Benda-Beckmann 2007). A property is also subject to contestation due to the enormous *economic* as well as cultural, *spiritual* and *emotional value* it may have for the property holders. For the ascribed values, property entails several *modes of protection*, depending on the context and the people. Property, values and modes of protection are not neutral or simple concepts. Instead, they are charged with situational and relational dynamics, past and present inadequacies, and confinement; but also with promise, desire and hope. The situational interrelationship of *value, property and knowledge protection* will be unraveled for each site in the chapters.

Fifth, the field was influenced and determined by my own position, first as a researcher in the contested field of bioprospecting, and second as a (white)[4] person from the Global North, in a country still affected by the vestiges of colonialism and Apartheid politics and biopiracy. The many diverse actors and sites, especially with regard to past and present political implications, struck me. Unaware that "bioprospecting is a minefield,"[5] it took me considerable time to adjust to the political diplomacy and cultural sensitivities that a study of bioprospecting requires. Initial

---

4   The terms 'black', 'white' and 'colored' are commonly used in South Africa and in themselves have no racist implications.

5   Quote from a conservation with Dr. Hutchings, a retired biologist at the University of Zululand in Empangeni, KwaZulu-Natal, October 2009.

fruitless interviews and an ostensibly secretive attitude and some rough encounters with interlocutors at the beginning of the research made me aware that the field was challenging, not only due to my own trepidation, but also due to bioprospecting contact zones (Pratt 1992), which constitute of historical influences, current politics and my interlocutors exposure to the field.

Finally, bioprospecting releases hopes, desires and motivations, ignited, among others, by global and national politics. Consequently, new forms of (cultural) agency (Coombe 2011) for indigenous peoples, NGOs, science and government may emanate from current political debates on ABS and the protection of (intellectual) property. The outlined trajectory of the different values attributed to medicinal plants and associated knowledge will lay open the correlations, juxtapositions and frictions that ensue in the contestation of property in terms of ABS and knowledge protection. Eventually, the outlined trajectory may unleash suggestions for a culturally appropriate *sui generis* protection system of intangible (intellectual) property. This is important because it contributes to ideas for future concepts of (indigenous) knowledge protection, also with regard to the United Nations Decade on Biodiversity (2011–2020) intended to "better understand the links between biological and cultural diversity and their implications for policy and actions at various levels, including different regional perspectives." Darrell Posey claims, "global trends that substitute economic and utilitarian models [e.g. TRIPS] for the holistic concept of the 'sacred balance' need to be reversed" (Posey 2002a 3). Although I agree, I would nevertheless argue that instead of a reversal, we need to develop a better understanding of knowledge practices, production, protection and the relationship of these to customary law, the surrounding environment and the larger community. This would add insight to future models of indigenous knowledge protection, beyond common IP protections, and beyond the reverse of current IP-models, to enable new models. This book thus contributes to a better understanding of bioprospecting in South Africa and to future solution for indigenous knowledge disclosure and protection in the wider field of bioprospecting in Africa and beyond.

The Crucial Moment: The Disclosure of Knowledge

The first time I came into contact with the implications of knowledge disclosure was at an excursion to the South African Government's Department of Science and Technology (DST) and the Council for Scientific and Industrial Research (CSIR), both in Pretoria, in February 2009. The director of the Indigenous Knowledge Health Systems Lead Program (from now on IKS Lead Program), Dr. Matsabisa, invited me to join the excursion, which was planned for a Chinese delegation from the Guangzhou University of Chinese Medicine (GUCM). The three Chinese representatives had come to South Africa to negotiate bilateral research exchange on medicinal plants with anti-malarial properties. The two days in Pretoria were packed both with meetings with stakeholders from South African research institutes working in the field of bioprospecting, as well as with an aura of political significance and sensitivity, which was already evident at the entrance gate of the DST, where we were exhaustively screened and registered before we could finally enter the highly secured governmental compound. At the time, I was still a novice in the research field and felt ungainly with regard to my performance as an anthropologist in this highly politicized environment. How much information would people want to reveal to me as an inquiring ethnographer?

Soon after the first meetings, the IKS Lead Program Director, Dr. Matsabisa, rendered possible an interview for me with Mr. Sechaba, CEO of the 'Innovation Hub' in Pretoria and a legal expert working on patent law, innovation and traditional medicine. The Innovation Hub assembles innovative knowledge and technology for scientific innovation. Mr. Sechaba advises the government and research institutes on intellectual property (IP) law, knowledge protection, and ABS agreements. In an interview, he introduced me to the challenges that bioprospecting bestows on its actors. With regard to the politically and legally much debated and as yet unresolved question of how to protect traditional knowledge and fairly share the benefits arising from traditional knowledge-based products, Mr. Sechaba simply suggested: "Patent it or keep it secret"; a shortcut answer for a much more complex situation.

> **BR:** Could you briefly give me an example of the major challenges in the protection of traditional knowledge?
>
> **MS:** Well, if a healer says his medicine is effecting a reduction of the viral load and they [HIV patients] are getting an increase of the CD4 count.[6] That is [a claim for] evidence that this thing [the traditional medicine] is doing something. But is it acting as an immune booster or is it acting as... What is it acting as? So from a patenting point of view, you would then proceed to patent. But it is not so straightforward, because the [plant] species also performs within the ambit of the [South African] Biodiversity Act, which then governs how indigenous plants and other things are processed in the country. And then you have to get [bioprospecting] permits [from the Department of Agriculture and Tourism] and all sorts. So from

---

6   Viral load indicates on the amount of the HIV virus in the blood. CD4 cells are a type of white blood cell that play a major role in protecting the body from infection, and are the most important indicator for HIV patients of the progression of the infection and how well the immune system is functioning. See i.e.: "Fact Sheet 125: Viral Load Tests", AIDS InfoNet, January 23, 2019 (www.aids
infonet.org/fact_sheets/view/125).

a healer's point of view: What is the value of a patent, because a patent is a commercial tool?

BR: Hmm, so what does that mean for the traditional healer?

MS: For the healer, it is in essence getting acknowledged that he provided the basis for scientific development. Because that traditional healer could approach someone like Gilbert [Dr. Gilbert M. Matsabisa, IKS Lead Program] or similar people and will say, "I've got this, but I don't understand the science behind [it]." And then Gilbert and his team start to analyze the medicine and eventually find the active compound.

BR: But that takes years.

MS: Yes, it takes years, but the basis is that particular disclosure. Therefore, there is then some benefit that could be brought back to that particular traditional healer. But to my mind, the patenting system is not very ideal for traditional medicine.

In this small excerpt from the 45 minutes interview I had with Mr. Sechaba, he hints at the crucial moment in bioprospecting, the *moment of knowledge disclosure*. Without the disclosure of knowledge, the protection of this knowledge and the sharing of arising benefits would basically be irrelevant. The giving away and the protection of knowledge have always been relevant in the history of bioprospecting. But it has become an increasingly (political) challenge with the rise of IP law in the global knowledge economy and with the growing international recognition of the urgency to protect rapidly declining global biodiversity. Indigenous knowledge has been recognized as a source when it comes to the utilization of biological and genetic resources, and is progressively being acknowledged as an important part of cultural heritage and identity. Indigenous knowledge in the context of bioprospecting is thus torn between the two poles of utilization and protection.

Ideally, it ought to be a voluntary decision of the knowledge holder(s), in this case traditional healers, to disclose knowledge to interested parties, i.e. researchers or companies. Historically, indigenous peoples might have been less aware of the fact that they could have chosen *not* to disclose knowledge. Today, (some) traditional healers in South Africa seem (more) conscious of the value of their knowledge and the fact that they can refuse disclosure, or at least demand appropriate and fair compensation for the exchange of natural resources and knowledge. This may be the result of the vastly changing biodiversity and human rights landscape since the end of World War II. The global Convention on Biological Diversity (CBD, 1993) and the South African National Environmental Biodiversity Act (NEMBA, 2004), for instance, propose that there should be fair ABS agreements between all parties in case traditional knowledge is involved in the development of a new product. This prospect of potential benefits may have motivated and fortified the voluntary disclosure of valuable (medicinal) knowledge by traditional healers.

Nevertheless, traditional healers still have to meet particular rules of knowledge exchange, sharing and protection that are embedded in a web of socio-cultural, symbolic and spiritual meaning. Accordingly, it might not always be easy for traditional healers to disclose sacred and secret knowledge to scientific or other interested institutions. They might be torn between their own intrinsic rules of knowledge sharing and protection and their hopes for monetary and/or non-monetary benefits, as well as for more political acknowledgement and empowerment in post-Apartheid South Africa. But as George Simmel has stated, wherever there is secrecy, there is the "probability of betrayal (…) The keeping of the secret is something so unstable, the temptation[s] to betrayal are so manifold, in many cases such [a] continuous path leads from secretiveness to indiscretion" (Simmel 1906: 473). Disclosure might also 'simply' be motivated by the wish to share valuable medicinal knowledge that might combat threatening diseases like malaria, HIV/AIDS, tuberculosis, cancer or diabetes, also in light of the idea that research is fundamentally good for humanity and that participation should be rendered "an act of gift-giving or donation rather than secured by undue inducement, that is luring people to participate in research by offering direct returns for their involvement" (Nakazora 2015: 109; see also Merz et al. 2002). And in fact, medicinal plants or a plant mixture may well yield medicinal benefits for millions of people worldwide. Examples such as *Pelargonium sidoides*, available on the market as the respiratory infection remedy *Umckaoloabo®*, or *Artemisia annua*, as Artemisinin in the anti-malaria product *Coartem®*, have been scientifically verified for their medicinal value (cf. Meier zu Biesen 2010, 2013). The role of natural products in new drug discoveries should thus not be underestimated; indeed, of all prescription drugs on the market, it is known that at least 25% derive from plants (Mander & Le Breton 2006: 3).

In this context, medicinal plants play a major yet ambivalent role. Given the high demand for natural resources by the (medicine/pharmaceutical) industry, medicinal plants have often been overused. Garret Hardin's article 'The Tragedy of the Commons' (Hardin 1968) has often been criticized for mistaking the commons to mean open access to resources, which are then abused mainly for self-interest, which stands against the idea of a commons implying the controlled use of resources. Typical threats to knowledge and natural resources as commons are commoditization or enclosure, pollution and degradation, and unsustainable practices (Hess & Ostrom 2011: 5). In contrast to the abuse of the commons, the tragedy of the *anti-commons*, a term adapted by Michael Heller in 1998, lies in "the potential under use of scarce scientific resources caused by excessive intellectual property rights and over patenting in biomedical research" (Heller 1998, cited in Hess & Ostrom 2007: 11). Through (political) restriction to access to resources, research on plant material may be prohibited. This is a 'tragedy' in the sense that valuable resources that could be used to treat some of the most prevalent diseases such as HIV/AIDS or tuberculosis may remain undiscovered. The dilemma between the tragedies of the commons and the anti-commons reflects the tension between the use and abuse of common resources. On the one hand, resources should be protected, while on the other, over-protection undercuts potential research and the development of new, valuable products.

At the moment of knowledge disclosure, however, the future of a medicinal plant and the associated knowledge is unpredictable. It might end up in a research and development process, and drop out of it for lack of valuable results, or it might be further developed and enter the global market as a new product. In the latter case, it is the *bare information* (Parry 2004: xviii) of the plant, as processed by scientific practices, that leads to the product. In case traditional knowledge was involved in this process, it serves as an information-delivering and path-directing resource. Generally, only global corporations or state-funded institutions can afford the cost-intensive processes of research and development, product development and subsequent patenting. A traditional healer, or a community of traditional healers or other indigenous knowledge holders, would hardly be able to finance these processes, let alone understand the complexities, rhetoric and application of the processing and control of patents.

Disentangling the value of indigenous knowledge from the financial costs that scientific research invests in a new product is, likewise, almost impossible. The value of intergenerational and community-shared indigenous knowledge is generally difficult to estimate in economic terms. Mr. Sechaba shared the following concern:

> (...) in terms of traditional medicine, what you find quite often, I mean, I have sat with a number of traditional healers. One of them, a lady, would tell me: "I go to a certain place to pick up my plants, I go at certain times of the day." That I understand, because it is biology and all kind of things. She continues: "At times, I am told by the ancestors and the spirits in the dreams to pick up the plants in a particular manner, or prior to picking up the plants I must not sleep in the same house as my husband. Now, there is no scientific basis for that. These are the sorts of things you cannot prove, what the efficiency is, how is it affected by those things that she has been told in the dream, the things that she must not do. So, there is a bit of mysticism the whole thing. But let's assume that one can be able to commercially translate the mixture into something that multiple people could use, so therefore there is a commercial case. Then a patent system would work for that particular traditional healer, because then they can police it. If they cannot police it, then there is not much value in it.

The final product of scientific investigation and development, and the comprised indigenous knowledge with its practices and spiritual background (such as the integration of information received from ancestors), so far inevitably falls under the protection of IP law. IP law is a globally applied economically oriented knowledge protection scheme that only protects individually held inventions, and thus leaves out the collectively held and culturally embedded knowledge of traditional healers. Darell Posey points out that IP rights:

> (...) are intended to benefit society through granting of exclusive rights to 'natural' and 'juridical' persons or individuals, not collective entities such as indigenous peoples. As the Bellagio Declaration[7] outs it: Contemporary intellectual property law is constructed around the notion of the author as an individual, solitary and original creator, and it is for this figure that its protection is reserved ... [T]he laws cannot protect information that does not result from specific historic act[s] of 'discovery'. Indigenous knowledge is transgenerational and community shared. Knowledge may come from ancestor spirits, vision quests, or orally transmitted lineage groups (Posey 2000: 195).

But as Dutfield argues, many submitted patent cases are "spurious inventions" and can therefore be implicated in 'biopiracy', which "normally refers either to unauthorized extraction of biological resources and/or associated traditional knowledge from developing countries or to the patenting of spurious 'inventions' based on such knowledge or resources without compensation" (Dutfield 2004: 52). Since such 'inventions' originally derive from indigenous knowledge and/or natural resources, they can only partially be claimed to be inventions. Critical voices claim that when the indigenous knowledge behind such spurious inventions is not acknowledged, the patent on this invention is based on biopiracy, the uncompensated taking of natural resources and its associated knowledge (Shiva 1997, 2007; Frein & Meier 2008).

The term biopiracy is controversial, however. It remains unclear how to differentiate between legitimate and unfair exploration and remains only vaguely defined until today (Dutfield 2004, 2006). The first to frame the term biopiracy was the Action Group on Erosion Technology and Concentration (the ETC Group): "Biopiracy refers to the appropriation of the knowledge and genetic resources of farming and indigenous communities by individuals or institutions who seek exclusive monopoly control (patents or intellectual property) over these resources and knowledge" (ETC Group[8], undated; cf. Oguamanam 2012: 39). Vandana Shiva, a human

---

7   The Bellagio Declaration of 1993 is a resolution aimed art reforming IP laws in order to strengthen works of cultural heritage and biological heritage and the biological and ecological knowhow of indigenous peoples. It was adopted at the Bellagio Conference "Cultural Agency/Cultural Authority: Politics and Poetics of Intellectual Property in the Post-Colonial Era" on March 11, 1993. For the content of the Declaration, see: http://college.cengage.com/english/amore/demo/ch5_r2.html.

8   See: www.etcgroup.org/content/issues.

rights activist and strong voice in the fight against current IP law, has in turn defined biopiracy as "the patenting of biodiversity, its parts and products derived from it on the basis of indigenous knowledge" (Shiva 2007: 275).

In the current neoliberal global economy, the pharmaceutical and other industries, as well as research institutes, biotechnology companies, universities and governments, are, nevertheless, all keen to protect their means by holding patents that are often worth billions of dollars. These developments signify an intensified commoditization process of knowledge and nature and the privatization of these resources (Castree 2008) in the global market economy, with knowledge and information being of incommensurable value (Oguamanam 2012). Through the procedures of international institutions and the patenting system, the patenting process is, however, a one-way road from the South to the North (Mgbeoji 2006: 13), a situation that forces a legal and economic hegemony or "information feudalism" (Drahos & Braithwaite 2002) on indigenous peoples. Once a patent is granted, the patent holder has the individual right to the product. This was defined in the World Trade Organization's (WTO) agreement on Trade-Related Aspects of Intellectual Property Rights (TRIPS), defined in the Uruguay Round of the General Agreement on Tariffs and Trade (GATT) in 1994. Under TRIPS, individuals and groups who claim to have 'discovered' or 'invented' something are given a monopoly over the commercial development of their innovation for a period of 20 years. Anything that is not protected by IP law is, according to TRIPS, considered to be in the 'public domain', and can thus be exploited by anyone without concern for the needs of the original knowledge holders or the sharing of any revenues (Tedlock 2006: 256).

Accordingly, the definition of ownership over 'spurious inventions' or 'mixed-knowledge products' – products that include both traditional and scientific knowledge – is not easy and often leads to contested battles over ownership rights and benefit sharing. The most prominent South African examples of such ownership battles are the cases of *Pelargonium sidoides* and *Hoodia*. The *Basmati*[9] and *Neem* cases[10] are further examples of ownership battles that have ended in indigenous communities having to buy their own heritage from the producing patent-holding companies. Mr. Sechaba's question above – what is the value of a patent from a healer's point of view? – is worth revisiting here. According to Vandana Shiva, the value of a patent is primarily of a commercial nature. It is meant to protect the

---

9   In 1997, an American company (RiceTec) acquired US Patent No. 5,663,484 on Basmati lines and grains and thereby had the right to appropriate a globally recognized name and threaten the livelihood of many Punjabi farmers who live on the export of basmati rice (Mgbeoji 2006: 15).

10   Around 90 patents were claimed on diverse Neem products (mostly by US companies), which made the trade in Neem by local farmers or communities almost impossible. However, some patents can be challenged. See for example "India wins landmark patent battle", March 9, 2005 (http://news.bbc.co.uk/2/hi/ science/nature/4333627.stm).

commercial value of a commodity, or a commodity-to-be (e.g. a chemical compound). It does not, however, suggest anything about the reimbursement of the value of indigenous knowledge incorporated in the invention and subsequent product. This can, Shiva argues, be framed as a human rights violation. This violation and the long-term influence of biopiracy are not compensable. The unequal relationship between knowledge holders and knowledge users continues until today; yet it does show new implications in terms of ABS politics.

There have been and still are many other global, national and local attempts to find appropriate solutions for the protection of indigenous knowledge and the fair sharing of benefits arising from mixed-knowledge products. Mr. Sechaba, however, suggested a simple solution for the unsolved question of how to protect traditional knowledge:

> **MS:** Ya, so, going back to the question you asked, what is the alternative? The alternative, in essence, is either patent it or you keep it secret. (...)
> **BR:** So there isn't another solution yet?
> **MS:** There isn't really a solution. I think one uses multiple means of protection. For me, it comes down to what is the purpose of protection? That is the crunch.

While secrecy may indeed be the best way to protect knowledge, it may not always be the most appropriate. Alternative solutions are being investigated, though these solutions are brittle, fragmented and context dependent. At the same time, however, they may release new synergies and agencies engaged in, for example, human rights debates and local and national environmental and knowledge governance systems. Potential involvement in fair ABS agreements also releases different hopes, ranging from mere financial reward, the building up of a scientific reputation, to helping people in need move towards political empowerment. The moment of knowledge disclosure thus includes layers of "law, ethics, morality and fairness" (Mgbeoji 2006: 12), human rights claims, and concern over questions of cultural heritage and identity. These emerging elements in the moment of knowledge disclosure will be analyzed, without forgetting that the hopes involved in this moment may (often, though not necessarily) remain illusory.

The Promises of Bioprospecting: Hope or Just An(other) Illusion?

The cosmetic product that was expected to develop from the plant material that the Kukula Healers exchanged with the cosmetic company Godding & Godding never materialized and a subsequent benefit sharing agreement was never negotiated. This stands as an exemplary illustration of the many 'dead-end roads' in bioprospecting. And yet the plant exchange also vividly exemplifies how bioprospecting is a field of hope (cf. Crapanzano 2003, Brown 2006, Hirokazu 2004, 2006, Novas 2006,

Rutert 2012). The exchange was originally intended to open the way for upcoming cosmetic products. On the healers' side, it was nourished by the seductive hope of knowledge disclosure that might lead to engagement in the sharing of future benefits, as purported by the rhetoric of the Convention on Biological Diversity (CBD) and other international political statements/agreements. This is the tricky element in bioprospecting, as it opens potential pathways and possibilities, but hardly ever reaches its politically claimed goals.

Nevertheless, medicinal plants and associated knowledge are a form of *ecological, economic* as well as *emotional capital* (cf. Bourdieu 1986) for indigenous peoples, scientists, NGOs and states alike. Despite the general economic rhetoric and hegemonic forms of capitalization attuned to bioprospecting (Takeshita 2001: 264), emotional attachment, social relations, cultural heritage and identity, and political articulations all become contested in a similar way to the commoditized results of bioprospecting activities, i.e. the pharmaceutical or cosmetic product. But even then, the question arises of how much of this suggested 'empowerment politics' is in fact created with the intention of making indigenous peoples ally with bioprospectors in order to ultimately feed the economic market (Takeshita 2001). In other words, how much are indigenous communities being 'instrumentalized' as so-called 'stewards of their resources' and 'new custodians of environmental protection' – rhetoric promoted by international agencies like the United Nations and NGOs – while nevertheless remaining unequal partners in bioprospecting interventions? Bioprospecting and the emerging associated form of agencies, expelled i.e. in developing a BCP might simply be another tool in the attempt to conform indigenous peoples to dominant political discourses and adjust them to the neoliberal market. This raises the question of whether forms of agencies that emerge from bioprospecting, like the development of a BCP, are simply another example of economic interests being dressed up in the 'magic cap' of self-empowerment for indigenous communities, sustainable development and the conservation of biodiversity, as proposed in the Convention on Biological Diversity. Can – and do – actors involved in bioprospecting appropriate the market chains that bind them (Radin & Sundar 2004)?

Indigenous communities may use current bioprospecting politics not only to increase economic benefits, but also to proliferate their power and political influence. Simultaneously, states face the challenge of how to harness indigenous culture as part of their cultural heritage, in order to consolidate national identity on the one hand, and build a sustainable economic future on the other (Ostergard et al. 2006). This is nowhere more saliently expressed than in the call for an 'African Renaissance', as proclaimed by Thabo Mbeki, President of South Africa from June 1990 to September 2008, in 1998. The African Renaissance was a double call for the revitalization of African values and the reinforcement of the South African national economy[11]. Medicinal plants and indigenous knowledge could therefore ostensibly provide the means for local and national identity creation as well as economic progress. In this context, different "regimes of values" (Appadurai 1986) converge. On the one hand, considering the huge impetus to market plant products and related indigenous knowledge(s), one inevitably has to speak of the "commodification of culture" (Appadurei 1986; Geschiere & van Bimsbergen 2005). Jean and John Comaroff argue in their seminal book 'Ethnicity, Inc.' (2009) that in the current neoliberal world order, everything sooner or later falls within the scope of capitalism and is thus considered for commoditization. Heritage, culture, ethnicity, identity, the Comaroffs condense indigenous public activities and enterprises into an "identity economy" in an "identity industry" (Comaroff & Comaroff 209: 22ff.).

However, I suggest looking more precisely at the meaning of value attached to plants and knowledge in each context, to give more space to interpretation beyond the 'commodification of culture' discourse and to open up space for other synergies. Aside from economic value, other no less influential regimes of value – such as *emotional values*, including the *emotional value of cultural heritage and property*, which entail *inherent passionate interests and desires* (Latour & Lépinay 2010) – need to be included in the analysis. They express themselves in emotionally loaded, sometimes resentful, discourses concerning plants and related knowledge, and are for the final analysis as important as the *scientific value* or *biovalue* (Waldby 2002) that are so often propagated by scholars from science and technology studies (STS)[12]. All values are ultimately bound to a constantly changing *political value*, as expressed in ongoing political discourses within government, traditional healers' organizations, NGOs or 'simply' around the fire in village homes.

Following the trajectory of plants and knowledge through different sites and situations may not only enrich our analytical understanding of concepts on tangible and intangible property and its value. It may also bring about suggestions for the widely discussed and as yet unresolved issue of how to negotiate fair ABS agreements. ABS agreements are supposedly meant to balance out inequalities and

---

11   The term 'African Renaissance' was first developed by Cheikh Anta Diop (2000) in a series of essays, collected in the book 'Towards the African Renaissance: Essays in Culture and Development, 1946–1960'. William Makgoba (1999) published another volume on the African Renaissance, with a prologue by Thabo Mbeki. The term should be considered critically, as it actually creates what it tries to oppose, since it takes as its reference the European epoch of the Renaissance, which is known to have been the historical beginning of colonialism (ibid.). The debate does, nevertheless, certainly demonstrate an invigorated African self-consciousness and identity.

12   Biovalue stands analytically shoulder-to-shoulder with similar terms such as biocapital (Sunder Rajan 2006) and bioeconomics (Rose 2001, 2008), which define the often-promoted (within STS) capitalization or fetishization of 'bio' in socio-techno-economic processes and relations (Birch & Tyfield 2012: 3).

redistribute benefits generated in the neoliberal market. The idea of ABS is thus fundamentally rooted in the economy, similar to IP law. But the notion of property ensures a wide array of other modes of *protection*, ranging from *secrecy* to protection via *customary laws* or other *sui generis modes of protection*, depending on the (cultural) context. This raises a number of questions. How can indigenous knowledge be appropriately valued in an economy-based value system? And how can benefits be shared equitably and fairly (cf. Millum 2010) when values in indigenous communities are assessed differently to the values of business companies or a biochemical laboratory? Is 'fair sharing' even possible? These questions cannot be answered fully within the scope of this book, but they can serve as a contribution towards finding improved solutions for ABS and knowledge protection in the field of bioprospecting in South Africa.

Outline of Chapters

Drawing on this background, this book scrutinizes the promises and chances, challenges and illusions, of bioprospecting in South Africa by focusing on the interrelatedness of traditional medicinal plants and associated (indigenous) knowledge, and the anchorage and valorization of both in indigenous communities, in biochemical research, and in customary law and in ABS politics and intellectual property law. Each of the chapters tells stories of connections and disconnections, of translations and the 'untranslatable'. At first, the stories may not appear to conjoin, seemingly exposing too many loose ends and disjointed connections. But the case studies and examples of the different field sites illuminate the values ascribed to plants and knowledge, which, once in interaction, produce new synergies and forms of agency, such as local development and community empowerment. But does bioprospecting really open up so many spaces of national and local (economic) growth and development, as is promoted, or is the rhetoric louder than the reality? And in how far is this hoped-for-growth entangled with the attached and produced values of medicinal plants and associated knowledge as property? Questions, this book aims at answering in the eight chapters.

Chapter one – this current chapter – opened with a short vignette presenting a moment of knowledge disclosure between stakeholders engaged in the field of bioprospecting. The chapter depicts the core actors and unfolds the main challenges of the field. After having shed light on the context and laid out the aims and setting of the book, the second chapter will continue with the theoretical and methodological contextualizations.

Chapter two first introduces into the timeframe, different sites and challenges of the 20 months of multi-sited ethnographic fieldwork. The chapter then discusses and reflects on the methodological framework that constitutes of multisited ethnography and actor-network-theory (ANT). These methodological approaches require further theoretically elaboration, here provided with main analytical concepts of this book, value and (intellectual) property. In addition, the often-discussed issue of the commoditization of culture, as 'the only' driving factor in the field of bioprospecting, will be questioned.

Chapter three draws a picture of bioprospecting from the beginning of colonialism through Apartheid times, and then on to the political, economic, legal and socio-cultural context at present. By using the approach of "studying through" (Reinhold 1994, Shore & White 1997), I argue that politics influence the economy and the other way round, and this interaction also influences the actors, i.e. indigenous peoples and communities, involved. Therein, the term 'indigenous' demands thorough scrutiny. I refer to this interaction as bioprospecting "contact zones" (Pratt 1992). Furthermore, reflections on emgerging intersubjective encounters in the field elucidate my own positionality as a (white) researcher from the global North.

Chapter four analysis the value of knowledge and plants for traditional healers, also by reflecting on the ancestors as an important category for knowledge protection. Plants and knowledge production and protection stand in relation to the surrounding environment and the communities the healers live in. Who is involved in this web of relations? How is knowledge held and who is entitled to hold the rights to knowledge and plants? And how are these rights and relations anchored in the broader community? Hence, plants and knowledge will be investigated as properties in relations and translation. By looking at these relations in healers' communities in three different geographical (and cultural) regions of South Africa – the Eastern Cape; KwaThema/Johannesburg and Mpumalanga Province – the ascribed values of plants and knowledge will be elucidated to understand their contestation in current ABS and IPR politics.

Chapter five continues with the trajectory of medicinal plants and knowledge by moving to the Indigenous Knowledge Lead Program's biochemical laboratory in Cape Town to investigate the translation of values from cultural and spiritual values to scientific values. The chapter investigates the embeddedness of plants and knowledge at the IKS Lead Program and its laboratory, which is specialized in the biochemical analysis of medicinal plants and the promotion and support of indigenous knowledge systems. Further, the chapter also looks at additional assignments of the IKS Lead Program to understand in how far "indigenous knowledge systems" are eventually integrated in the overall scientific agenda.

Chapter six then treads into the field of access and benefit sharing and its challenges. ABS is based on the idea that one particular value can be (monetarily or non-monetarily) substituted or exchanged for another. The chapter will give voice to people who work with medicinal plants (e.g. traders, independent researchers, NGOs) and who are affected by the current ABS legislation.

Chapter seven continues illuminating the other side of the ABS coin, the hopes, aspirations and agencies that emerge from ABS. It therefore elaborates on how property relations help indigenous communities, here the Kukula Healers, to determine their rights to their knowledge and their stewardship over the environment they live in and the medicinal plants they use.

Chapter eight finally brings all of the different, in the book elaborated values that emanate from the field of bioprospecting together to the question of what the value of medicinal plants and indigenous knowledge in the different sites convey about (i) a culturally adequate *sui generis* knowledge (intellectual property) protection system in a multi-ethnic and biodiverse country such as South Africa, and (ii) values that move beyond the 'commercialization of values' approach. It reveals that the contestation over property in the field of bioprospecting of medicinal plants in the final analysis provides much more than mere economic and scientific values and incentives and offers solutions for new elaborated forms of ABS and *sui generis* knowledge protection schemes within and beyond common intellectual property law.

Chapter II
Methodological, Theoretical and Spatial Reflections on Bioprospecting as a Field in Translation

> Every ethnologist is capable of including within a single monograph...the distribution of powers among human beings, gods, and non-humans, the procedures for reaching agreements; the connections between religion and power; ancestors, cosmologies; property rights.
> Bruno Latour (1993: 14)

Introduction

This chapter concerns the methodological, theoretical and spatial framework of the thesis. By following medicinal plants and associated knowledge through different sites, I engage with the transformation and (not always) linear translation (Buzelin 2007; Callon 1986a; Faquar 2012; Fischer 2012; Latour 2005; West 2005) of concepts of tangible (medicinal plants) and intangible (knowledge) property and attributed value, by using multi-sited ethnography and actor-network-theory to being the different actor – human and non-human – together in a web of translation.

The chapter starts with a detailed introduction of the sites of the research, followed by an overview of the main methodological and theoretical approaches applied in the course of the chapters. It then concludes with an introduction of the plant *Sutherlandia frutescens*, as an illustrative case that demonstrates why bioprospecting in South Africa is a scattered and oftentimes difficult to grasp field and why, instead of choosing one particular plant – in the tradition of 'following a thing' (cf. White et al. 2002) – I chose to engage with discourses on value and property and analyze them according to site and situation.

The Framework: Multiple Sites and Temporalities

Figure 1 Map of South Africa showing the main research sites[a]

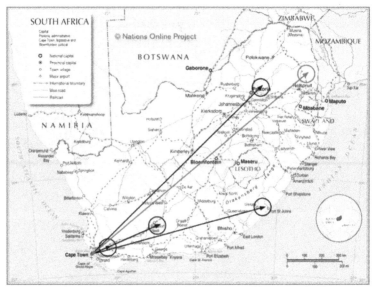

Sorce: Nations Online Project (www.nationsonline.org/oneworld/map/south_africa_map.htm).

The above map illustrates the scattered but nevertheless congruent and partially connected research sites. As will be shown later on, each of the sites is somehow connected to the others, or at least builds up on previous sites. This gives credibility to the attempt to make multi-sited ethnography a mindful and successful project.

Sites, Movements and Impressions: First Research Phase

In total, I conducted twenty months of multi-sited ethnography in South Africa, split into two research phases. In the first research phase (January 2009 – Febru-

---

a   Circles in black represent the main research sites of the first research phase. Black arrows represent movements from Cape Town to the sites De Dorrns close to Worcester, Beaufort-Wet and the Eastern Cape/Mthatha. The red circle and red arrow represent the main research sites during the second research phase: Cape Town and Bushbuckridge Municipality, Mpumalanga and Limpopo Province.

ary 2010), I was mostly positioned in Cape Town[1]. Established in 1652 by Dutch sailors and traders, Cape Town is South Africa's oldest city, often called 'the mother city'. Before the invasion of Dutch settlers, San and KhoiKhoi groups inhabited the rugged interior of the country. With the Dutch, and later the British, invasion, land claims were soon established as land rights, in favor of the white invaders. Until today, the city is segregated with a mostly white city center circling around the city's harbor, followed by housing for the colored population and then the huge townships in the Cape Flats area, which are predominantly populated by black and colored citizens. The population census of 2011 stated that of Cape Town's population, 38.6% were of black origin, 42.4% colored, 15.7% white and 1.4% Asian[2]. The segregation that began early in the history of the city is based on inequality structured along racial lines, with the highest poverty rates found in the informal settlements of the Cape Flats.

Cape Town is home to the country's legislative institutions, hosting the national parliament as well as an increasing number of national and international companies (Lemanski 2007: 451), and one of the leading medical research institutes in South Africa, the Medical Research Council (formerly MRC, since 2014 SAMRC). The MRC headquarters is situated in the northern suburbs of Cape Town, in Tygerberg/Parrow. The Indigenous Knowledge [Health] Systems Lead Program, to which I was affiliated during my research, is a sub-unit of the MRC. The IKS Lead Program's laboratory was established in 2004/5 on a former military compound in the Driftsands Nature Reserve close to Delft. Delft is a huge township approximately 40 km north of Cape Town. I regularly commuted between the laboratory in Delft, the IKS office in Tygerberg/Parrow and Rosebank/Rondebosch in the southern suburbs, where I found accommodation in the house of a white, Afrikaans-speaking woman, who coincidently was a trained traditional healer.

At the IKS Lead Program's laboratory, I mainly observed the biochemical analysis of medicinal plants, which turned out to be a tedious and slow process. It takes weeks, months and sometimes years to search for the needle in the haystack: a new chemical compound, a new method or application for a medicinal plant, or a new medicinal plant mixture consisting of different plants from different regions in the country and beyond. Over the course of the year that I spent at the IKS laboratory, I learned about the technical equipment and biochemical substances used there, about biochemical methods and procedures, and about the language used in the process of scientific analysis. I observed the work of the scientific and

---

1   In-depth information on the larger environments (Cape Town and the Western Cape, the Eastern Cape and Bushbuckridge Municipality in Mpumalanga Municipality) will be provided in this and the relevant chapters.

2   City of Cape Town (2011): 2011 Census – Cape Town (www.capetown.gov.za/ en/stats/Documents/2011%20Census/2011_Census_Cape_Town_Profile.pdf).

non-scientific staff members and interviewed students, post-doc researchers and visiting researchers.

Nevertheless, I came to realize that much of the work and processes at the laboratory would remain inscrutable to me. First, I was a novice with regard to biochemistry. Much of what was said at the laboratory remained unknown and alien, even though I learned a fair bit about biochemestry. Second, the disclosure of plant names was actually prevented by the strict rules on anonymization and secrecy, even to the young researchers themselves, who, in publications or presentations, used pseudonyms for the plants they were working with. Competition is high in the field of biochemical analysis of medicinal plants and researchers carefully guard their research results against scientific piracy. Only when a new chemical compound is eventually patented is the plant's name disclosed to the public.

After weeks of observing and waiting for something interesting or important to happen, I noticed what Ulf Hannerz poignantly highlighted when he questioned "What do you do when 'your people' spend hours alone at a desk, perhaps concentrating on a computer screen?" (Hannerz 2003: 366). Most of the time, the young students were sitting behind their computer screens, playing computer games, writing research reports or filling up silicon-filled gravity chromatography columns with new medicinal plant extracts. In order for 'something interesting and important to happen' and to gain a more comprehensive understanding of bioprospecting beyond scientific processes, I had to speak to other stakeholders. And so I decided to follow medicinal plants and indigenous knowledge out of the laboratory. As Bruno Latour suggests:

> ...sociologists of scientific practices should avoid being shy and sticking only to the level of the laboratory (for this level does not exist) and being proud of diving inside laboratory walls, because laboratories are the places where the inside/outside relations are reversed. In other words, since laboratory practices lead us constantly inside/outside and upside/down, we should be faithful to our field and follow our objects through all their transformations (Latour 1983: 160).

The original idea of the initial research proposal for this project was to follow a plant from its place of origin – a traditional healer in a local community – to the laboratory and into intellectual property and ABS discourses and its challenges. This idea was upheld, but in a much less linear way than initially proposed. Instead, the 'reality of the field' revealed that this transition is much more scattered, disrupted and complex than a journey from A to Z. For example, I tried to follow a plant, whose name was, to my own surprise, disclosed to me at the laboratory as *Dicoma anomala* (DA), but I soon lost track of it, as it was neither connected to an indigenous community or traditional healer nor involved in any political or legal debates. Instead, it was commonly known as a common ground-creeping plant from northern South Africa and was lengthily described in the book 'Medicinal Plants of Southern Africa' (van Wyk et al. 2009). Only much later, after the first research year, did I learn that DA had eventually been submitted for a patent[3].

Plants that were totally anonymized *inside* the laboratory could hardly be traced *outside* of the laboratory. For instance, a plant mixture under analysis at the laboratory called PHELA (isiXhosa: health) consisted of four different plants originating from four different countries outside of South Africa (Sehume 2010: 4–5). Tracing these plants to their place of origin would have been virtually impossible. Due to the lack of traceability and in order to adhere to the anonymity of the plants, I finally decided to focus on *the discourse of the value of medicinal plants and associated knowledge* at each site, and how this value changed and was re-evaluated in the trajectory from site to site. I therefore did not focus on one particular plant from A to Z, but instead regarded medicinal plants and associated knowledge conceptually as multiple and often fragmentary 'actors' in these discourses.

Using a 'radial data generating system' based on snowball sampling in order to find new interview partners on the basis of already existing contacts, I collected supplementary data and conducted interviews outside of the laboratory, from sources and interview partners both dependent and independent of the IKS laboratory. When the IKS Health Director Dr. Matsabisa was present at the IKS Lead Program, he occasionally invited me to join official meetings or (telephone) conferences at the main office of the MRC headquarters. In addition, I was invited to attend three trips to follow up on medicinal plant claims made to the IKS Lead Program by traditional healers and other South African citizens. The journeys brought us to Beaufort West, Worcester and Bonnivale, all situated in Western Cape Province. I also joined a delegation of Chinese researchers from Guangzhou University of Chinese Medicine (GUCM) to the Department of Science and Technology (DST) and the Council for Scientific and Industrial Research (CSIR) in Pretoria. Also, after some negotiation, I was permitted to conduct interviews with employees at the IKS Lead Program *Sutherlandia* plantation site in De Doorns, a village in Breede Valley, 140 km north of Cape Town. I regularly went there from August 2009 to February 2010 to observe the plant growing process, help with weeding and interview the plantation site staff members.

In addition, Dr. Matsabisa declared Mirranda, his direct assistant, to be my own 'helping hand' and research assistant. She had trained as a traditional healer and was a bachelor student of anthropology at the University of the Western Cape. She was responsible for facilitating cooperation between traditional healers and healers' associations in Cape Town and other parts of the country and the IKS Lead Program. Together, we went to the Eastern Cape to interview traditional healers in the area around Butterworth and Mthatha. The Eastern Cape was formerly divided

3   http://innovation.mrc.ac.za/malaria.pdf (last accessed February 10, 2016).

into two homeland areas[4], Ciskei and Transkei, before it united to form Eastern Cape Province in 1994. Until today, the Eastern Cape is inhabited by 86.3% black, 8.3% colored, 4.7% white and 0.4% Asian people[5].

As said, the initial idea of the research proposal was to conduct research in the Eastern Cape by following medicinal plants from a project and community (the Tsolwana plantation site project) into the IKS laboratory. This soon revealed itself to be impractical, however, because the link between the Tsolwana plantation site project and the IKS laboratory hardly existed and was mainly based on administrative support. An exchange of indigenous knowledge with traditional healers never happened, mainly because the population in the area mainly consists of colored people, who do not engage in the tradition of the traditional healing practiced in back communities, but prefer to consult physicians or health clinics. In addition, when I briefly visited the Tsolwana project in April 2009, I learned that it had come to a standstill due to political inconsistencies between the IKS Lead Program and the Department of Science and Technology. I had to reconsider my research agenda, so I asked Mirranda whether she could help me to locate traditional healers to interview them about knowledge and property. Mirranda agreed and we conducted ten interviews with randomly chosen *sangomas* and *inyangas*. In addition, we visited two *izsangoma*, whom Mirranda knew from her training as a healer in the Eastern Cape. All of the interviews were semi-structured and subject to many spontaneous changes, as they were my first interviews on the protection of knowledge and concepts of property and values. I noticed that these were abstract terms that I had to break down into more 'hands-on', comprehensible concepts. For instance, instead of asking "What is property for you?" I started to ask "How do you learn about medicinal plants?" or "Who taught you to prepare *muthi*?" Although the interviews were insightful, I soon realized that I would have to stay longer in one local community in order to really understand such abstract and complex concepts as property and value. After five days with a healer in Mzanzi, a small village south of Butterworth, I came to understand that at best I would have to stay in a community that was already involved in an ABS agreement or at least knew about the broader debate on ABS and (intellectual) property protection. If not, data collection would be limited, not least due to language constraints (I address this language issue further below). At first I thought that the healers of the community in Mzanzi would be suitable, but my interactions with a healer there turned out to be challenging and

---

4   Under the Apartheid regime, the country was divided into homelands (also known as Bantu-stans, Bantu homelands, black homelands or black states), for the purpose of concentrating members of designated (black) ethnic groups into one territory.

5   Stats SA (2014): Mid-year Population Estimates (http://beta2.statssa.gov.za/pub lications/P0302/P03022014.pdf).

furthermore, although the healers knew about the value of their knowledge, they knew little about ABS politics.

Generally, many of the activities that I joined under the auspices of the IKS Lead Program were accompanied by a feeling of unease. My 'official position' as an IKS associate, and the etiquette and reticence that was implicitly demanded within a governmental program, sometimes inhibited my own intuitive contact with people. I experienced my interlocutors as more reserved and financially more demanding when I conducted interviews in the name of the IKS. I was therefore glad to have also established research contacts independently of it. This independence enabled me to obtain different, less directed, more critical and broader perspectives on bioprospecting. I obtained these independent contacts with other stakeholders at conferences or workshops or through the recommendations and introductions of people working in the field of bioprospecting of medicinal plants. I interviewed a lawyer who had extensively worked with the San Council on the *Hoodia gordonii* case; two independent researchers who had conducted research on medicinal plants; two plant traders and herbal medicine suppliers; and five traditional healers from inside and outside Cape Town. In addition, I conducted two focus group discussions (FGDs) with traditional healers, one at the IKS Lead Program's main office and one in Lwandle, a township close to Summerset West, 40 km north of Cape Town, the latter through a contact that I received from a professor at the University of the Western Cape.

Making contact with traditional healers was not always easy, particularly in the highly politicized context of the Cape Flats, where healers were organized into different healers organizations that partially stood in competition with each other. The healers of Lwandle, for instance, belonged to a different organization to many of the healers that the IKS staff member Mirranda worked with. I realized that working with healers in connection with Mirranda on the one hand, and with the Lwandle healers on the other, would possibly get me caught in the crossfire. Furthermore, as my research focus was about concepts of property, and not about the politics of traditional healers and their organizations in the Cape Flats, getting involved in such a politically charged environment would have offered an entirely different (and potentially distracting) research context. Hence I visited the Lwandle healers a few times and interviewed them once, but I avoided seeking deeper and more regular contact.

Coincidentally, when I was still in Germany before the commencement of my first field stay, a friend recommended that I seek accommodation at the house of her friend Annelie. Fortunately for me, Annelie's backyard cottage was available for rent for the entire period of my first research year. While still in Germany, my email exchange with her revealed that she was a white Afrikaans-speaking woman trained as a traditional healer in the Nguni tradition by an isiXhosa-speaking healer in the Eastern Cape village of Mtambalala, a small village close to Port St. Johns.

When in Cape Town, Annelie invited me to visit her healer trainers (*magobela*), and to participate in the initiation ceremony (*goduswa*) of a traditional healer initiate (*ithwasa*) and in the daily life of a healer's family. Being connected to a private person who was a healer made contact with healers in the Eastern Cape much easier and less distant, compared to my contact with healers under the auspices of the IKS Lead Program. Annelie had been so profoundly engaged with the healers in Mtambalala in the year 2004 and hence was well accepted in both their family lives and community[6]. I would not have understood the practices of traditional healing if I had only relied on my contacts with healers related to Mirranda and the IKS Lead Program. Access to traditional healers in rural areas independent of the IKS Lead Program was also invaluable because it changed my own role significantly. While I was an official researcher in the name of the IKS Lead Program in the one instance, I changed into a friend when I was with Annelie. As a friend, I was less regarded as someone who potentially wanted to take knowledge or plants away. I did voluntarily contribute to the healer household in which I engaged in Mtambalala, but I was never forced to do so.

In total, I spent two months of the first research year in Eastern Cape Province: in communities around Mthatha and Butterworth, in Mtambalala close to Port St. Johns and in Mboyti close to Lusikisiki. Mirranda translated the interviews of the first encounters with the healer. Conversations and interviews that I had during my second series of encounters in Mtambalala, as facilitated by Annelie, were led in broken English, through gesture and on the basis of experience with healers I made during the trip with Mirranda. In Mbyoti, the interviews where translated by Dave, a white South African herbalist and *sangoma*-to-be and a friend of Annelie, who had lived in the Eastern Cape for 15 years and was fluent in isiXhosa. He introduced me to his friend and trainer Twasa in Mboyti[7], where I spent a couple of days gaining insight into traditional healing.

These two months offered valuable initial insights into the lives of traditional healers and their communities, the collection and to a limited extent preparation of traditional medicinal plants, the treating of patients, and the acquisition, sharing and protection of knowledge. But I realized that time was short and language barriers intrusive, even with the help of a translator. The language issue generally remained a problem throughout the twenty months of research. Although I had attended two intensive isiXhosa courses of four months in total at the University of Cape Town, I never advanced enough to speak the language and fully

---

6   The position of white people trained as traditional healers was discussed ambiguously by some of the black traditional healers. Some were against white people being *sangomas* because "they don't have our ancestors." Others claimed that anyone who has *amaNdlozis* (ancestral spitit) many train as a healer, irrespective of skin color.

7   Twasa is a nickname, which he earned due to his having undergone training for more than 15 years.

understand the interviews. Furthermore, to understand and make understandable abstract concepts such as property was particularly difficult. My knowledge of traditional healing practices was still in its infancy and the shortage of time and lack of language skills added to my gaining only a fragmented picture. I reconsidered and reformulated my research questions away from the abstract concepts of property towards greater tangibility. However, I was limited by the ethical restriction of not asking about specific knowledge on particular plants, as this could have been read as attempted biopiracy. I was thus caught between too abstract formulations and my access to information therefore remained limited.

My interview experiences alternated between fruitful and futile during the first research phase. Some interview partners, such as the traditional healers and scientists, had issues with trust concerning my position as a researcher from the Global North, in a politically apprehensive situation with regard to knowledge sharing. They were reluctant to be audio-recorded or to disclose specific information. Traditional healers, in particular those engaged in Cape Flats 'healing politics' or those connected to the IKS Lead Program as a governmental institution, were not always willing, or only reluctantly, to engage in interviews. I regard these 'futile' interviews as part of the dynamics of bioprospecting, because they too define the field as one that is still determined by past and present politics and issues of biopiracy. Interviews were generally important for me to formulate an interpretation of discourses on knowledge and the protection of property. But since the thesis concerns about both human and non-human actors, and since non-human actors cannot be interviewed, it was also equally important to include other non-narrative perspectives and data in the analysis, since such data also contributes to the picture of bioprospecting in South Africa.

After the two months of informative stays in local communities, I realized that I would have to stay with healers on a long-term basis in order to build up a good trust relationship and better understand the embeddedness of plants and knowledge in the everyday lives, rituals and environment of healers and their communities. The foundation for the long-term stay in Bushbuckridge Municipality developed coincidently towards the end of the first research year.

More Congruency: Second Research Phase

I spent most of the second part of the research project in the Bushbuckridge area in northeastern South Africa (November 2011 – May 2012). Spread across parts of two provinces (Mpumalanga and Limpopo), Bushbuckridge lies within the Kruger to Canyon (K2C) region, which the United Nations Educational, Scientific and Cultural Organization (UNESCO) has declared a biosphere reserve. The day I arrived in the area, Marie-Tinka, a member of the K2C Management Committee, which is responsible for environmental, tourist and community-based activities in the K2C

Biosphere Reserve, picked me up and took me to acclimatize at her lodge next to the Blyde River, about 15 km from Hoedspruit, Maruleng Municipality. Marie-Tinka introduced me to the K2C region with its particular colonial history, its multiple ethnic groups and impressively wide range of different landscapes and rich biodiversity. She also introduced me to the dangers and threats of the area. She insistently tried to convince me not to stay 'there' over Christmas, as she claimed that alcohol abuse and violence increase dramatically over Christmas. This 'there' was the area where the healers, my main research participants, were living, and which is located in the former homeland of Gazankulu in Bushbuckridge Municipality. While Maruleng Municipality, and Hoedspruit in particular, is dominated by white Afrikaans-speaking farmers, Bushbuckridge Municipality is mainly inhabited by black citizens. It struck me that even though I knew it was meant for my own safety, I was being confronted with statistics on the increase in violence and rape over Christmas on my very first day. Was this a realistic concern or was it based on centuries of racial difference between black and white citizens in South Africa? Did I really have to confine myself and be worried about my safety? I listened to Marie-Tinka, but decided to trust my own intuition.

Five days later, when I joined Marie-Tinka on an exchange of medicinal plants in Thulamahashe, I was surprised about how clearly the visible yet imaginary 'racial line' exposed itself through the empty, structured agricultural pastures and organized bushland in Maruleng Municipality on the one hand, and the hilly, sprawling and densely populated settlements of Bushbuckridge Municipality on the other. We left Maruleng Municipality early in the morning. Right behind Klaserie, a small settlement of houses at the provincial border between Limpopo and Mpumalanga, we traversed into Bushbuckridge Municipality, where the potholed roads were crowded with people, cows, goats and the incessant traffic of minibuses, street vendors were selling tomatoes, onions and butternut squash along the roadside, and tinny music shrieked out of music boxes in Pakistani shops. The area where I would conduct my research for the coming six months triangulated between Acornhoek in the north, Thulamahashe in the south, and Hluvukani and Welverdiend in the east.

In Apartheid times, the area was part of the homeland of Gazankulu, allocated to the Shangaan Tsonga people, a marginalized ethnic group in South Africa (Dovie et al. 2005). To the east, it borders the famous Kruger National Park with the road to Orpen Gate, one of the park's main access gates. The road also constitutes the border between the two municipalities, as well as between Limpopo and Mpumalanga Province. Further to the west, the area is framed by the watershed and forest of the Drakensberg Escarpment, the southernmost extension of the great African Rift Valley and mountain system (Thornton 2002: 1). The Blyde River canyon serves as the western border of the K2C Biosphere Reserve. The provincial town of Bushbuckridge, from which the municipality derives its name, rests on the ridge of the Drakensberg Escarpment. From there, the landscape rolls down into the central Lowveld, with bushy mountains, watersheds covered in green pastureland, savannah and dry thorny bushland.

Before the middle of the 20th century, much of the Lowveld was known to be uninhabitable 'fever country'. Sleeping sickness and malaria posed major threats to the white settlers in the 18th century, who would not cross the 'fever border' and thus designated the hot and dry area to the black population. The designated border between white and black areas is thus a relic of this past health-based border. Historically, the area transformed from an ethnically uniform agricultural society into a melting pot of different ethnic groups, and consequently a region of many interethnic traditions and customary laws, but also of tensions, insecurities and inequalities produced through the force of labor migration and high unemployment rates. With the enforcement of the Natives Land Act of 1913, restricted property (land) rights in the homeland areas and subsequent migration movement (e.g. to Johannesburg) influenced social and cultural life. This continued with the official beginning of the Apartheid era in 1948. The then Afrikaner government introduced homeland politics, which allocated the Bushbuckridge region to the Northern Sotho (Bantustan Lebowa) and to the Shangaan (Bantustan Gazankulu). As a result, the social infrastructure of the homelands changed drastically. Village conglomerates were consistently replaced by family cells, which usually consisted of the family homestead, fields and a large number of cattle. In the 1970s, Shangaan war refugees from Mozambique (Ziervogel 1954: 107) settled in the area, and the constant movements of labor migrants to and from the area brought new influences and changes. The dependency of local people on the remittances of migrant men (Niehaus 2005: 195) was high. This rapidly changing situation destroyed much of the 'traditional' way of life, and also simultaneously fueled the fear of witchcraft; young anti-Apartheid comrades conducted witchcraft eradication campaigns to cleanse rural areas of "immorality, misfortune, and evil" (Niehaus 2001: 130–155; Ritchken 1995). Through all of these influences and movements, the K2C area is, next to the bigger cities, probably one of the most ethnically and politically-historically heterogeneous areas in South Africa. The main languages are Pedi, Pulana (a mixture of Pedi, Swazi and Tsonga), Tsonga (originally spoken in Mozambique), Swazi and Sotho (Thornton 2002: 15). Most inhabitants speak at least two or more languages and passively understand most of them. Intercultural marriages and interwoven cultural practices (such as undergoing initiation rituals) are part of daily life.

Staying 'There' With Its Assets and Drawbacks

After deciding that living 'there' would not impose any threat to my personal security, I moved to Share/Hluvukane in Bushbuckridge Municipality, Mpumalanga Province, to live with the CEO of the Kukula Healers, Rodney Sibuyi. The Kukula

Healers became the center of the research during my second research phase. From this base I conducted participant observation and interviews with twenty members of the Kukula Healers; traveled to other areas such as the neighboring Maruleng Municipality to conduct interviews with the K2C committee member Marie-Tinka and the owner of the cosmetic company Golding & Golding; conducted interviews and/or informal conversations with other stakeholders such as the chief and *induna* (sub-chief) of each village in the area; was present at almost every meeting of the Kukula Healers; and helped to organize cooperation between the K2C committee, Natural Justice and the Kukula Healers, as well as other activities and celebrations. I basically became a participant in all of the Kukula Healers' activities for the entire duration of my stay.

The collaboration with Rodney Sibuyi as my research assistant was invaluable. His position as a highly respected healer, as CEO of the Kukula Healers, as a local businessman and a leading figure of the community of Share/Hluvukane, with his huge network of friends and relatives stretching from Hluvukane to Johannesburg, meant that many doors were opened to me with invaluable hospitality. As it was generally difficult to find a person fluent in English and the local languages, Rodney also translated all interviews that we cooperatively conducted from xiTsonga or seSotho into English. The flip side of this close cooperation was that Rodney had an enormous influence on the data generating process. I did not speak any Shangaan, aside from a few sentences and expressions that I learnt during fieldwork. It was virtually impossible to find any printed, online or taught Shangaan language courses, either in the region or in Johannesburg. The only source I could find was a schoolbook for children with translations from Shangaan to English. Luckily, to some degree I could rely on English, given the fact that many people in Bushbuckridge Municipality periodically migrate to work in Johannesburg, which means that many people speak at least some English. The quality of English was generally low, but was (among the younger generation at least) to a limited extent existent.

Although Rodney's position was invaluable, I also realized that I would have to take the perspectives of other Kukula Healers into account. I thus also spent a couple of days with the families of other Kukula Healer members (i.e. Adah Mabunda and Mama Rose). Language and infrastructural constraints prevented me from staying on a more long-term basis. Although some of the healers spoke a few words of English, it was not enough to lead a proper conversation on knowledge healing practices and concepts of property. I therefore stayed most of the time at Rodney's house and relied on his assistance as a translator. His dominant opinion could be balanced out by the many interviews I conducted with other Kukula Healers. Generally, I felt safe and welcomed in Bushbuckridge Municipality from the day of my arrival until my final day. Rodney repeatedly introduced me as someone 'who knows' about traditional healing and who is 'like us', for "she can even eat our food" (trying *Mbopane* worms, a regional delicacy, and eating *papp*, the ty-pical starch-rich maize meal, seemed proof enough of my local adaptability) and "can work on the field" (I sporadically helped Rodney to harvest beans and collect the cows from the common grazing land). What seemed normal to me, a person who had not grown up under the Apartheid regime, was special in a highly segre-gated area, where white and black citizens hardly intermingled on a private basis. A white person who voluntarily worked in the fields was not at all common in the former Bantustans. Furthermore, the long-term, successful and respectful coope-ration between Natural Justice, the K2C committee and the Kukula Healers might have added to the overall positive attitude towards me.

In addition to the six months in Bushbuckridge Municipality, I attended a workshop on the development of the 'code of conduct' of the Kukula Healers at Wit-watersrand University Rural Facilities near Orpen Gate (February 2012); an interim workshop on intellectual property in Nairobi (March 2012) hosted by the Open AIR network; and a workshop on the 'traditional knowledge commons' in Cape Town (May 2012), hosted by Natural Justice. These workshops were all related to my sub-ject and were thus insightful. Finally, after I had stayed in Bushbuckridge for the huge celebration of the Kukula Healers in May 2012, an event that the healers had been preparing for during the entire time of my stay, I went back to Cape Town. When there, I conducted final interviews with five members of Natural Justice. At the beginning of June, six and a half months after my arrival, I returned to Germa-ny.

In March 2013, I returned to Bushbuckridge Municipality for a brief follow-up visit, where I spoke to earlier research participants (Kukula Healers, K2C commit-tee members, Golding & Golding representatives), and in December 2013, I parti-cipated in a huge intellectual property conference, again hosted by the Open AIR network in Cape Town. At the conference, a book was launched with a chapter that I had co-authored, largely based on my research results. In addition, I actively con-tributed to a video[8] and delivered information for an Open AIR briefing note on traditional knowledge. Data from the second research phase were thus based on interviews, participant observation and regular and active participation in work-shops and conferences, as well as active participation in the meetings of the Kukula Healers. Finally, over time and with growing knowledge, I also became inaugurated into the work as a healer's apprentice, even though I had not initially intended to train as a healer. In this sense, the 'triple role' of participant observation, active par-ticipation and the ascribed role as a healer's apprentice combined to bring about very close and active access to the field (this closeness will be critically reflected

---

8   "Managing Benefits from Traditional Knowledge (TK) in Bushbuckridge, South Africa", No-vember 11, 2014 (www.youtube.com/watch?v=Ve8i-akzCOk).

on in chapter III, in light of the criticism of the possibility of 'going native'). Taking fieldnotes, collecting grey literature and reviewing the transcripts of speeches given during workshop and conferences, as well as looking at leaflets, maps and other additional information such as policy papers, supplemented the assemblage of data that I gathered around the two starting points – the IKS Lead Program and the Kukula Healers in the K2C Biosphere Reserve – with the main research attention being on the value of medicinal plants as tangible property and associated knowledge as intangible property.

The data analysis process turned out to be difficult due to the many different geographical areas and research subjects. The manifold interviews with very different stakeholders at first showed little congruency and the regions had few to no similarities. However, things began to become clearer as I started to organize the data into thematic clusters such as: concepts of tangible and intangible property; the protection and disclosure of knowledge; the sharing of benefits; and the hopes, desires and politics arising from bioprospecting. I realized that I would have to integrate these themes, some with more and some with less emphasis, in each chapter, but primarily in relation to the two main research centers: the IKS Lead Program and the Kukula Healers. However, all of the other stakeholders and actors (such as the government, NGOs or traders) must also grapple with these themes, and their stances will be inserted where relevant in each chapter.

Bioprospecting Assemblages: Method (as) Theory

Following the previous section, which dealt with the sites and some of the challenges that I came across in the field, the following section describes how these sites can be meaningfully brought together with the help of multi-sited ethnography and actor-network theory.

Multi-Sited Ethnography: Capturing Spatial Multitude

E.E. Evans-Pritchard, Bronislav Malinowski and Margaret Mead, the 'forefathers and -mothers of anthropological fieldwork', spent considerable time, often two years or more, understanding one entire cultural group and its social life. Things have changed since these 'old masters' studied the 'natives' on such a long-term basis. Hardly any ethnographic research today is conducted in the old classic style (Faubion & Marcus 2009; see also Gupta & Ferguson 1997; Rabinow 2005; Strathern 2004). Even studying a seemingly 'closed society' would sooner or later imply getting in touch with the global world (e.g. via telecommunications or commodities).

Contemporary societies are "invariably, inevitably, and self-evidently located within larger wholes" (Falzon 2009: 5).

A number of theoretical and methodological approaches have dealt with these larger wholes. Studies of global-local discourses and relations, transnationalism and migration deal with things and persons in motion. Ong and Collier defined the term *global assemblages* to explain "new material, collective, and discursive relationships" in a globalized world (Ong & Collier 2005: 4; see also Dilger et al. 2012). Bioprospecting is a transnational phenomenon, as the *Hoodia* case, with the involvement of at least three neighboring African countries and exports from China and to the US as well as Europe, tells. None of these approaches to global phenomena engage, however, with the limitations that this research faced, with the short time periods at each site and the sites' spatial disjointedness and occasional incongruence. I therefore drew on multi-sited ethnography from the first instance. It was George Marcus (1995) who nailed the turn away from conventional ethnography on the door of the 1995 Annual Review of Anthropology (Falzon 2009: 1). Marcus proposed multi-sited ethnography as a methodological tool to examine the flow of things or ideas through different geographical and/or social locations and sites. He asserted that

> multi-sited research is designed around chains, paths, threads, conjunctions, or juxtapositions of locations in which the ethnographer establishes some form of literal, physical presence, with an explicit, posited logic of associations or connection among sites that in fact defines the argument of the ethnography (Marcus 1995: 105).

The object of multi-sited ethnographic research is ultimately mobile and multiply situated, and has a comparative dimension that is integral to it, in the form of juxtapositions of phenomena that may usually appear to be "worlds apart" (ibid.). Falzon, in a similar vein, asserts that "the essence of multi-sited research is to follow people, connections, associations, and relationships across space (because they are substantially continuous but spatially non-contiguous)" (Falzon 2009: 1).

The focus of attention shifts from full concentration on one element (e.g. ethnic group, company, laboratory) to an alternating focus; in the context of this research, to the altering *theres* enclosed in the multiplicity of the entanglements of plants and knowledge in South Africa, a biodiverse country with a complex political history that reaches into the present. To capture the multiplicity or complexities (Law & Mol 2002) is, therefore, a methodological challenge[9]. According to Hannerz, multi-sited or multi-local ethnography involves "Being there ... and there ... and there" (Hannerz 2003: 201), which soon turned out to be a reality in the context of my

---

9   For a discussion of the challenges with regard to 'contexts' and 'sites' in medical anthropological research, see also Dilger & Hardolt (2010).

research. I was *there* (at the IKS Lead Program and its laboratory) and *there* (with healers in the Eastern Cape) and *there* (with the Kukula Healers in Bushbuckridge Municipality). I was also *there* and *not there* (Chung 2009: 65f.), because my *being there* excluded *being in another there*. At every *there*, I gathered a mere glimpse or a piece of a puzzle that was supposed to be my field, and of which I was hoping to gain a coherent picture in the end. The long time period I spent in Bushbuckridge during my second research phase, however, assembled the picture that would have looked much more scattered without it.

To connect the sites, *translation* between the sites and their actors was vital and necessary. This function traverses the primary, dualistic 'them–us' (local people–ethnographer) frame of conventional ethnography and requires "considerably more nuancing and shading as the practice of translation connects the several sites that the research explores along unexpected and even dissonant fractures of social location" (Marcus 1998: 100–101). Such unexpected and dissonant fractures were regularly at stake in the first research phase; for instance, between the IKS Lead Program and some traditional healers, and, more subtly, in the second research phase between the Kukula Healers and the K2C committee.

Some critical voices say that multi-sited ethnography is simply a buzzword, "since its signification and ramifications are (not) explored by many of its users... (who) use it mechanically" (Hage 2005: 464). During and after the research, I wondered whether ethnography's richest offerings – depth or the Geertzian (1973) "thick description" – could be generated at all through the horizontalism that multi-sited ethnography almost inevitably leads to. Taking into account the reasonable critique of multi-sited ethnography, I drew the conclusion that concentrating on *translation processes* is the most suitable way out of potential superficiality. In addition, I resolved that depth is a matter of definition. It depends on the overall research question that is to be answered by the data, where the actual data is generated, and how the data corresponds to data from the other sites. By focusing on the value of medicinal plants and associated knowledge(s), and by putting the attention on the two core centers of research, I avoided mere 'horizontal site hopping' by bundling floating data and thus providing some vertically deep data. Nevertheless, I also came to realize that my interpretation of multi-sited ethnography as a methodological framework required an extension to capture and give space not only to the sites but also to the human and non-human actors within the research to understand processes of translation.

Actor-Network Theory: A Theory Is not Always a Theory

Initially, actor-network theory (ANT) developed out of science and technology studies (STS), which aims to explore how social, political and cultural values affect scientific research and technological innovation, and how these in turn affect society,

politics and culture. The aim was to understand processes of technological innovation and scientific knowledge creation (Latour 1985, 1987, 2005; Latour & Woolgar 1986; Knorr-Centina 1995; Star & Bowker 1999) by looking at scientific practices and actors in networks of routes and connections, in processes of *translation*
(Callon 1986). As a result, one of the key questions posed by actor-network theory was "How can we describe socially and materially heterogeneous systems in all
their fragility and obduracy?" (Callon 1980, cited in Law 2009). In these systems,
an 'actor' or 'actant' is "anything provided it is granted to be the source of an action" (Latour 1997: 4). In ANT, every actor or actant, human and non-human[10], has
agency, irrespective of its material form or use. By giving space to non-human actors, ANT challenges the typically anthropocentric or socio-centric stance within
social science that often deliberately leaves out the non-human world, or only allows it to play a side role. The semiotics of things in ANT is not related to meaning
but is rather construed as path building, or order making, or creation. Things and
human beings "circulate, mix with one another, solidify and dissolve in the formation of more or less enduring things" (Ingold 2011: 16). It is not an actor that
produces reality, but it is "an actor whose definition of the world outlines, traces,
delineate, limn, describe, shadow forth, inscroll, file, list, record, mark, or tag a
trajectory that is called a network" (Latour 1996: 14). Multiple actors associate in in-
definable groups wherever and whenever they meet, drift apart, act and react. One
may rightly ask whether the non-human 'can speak' in the same way as the human
(cf. Spivak 1988; Mitchell 2002), and thus question whether non-human actors do
indeed have agency per se; but the relevance lies more in the interstices, the agency
that is produced in the interaction between human and non-human actors. Advocates of ANT – Bruno Latour, John Law, Michel Callon, Annemarie Mol – propose
thinking beyond the common dialectic of the social versus the material/objective,
sociology versus natural science or culture versus nature, and instead integrating
them in an assemblage of actors that *reassemble the social* (Latour 2005). Moreover,
there is never just one network or assemblage but many assemblages and multiple
realities that create a specific situation. Although the name actor-network theory
suggests a theoretical approach to capture these multiple realities, it is rather a
methodological and descriptive approach to data:

> [T]he actor-network approach is not a theory. Theories usually try to explain why
> something happens, but actor-network theory is descriptive rather than founda-
> tional in explanatory terms, which means that it is a disappointment for those
> seeking strong accounts. Instead it tells stories about 'how' relations assemble, or
> don't (Law 2007: 2).

---

10   Some scholars critically reflect on the term 'non-human' as being similar to 'non-white', since
      "it implies the lack of something" and is grounded in human exceptionalism (Helmreich 2010:
      555).

For its intangibility, which is that non-human actors have equally strong agency, and its lack of a clear structure, ANT has often been criticized. Sandra Harding (2003) has claimed that ANT dismisses basic social factors such as race, class, gender and post-colonialism. By ignoring these basic categories of social science, ANT is unqualified to challenge the power of racism, patriarchy or euro-centrism. David Bloor (1999) and Sal Restivo (2010) have criticized ANT on similar grounds, noting that ANT vocabulary and analytical tools cannot challenge power structures but can only describe them. For others, the proposition that non-human actors have the same agency as human actors is difficult to accept. Collins (1992) asserted that non-human actors have no 'social life' worth detailing (see also Collins 2010: 140). Others have argued that while non-humans do not possess the level of agency imputed by ANT, they nonetheless exercise a limited "causal agency" (Bloor 1999: 91). Latour rejects the claim that ANT-based research should provide any kind of framework (Latour 2004b: 67). Instead, he offers to just describe the gathered data. I endorse his approach to 'just describe' the realities that are composed by human and non-human actors and regard this approach as highly valuable to explain the creation of bioprospecting contact zones from past to present, which are constituted of people, plants and politics. However, 'just describing' would probably not do (enough) justice to the theoretically complex concepts of property and value.

In the context of this research, ANT is a tool to explore and *describe* the different realities of medicinal plants and knowledge and their value, and the *translation*[11] processes from one site to another, and elucidates forms of *agency* emerging from the interplay of non-human actors – chemical compounds, a plant, a technical or mechanical device – and human actors – scientists, healers, or lawyers that associate, de-associate and re-associate with groups (Latour 2005). Without translation, the actors cannot speak to each other. Translation is "a process in which actors construct common meanings and continuous negotiation to achieve individual and collective objectives by means of he driving force of "interessement" (Wolf 2007: 23, see also Callon 1986a; Latour 1987; Star & Griesemer 1989). The knowledge attached to the plants and human actors form assemblages. The translation processes that happen between the actors and discourses in the assemblages are ongoing, but by no means undisturbed and linear. They are fragmented and full of ruptures and misleading ends. They might even fail (Callon 1986b). Still missing, however, is an analytical framework of medicinal plants and associated knowledge

---

11   Translation has always played an important role in anthropology, but with different implications: the translation of languages; the translation of data into an ethnographic text; the translation of worlds as an epistemological principle; the translation of emergent, manifold ontologies (Hanks & Severi 2014). For this book, the latter is of particular importance, since property is followed into different ontologies and thus demands translation between these ontologies.

as tangible and intangible property, and the discourses of value attached to them. The subsequent section is thus concerned with the interplay of the core analytical concepts of this thesis: property and value.

Property and Its Value: A Tricky Match

The Oxford Dictionary (2013) defines *property*[12] as "a thing or things belonging to someone; possessions collectively" and "the right to the possession, use, or disposal of something; ownership: rights of property." These short summaries depict central qualities of the term 'property', something that "always belongs to someone who then owns the right to something, but not the thing itself" (Hann 1998: 4). The right to something changes with transactions, exchanges, social obligations and social relations. "Property relations are consequently better seen as social relations" (ibid.). Perceptions of property were always culturally and historically variable (Hann 1998: 3). Although an individual or group can own an object and refer to it as 'personal' property, this property is nonetheless subject to constant negotiations within the institutional and cultural context. Property is involved in a wide variety of social phenomena, in cultural ideals and ideologies, in legal institutions, in social relationships and socio-moral practices. Property is, therefore, not an isolated object that must be regarded as formalized in legal codes, but an object integrated into "the institutional and cultural context within which such codes operate" (ibid.: 7).

"Property in the most general sense concerns the ways in which the relationships between society's members with respect to valuables are given form and significance" (Benda-Beckmann et al. 2007: 14). Property is thus always enclosed in a "bundle of rights" (Main 1986, cited in Hann 1998: 8). Although an individual or a group can own an object or knowledge and refer to it as 'personal' property, this property is nonetheless part of constant negotiations within the institutional and cultural context. The plant and knowledge exchange of the Kukula Healers, for instance, included much more than the mere exchange of goods. Rather, it was an exchange of cultural property that was attached to very specific rules of sharing.

In this context, property needs to be defined beyond objectification. Intellectual property cannot be objectified the way a material object can be[13]. Both tangible and intangible property are embedded in complex webs of social encounters, power

---

12   For the history and philosophy of intellectual property, see Drahos (1999, 1996).

13   Many scholars have worked profoundly on the 'problems' of intellectual property and intangible property. It goes beyond the scope of this thesis to deal with all of these problems in detail. For more information, see: Anderson (2009); Brown (2003); Coombe (1995, 1998a+b, 2001, 2009); Bell & Patterson (2008); Drahos & Frankel (2012), Nicholas et al. (2010); Strathern (1988, 1999a+b, 2000a, 2004).

relations and historical circumstances (Nicholas et al. 2010: 119). When today (intellectual) property such as indigenous knowledge of a medicinal plant is involved in a patenting process, it traverses a whole range of property relations, from collectively held, culturally embedded property – as is the case in healers' communities – to individually claimed and defined property in globally accepted policies. In these shifting relations, the values attributed to the property also change.

Value, according to David Graeber (2001), is an ambiguous term that lacks a precise definition. It is mostly defined in economic terms as "the degree to which objects are desired, particularly, as measured by how much others are willing to give up to get them" (Graeber 2001: 1). From a sociological perspective, value is defined as a "conception of what is ultimately good, proper, or desirable in human life" (ibid.). In the anthropological literature, value has been commonly analyzed in economic terms. In 'Culture and Practical Reason' (1976), Marshal Sahlins differentiates the term value into "the price of something or the meaning of something (…) – even where market exchange is specifically absent. The people are nevertheless economizing their resources: it is just that they are interested in "values" other than material – brotherhood for example" (Sahlins 1976: 213f.). The economic perspective often links value to things as commodities (Appadurai 1986; Kopytoff 1986; van Binsbergen & Geschiere 2005). In the Marxist tradition, commodities are goods or products purely intended for exchange in the "institutional, psychological, and economic condition of capitalism" (Appadurai 1986: 13). This production focused approach to commodities leads to a dead-end, claims Appadurai. Instead, he suggests looking at commodities as things with a social life, with a trajectory from "production, through exchange/distribution, to consumption" (ibid.). This enables seeing "commodities as objects of economic value (…) with use value that also has exchange value" (ibid.: 3).

Objects of cultural heritage such as medicinal plants and associated knowledge are, however, objects that acquire value by circulation and transmission from one generation to another. Hence they are objects with a (past) social life, not a commodity in the first instance. They only become commodities when they are involved in a kind of monetary exchange, such as in the form of *muthi* being given by a healer to a patient or when *muthi* is involved in a pharmaceutical product. Considering the huge financial impetus of plant products and related indigenous knowledge(s) in the local, national and global economy, one inevitably has to speak of the commoditization of (cultural) property, an argument purported by the Comnaroffs, who said that everything will fall under the guise of capitalism and commoditization or economic value. Heritage, culture, ethnicity, identity, the Comaroffs condense indigenous public activities and enterprises into an "identity economy" and "identity industry" (Comaroff & Comaroff 2009: 22ff.). According to this argument, disclosing knowledge is an economic venture.

The renaissance in global politics of cultural heritage and identity indeed encourage nation states and indigenous communities to consider the marketing of products of heritage value. Heritage has, in recent times, obtained increasing recognition by global institutions, NGOs and world markets through the profiling and branding of local culture for the globalized, neoliberal consumer system (Herwitz 2012: 5). But to consider another view, the value of something immeasurable like an 'aura', the appearance of a magical or supernatural force arising from something's uniqueness (similar to mana)[14] (Benjamin [1936] 2008), is almost impossible to estimate in economic terms. Bruno Latour and Antonin Lépinay assert that "because value is a highly psychological dimension, and one that depends on belief and desire, it is quantifiable because it possesses a certain intensity.

> It [value] is a quality, such as color, that we attribute to things, but that, like color, exists only within us by way of a perfectly subjective truth. It consists in the harmonization of the collective judgments we make concerning the aptitude of objects to be more or less – and by greater or lesser number of people – believed, desired or enjoyed (...) (Latour & Lepinay 2010: 8).

Value in this sense is an emotional interplay of hopes, desires, ideas and volitions, which change depending on new movements, opinions and ideas. It is a subjective measure that is defined by the number of people who attach emotional value to the object.

> It remains true that value, of which money is but one sign, is nothing, absolutely nothing, if not a combination of entirely subjective things, of beliefs and desires, of ideas and volitions, and the peaks and troughs of values in the stock market, unlike the oscillations of a barometer, could not even remotely be explained without considering their psychological cause: fits of hope or discouragement in the public, propagation of a good or bad sensational story in the minds of speculators (ibid: 21).

Accordingly, different "regimes of value" (Appadurai 1986) converge in the field of bioprospecting. Aside from economic value, further regimes of value such as the *emotional value* of cultural heritage and identity, expressed in terms of desire (Deleuze 1997), hope (Crapanzano 2003, Brown 2006, Hirokazu 2004, 2006, Novas 2006, Rutert 2010) and passionate interests (Latour & Lépinay 2010) must also be taken into account in the analysis. These values comprehend "culture as a resource" (Yandice 2003, cited in Coombe 2009: 394) of the present as well as the past. Protecting

---

14   *Mana* is a word coming from Austronesian languages meaning "power, effectiveness or prestige", with power mostly having a supernatural cause. In the anthropological literature *mana* has been widely discussed (cf. i.e. Keesing1984, Mauss 2007, Tylor 1871, 1974).

these resources also induces claims of (political) advocacy over heritage. They ex-press themselves in sometimes emotionally loaded and resentful public discourses about knowledge and knowledge protection. These values are as important as the *scientific value* or *biovalue* (Waldby 2002) produced in laboratories, or as the *political value* expressed in ongoing political discourses within the government, in traditio-nal healers' organizations, in NGOs or 'simply' around the fire in village homes. Against this background, I oppose the Comaroff & Comaroff "identity economy" line of reasoning by arguing that cultural heritage and identity are bound to more than the mere adjustment to global political buzzwords and a selling out of culture on the economic market (Herwitz 2012: 6). The economic market clearly determi-nes and may be the driving force in the value ascription of property, but it is ne-vertheless just one side of the many-sided value coin. Who defines what is valuable? What happens when these different concepts of property and different regimes of value come into contact, as is the case in the attempt to protect indigenous know-ledge under IP law? And how, against this background, can ABS agreements be negotiated adequately and fairly?

The Exchange of Values

When looking at the above questions, it soon comes to mind that the value of pro-perty is not only susceptible to different "regimes of value" (Appadurei 1986) but is also subject to situational exchange economies. A property that has an aura is differently exchanged compared to a commodity. Therefore, the differentiation bet-ween *gift exchange* and *commodity exchange* (Osteen 2002; Tsing 2013) is useful here. In *gift exchange*, the property given away by an owner is imbued with the identity of the owner, which causes the gift to have power, or an aura, that compels the reci-pient to reciprocate. This exchange inevitably leads to social bonding and deepens social relations and obligations (Mauss 1954] 2011). It is inalienable, only transfera-ble within the ties of a family or clan, in a liaison of things and persons (Gregory 1982; Weiner 1985, 1992). In 'The Gift' ([1954] 2011), Marcel Mauss claims: "Hence it follows that to give something is to give a part of oneself (...) one gives away what is in reality a part of one's nature and substance, while to receive something is to receive a part of someone's spiritual essence" (Mauss 1954: 10). A healer apprentice, for instance, may show gratitude to his/her ancestors by sacrificing a chicken, in return for specific knowledge received in training. *Commodity exchange*, by contrast, describes the alienation and autonomy of individuals in market transactions, and the strict distinction between things and persons during exchange (Mauss [1954] 2011: 46–47). It is the spiritual essence, or the aura, and its immeasurable value, that makes the exchange of plants and knowledge so convoluted. Finding an ade-quate answer for the substitution or compensation of accumulated value by mere economic transaction remains so far unsettled.

It has also been widely discussed whether societies rely predominantly on gift exchange or on commodity exchange, with indigenous communities often being interpreted as gift economies and Western societies as commodity economies. This distinction has, however, been rejected as ethnocentric. Appadurai suggests that "the exaggeration and reification of the contrast between gift and commodity in anthropological writings has many sources," one being "the tendency to romanticize small-scale societies and proclivity to marginalize and underplay the calculative, impersonal, and self-aggrandizing features of non-capitalist societies" (Appadurai 1986: 11). Instead, a more refined look at gift exchange in Western societies (Carrier 1990; Cheal 1988; Miller 2001) emphasizes that many exchange transactions have characteristics of both the gift and the commodity economy, which act and react to one another (Appadurai 1986: 11; Carrier 1992: 20; Parry 1986: 465; Bloch & Parry 1989: 8; Tsing 2013). Anna Tsing went as far as to propose that commodity exchange could not exist without gift exchange (Tsing 2013; see also Bloch and Parry 1986).

In most South African indigenous healers' communities, gift exchange is interrupted by the influence of commodity exchange. Most healers are economically reliant on their 'business' as healers. The money they receive for their healing services comes from and flows back into the economic market. But it is not solely a commodity exchange, since commodities at some stage in their biography transgress onto the stage of gift exchange; that is, they take on the personalized, relational, inalienable aspects of the gift. Plants and knowledge move in and out of the gift exchange status into the (yet to be negotiated and achieved) commodity status, a movement that causes the most challenges in the field of ABS and knowledge protection.

Research Challenges and Resolutions

Another complex issue when it comes to estimating the value of knowledge and plants is the fact that medicinal plants are not 'just' plants. Plants are multiplicities. They grow in specific environments, dependent on climate, soil, altitude, humidity or aridity. The use of plants by traditional healers thus also depends on the plants themselves. Some plants grow almost everywhere; others are very picky about their local preferences. Once one community claims healing knowledge based on a plant, other communities may come forward and do the same. This adds to the political confusion over how to share benefits with one community or healer, when the neighboring community has similar knowledge. And this is not only a political challenge, but poses a challenge for research as well.

The entire of this research, from the first phase starting in January 2009 up to the end of the second research phase in May 2012, was challenged by multiple conceptions and approaches to *muthi* and knowledge. The infinite entanglements and discourses that medicinal plants and indigenous/traditional knowledge produce made it difficult at first to find the red thread running through the research. By taking the example of the plant *Sutherlandia frutescens*, below I will show why the original idea – to follow one particular plant – soon turned out to be completely impractical. *Sutherlandia*, a very common shrub widely known and used in the Western Cape and beyond, is the plant that I encountered most across the many different sites and discourses. It was the only plant that somehow complied with the original research idea, but the multiplicity of *Sutherlandia* made me aware that a linear process of following *one* medicinal plant would be virtually impossible. *Muthi* is basically not singular, but manifold.

Originally, the word *muthi* stems from the Nguni root *thi*, meaning 'tree' (Ashforth 2008: 212). *Muthi* does not just encompass medicinal plants, but includes a universe of thoughts, knowledge(s), emotions and material matter. In the South African context, everything from substances such as animal parts and fats, stones, salt, oil, chemicals or over-the-counter and patented medicines (Cocks and Moller 2002) can be referred to as *muthi*. *Muthi* can be collected by healers or can be bought at *muthi* markets in the bigger cities, such as Johannesburg's Faraday Muthi Market or at Victor Market in Durban, at *muthi* stalls along the roadside, at bus terminals or from *muthi* hawkers. *Muthi* is part of the everyday life of the black population and is used for daily internal and external cleansing and purification, as much as for rituals (such as house cleansing) and ceremonies (for initiation, for instance). In most white South African households, *Sutherlandia frutescens* or other medicinal plants such as fennel, chamomile and buchu are commonly *not* associated with *muthi*. A (medicinal) plant that simply grows in nature, unaffected by human influence, is also not (yet) *muthi*. *Muthi* needs to be manipulated and imbued with human power and imagination, and thus it is an ambiguous term, since power and imagination can be both positively and negatively used.

In his book 'Witchcraft, violence and democracy in South Africa' (2005), Adam Ashforth gave much space to the section 'Poison, medicine, and the power of secret knowledge. The dialectics of muthi'. Therein, Ashforth offers a local differentiation between two kinds of *muthi* by assigning colors of moral order: "In Zulu, *umuthi omnyama* (black muthi) is the harmful poison, and *umuthi omhlope* (white muthi) is the healing medicine" (Ashforth 2005: 133). The distinction between healing and witchcraft is basically a moral one (ibid.: 134). Black *muthi* is used for witchcraft and spells, while white *muthi* is applied for healing purposes only. Positive healing and cleansing can thus also be substituted by the evoking of evil spirits and misfortune, and it can even kill (Ashforth 2000). People who use black *muthi* are spoken of as witches. Because of the use of animal or human body parts and the power associated with *muthi*, it is stereotypically associated with '*muthi* murder'[15], 'witch-craft' or 'black magic', as well as with 'black' healing and the everyday lives and health seeking behaviors of black South Africans, which differ in many ways from the daily lives and health seeking behaviors of white South Africans. Traditional healers who know about *muthi* by virtue of their abilities and knowledge often refuse the term 'witch doctor' in order not to be defamed as a witch. However, when used positively, *muthi* can cure virtually everything. This is at least the impression that I had when roaming around the *muthi* markets and speaking to healers at the markets or in small *muthi* shacks along the roadsides in the Eastern Cape. *Muthi* offers protection against bad spirits, fills up bank accounts, brings back lovers and makes its user win the lottery – at least if you believe the small advertising leaflets distributed around the city centers of Cape Town, Johannesburg and Durban.

While this advertising strategy may seem manipulative and outlandish, *muthi* generally plays a significant role in South African indigenous communities. For traditional healers, *muthi* is part of their everyday lives and healing practices. *Sutherlandia*, the plant I followed across various sites, is but one of a countless number of medicinal plants. But it is as infinite in its representations and use as *muthi* is in general.

Scattered Muthi: Sutherlandia Frutescens

Sutherlandia frutescens (L.) R.Br (subs. microphylla) is a beautiful shrub with dark red flowers and dainty light green, hairy pinnate leaves; a powerful yet shy plant that blossoms from spring to summer. After flowering, the blossoms develop into bladder like paper pods (van Wyk et al. 2009), from which the English name for the plant, 'balloon pea', might originate. The shrub is widely known in South Africa by many different local names: *unwele* (isiZulu: hair), *insiswa* (Zulu: dispels darkness), *pethola* (Tswana: to change), *lerumo-leradi* (Sotho: spear of the blood), *cancer bush* (English), *kankerbos, wildekeer* (Afrikaans: cancer bush), (Afrikaans: wild herb), *rooikeurtjie* (Afrikaans: pick up the red flower) (van Wyk et al. 2009; Gibson 2011). The plant is at home in the semi-arid areas of the Western Cape and the semi-desert Karoo in the middle of South Africa, but also in Namibia, Botswana and in the less dry areas of the Eastern Cape. Wherever I travelled along the national roads, the dusty side roads or in the Swarteberg Pass, a magnificent mountain range between Swellendam and Outshoorn in the Western Cape, I saw single or clustered *Sutherlandia* plants, often growing in and among other shrubs.

---

15   Headlines in the daily news also contributed to a negative image of *muthi*: 'Case against muthi murderers postponed' (Andrew 2007), 'Healers slate muthi killings' (Makaner 2012) or 'Muthi, mobs and murder in Mpophomeni' (Makhaye 2005).

Because of its extensive coverage, *Sutherlandia* is widely used by traditional healers, Rastafarians, bossiedoktors (Afrikaans: bush doctors) and allopathic clinicians. It has a long record of application dating back to the colonies in the Cape (Gericke 2001; Pappe 1850; Roberts 1990; Smith 1966). The plant was used for healing purposes by the Khoikhoi and San long before the colonizers' arrival, and until today it is known as a very potent plant with medicinal properties, used against internal cancer, common colds, diabetes, rheumatism, asthma, kidney disorders, urinary infections, stress and anxiety (van Wyk & Dugmore 2008; van Wyk et al. 2009). With its powerful healing properties, it assists the body to mobilize its own resources to cope with diverse physical and mental stresses. Known for its strength, it is used in the 'indigenous' realm as much as in the 'allopathic' realm. It is available in pharmacies all over South Africa as a crushed powder pressed into tablet form or as a liquid plant extract. I also saw pillboxes with *Sutherlandia* capsules at *muthi* markets and in the *indumba* (sacred space, usually in a hut, of a sangoma)of some traditional healers. I saw it being cultivated on the plantation site in De Doorns, Breede Valley and at the PROMEC unit[16], and growing as a common shrub along the dusty side roads and tarred main roads of the Western Cape.

The isiZulu word for *Sutherlandia* is *unwele*, meaning hair. Whenever I asked for *unwele* in mostly black contexts, such as the *muthi* markets or at a *sangoma*'s place, interestingly I hardly ever received the botanical species *Sutherlandia frutescens*, but always a different version and interpretation of a hairy type of plant. At Victoria *muthi* market in Durban, for instance, I was offered two different varieties of *unwele*, one a soft light green leaf and the other a harder dark green leaf. Both were proposed for different purposes, but neither were *Sutherlandia frutescens*. The light green plant "is good for HIV, you know. Drink it, make tea. But only take the light green version, the hard one is not good," explained the vendor at the market (Informal conversation with a female plant trader, Durban, October 2009). David, a traditional healer I met by chance at Pick 'n Pay in Musgrave shopping mall in Durban, said that *unwele* is well known and widely used among traditional healers in KwaZulu-Natal. A healer trained in the Griqua[17] healing tradition who lived in the Karoo told me that she knew about the use of *Sutherlandia* from her grandmother. As a child, she used to drink *Sutherlandia* tea against colds. But, she claimed, "it must be taken in big chunks, not as a powder, and with the plant having had little contact with human beings. Too much contact to human beings weakens the power of the plant" (Informal conversation with a healer, Beaufort West, June 2009). A researcher at the IKS Lead Program who had conducted extensive research on *Sutherlandia* at

---

16   The PROMEC (Program on Mycotoxins and Experimental Carciogenesis) unit is a research
      unit of the Medical Research Council (MRC) in Cape Town.
17   The Griqua people are a sub-group of colored people who live in the center of the country,
      mostly around Kimberly (Mountain 2003).

the University of the Western Cape told me that the quality of *Sutherlandia* products (capsules with *Sutherlandia* powder) diminishes the longer they sit on pharmacy shelves, a fact that is applicable to most phytopharmaceuticals (Informal conversation at the IKS laboratory, September 2009).

Sutherlandia is one of the few indigenous plants that has gone through a profound number of safety and toxicity studies at the Medical Research Council in Cape Town, the University of the Western Cape and the University of KwaZulu-Natal (Seier et al. 2002; van Wyk & Albrecht 2008)[18]. The MRC in Cape Town has conducted toxicity studies on *Sutherlandia* leaf powder (*sutherlandia microphylla*)[19]. The University of the Western Cape's International Center for Indigenous Phytotherapy Studies (TICIPS), in cooperation with the University of KwaZulu-Natal, also conducted safety and efficacy studies with people with a CD4 count above 250 and who were not on antiretrovirals (ARVs, drugs used in the treatment of HIV) (Oloyede 2011). The PROMEC Research Unit of the MRC has conducted research on the antibacterial and antioxidant activity of *Sutherlandia* (Katerere & Eloff 2005). David Katerere, a pharmacologist at the MRC PROMEC unit, has worked extensively on *Sutherlandia* and cancer (ibid.). In an interview he said: "It is the combination of all the compounds the plant entails that makes *Sutherlandia* so interesting. *Sutherlandia* is a generalist" (Interview at PROMEC unit, August 2009). Diana Gibson summarized the ambiguities of *Sutherlandia* in clinical research pointedly in the article 'Ambiguities in the making of an African Medicine: Clinical trials of *Sutherlandia frutescens (l.) R.Br. (Lessertia frutescens)*' (Gibson 2011; see also Oloyede 2010, 2011). The plant is particularly known as a potent immune booster helpful in the treatment of HIV/AIDS patients (Gericke 2001). Furthermore, researchers anticipate that further trials will show that use of *Sutherlandia* could delay the progression of HIV into AIDS, and actual disease remission is hoped for[20] (Harnett et al. 2005; Mills et al. 2005a+b). Nigel, whom I met at the Kirstenbosch Garden, Cape Town's botanical garden, told me that he had hundreds of records of the medicinal value of *Sutherlandia* at home. However, due to current intellectual property regulations and government politics, he was not able or willing to release the information.

Even though the many research results seem to indicate the high value of the plant, the government is not particularly interested in these results. Instead, it is proceeding with a 'biomedical path' (Interview with Nigel, August 2009) rather than following a 'public health path' that would support local knowledge systems and utilize existing local resources. This attitude somehow contradicts the political stance taken with the adoption of the IKS policy and the Traditional Health Practitioners Act, both from 2004. It shows how plants like *Sutherlandia* or *Hoodia* change the

---

18   www.sahealthinfo.org/traditionalmeds/sutherlandia.pdf (last accessed March 6, 2013).
19   www.sahealthinfo.org/traditionalmeds/firststudy.htm (last accessed March 6, 2013).
20   Sutherlandia and HIV/AIDS, January 24, 2019 (www.sutherlandia.org/aids.html).

politics of bioprospecting by offering their healing properties. These healing properties would go 'undiscovered' without generations of people who have used the plant, and who have invented and reinvented medicines.

Because of the healing properties of *Sutherlandia*, it has also become involved in contested discourses over who first came to know about these healing properties and who will thus gain the main share in case a product is eventually released on the international market. These are basically political processes, which show that knowledge is contested and that, at some stage, is subject to the assignment of artificial ownership in the global knowledge economy. Roger Chennels, a lawyer who advised the San Council in the *Hoodia godornii* case, envisioned that *Sutherlandia* might be the next plant to be discussed in terms of intellectual property rights. According to him, the San are the original holders of knowledge on *Sutherlandia*, because they were the first peoples in the Western Cape. In case a product deriving from *Sutherlandia* is patented and internationally commercialized, the San Council will most likely dispute the patent (Interview with Chennels, September 2009, Stellenbosch). However, though the San might have been the *first* to know about the healing power of *Sutherlandia*, it is in fact a very commonly known and widely used traditional plant, so any single claim over it will always be contested.

The example of *Sutherlandia* illustrates the assemblage configured around a medicinal plant and the ongoing interplay of plants, people and politics. I have gone into *Sutherlandia* so extensively in order to show how fragmented and ambiguous just one medicinal plant can be. In doing so, I also demonstrate why I chose not to follow one particular plant in the spirit of 'following a thing' (van der Geest et al. 1995; White et al. 2002) from its place of origin to a traditional healer's community to a laboratory and then into IP law. Instead, what I have shown is a glimpse of the multiplicity and complexity of medicinal plants and associated knowledge in the field of bioprospecting. Some plants have not yet been discovered, some have entered a laboratory where they are being anonymously analyzed and dissected, some plants are already being publicly discussed, and other plants, like *Sutherlandia*, are 'in the making', in the sense of transitioning from a common shrub to an internationally available phytomedicine and the new subject of an intellectual property rights discussion. Because of this incongruence and to resolve the challenges of being trapped in a story with countless open ends, rather than focus on one specific plant I chose to look at the discourses of property and value at each site, and occasionally related to specific plants, and to examine how property and value are translated between different sites.

Conclusion and Outlook

In this chapter, I illustrated the different contexts, sites and timeframes where medicinal plants and associated knowledge(s) are examined. These sites at first seem scattered and incongruent, but are connected through the discourses on the value of (indigenous) knowledge and medicinal plants. These values have different connotations and implications in each site, and for each stakeholder. The implied discourses on value are snapshots of the many discourses led in and about bioprospecting in South Africa in the years 2009 to 2012. The example of the medicinal plant *Sutherlandia frutescens* also underlines the fragmented and often open-ended field. *Sutherlandia* is embedded in divergent knowledge systems and geographical areas, has various botanical and culturally adapted names, and there are many stakeholders with different economic, political, legal and idealistic interests involved in its use. The contestation of the plant is dependent on its economic value as well as on its political, legal, cultural and emotional value. No value can be analyzed without considering the other values. The value of knowledge and plants also played an important role in my position as a researcher from the Global North. This role will be described in the next chapter, as it involves a number of intricate questions regarding the contestation of values in bioprospecting in South Africa's colonial and Apartheid past. I will argue that my own *positionality* in encounters between healers, *muthi*, ancestors, and myself enabled some deeper understanding of these contestations.

Chapter III
Ambiguous Contact Zones: Politics, Economy and the Ethnographer

> It is quite by accident and only from savage notions that we owe our knowledge of specific [medicines]; we owe not one of them to the science of the physicians.
> Moreau de Maupertuis (1752)

Introduction

"I expect that my potatoes will make you rich" (Brush 1995: 1). These words were said by a farmer in Tulumayo Valley in Peru, whom Brush interviewed in the 1980s on potato breeding. The farmer in Brush's article knew that his potato variety was valuable and could yield many benefits for whoever cultivated it. He also knew that his potato breed would not yield benefits for *him*, but for the person or institution – here represented by Brush as an anthropologist – who would take the potatoes to breed and trade elsewhere, most probably in the Global North. To claim his rights to 'his possession' did not occur to this farmer at this time. The message of the Convention on Biological Diversity (CBD) about "sharing in a fair and equitable way the results of research and development and the benefits arising from commercial and other utilization of genetic resources with the Contracting Party providing resources" had not yet reached the lives of indigenous peoples, including this farmer in Tulumayo Valley.

In 2009/10, traditional healers in South Africa seemed to be more aware of the fact that their medicinal plants and associated knowledge could potentially be taken away from them by others without the negotiation of a mutual benefit sharing agreement. 'Others' in this case were researchers or traders on the quest for valuable natural resources viable for commercialization. The assertive statement of a traditional healer whom I stayed with for a couple of days in Eastern Cape Province resonated with the humbler words of the Tulumayo farmer: "You are not going to take all our knowledge away!" she yelled at me, mistrustful after I was unwilling to pay an – in my eyes – vastly overrated price for her services. I heard this and similar articulations of mistrust from traditional healers in South Africa more than once, especially during the first research phase. It was never my intention to take their knowledge away and I always tried to reassure all of the healers that I would never ask them to reveal specific traditional knowledge if they did not volunteer it themselves. But as a researcher from the Global North, I was certainly just another person in a long history of people coming from far away to take their knowledge with the promise of coming back to share the benefits in the future, but never did so.

The following excerpt of an interview with Professor Kubukeli, a traditional healer and "flamboyant old man" (see also Wreford 2008: 10), conducted in Kayelitsha, the largest township of the Cape Flats, vividly depicts the twofold notion of prevailing mistrust and strengthened self-consciousness. Kubukeli, a man in his early 80s, is a well-known traditional healer in Cape Town, who likes to be known as Professor Kubukeli due to his vast experience as a healer and because he has trained numerous white people. As a healer representative of the Western Cape Province, he also contributed to the development of the South African Traditional Health Practitioners Act. To my question about to whom traditional knowledge belongs, he frankly answered:

> If you go far back, many decades. The only people who had knowledge on traditional herbs were the black people, the Hottentotts. And, eh, the Indians, on their side and the black Americans. Those are the people who had knowledge. I think they are the owners of traditional medicine. And, eh, then the people have travelled from afar, researching from the traditional healers, their way of healing or their way of using indigenous medicine. And in as much, well, it came in time, they go teaching the people, telling them that, well, once there is a book written on this thing or once we come back to you and will share the income of all this. That was never done! That is why the intellectual properties need to work, because these things belong to those people who have shared their knowledge with the researchers (Kayelitsha, Cape Town, February 2010).

Kubukeli was clear about the fact that the knowledge of indigenous people had been abused, both in the past and up until today. Hence his suggestion that "the intellectual properties need to work" is a logical conclusion, and is still one of the biggest challenges in the realm of bioprospecting. Until now, the taking of knowledge by unauthorized institutions or companies without fairly sharing the benefits remains an unresolved issue. Similarly challenging is finding a way to protect traditional knowledge, which in local healers' communities is protected within the boundaries of customary laws. These boundaries become blurred or even irrelevant when confronted with intellectual property law.

This chapter concerns the ambiguous (mis-)appropriation of medicinal plants and associated indigenous knowledge in South Africa from the colonial past until today. I propose looking at the history of bioprospecting in terms of *ambiguous contact zones* (Pratt 1992): relational encounters between different interest groups, natural resources and knowledge systems. In colonial and Apartheid times, natural resources and associated knowledge(s) were taken without any concern for redistributing something in exchange. When exchange did occur, it was mostly unbalanced; for example, alcohol and tobacco were given in exchange for natural resources. But the relationship between colonizers and the local population was not only characterized by disregard and abuse. As old colonial records recount, mutual respect and gratitude was also part of the encounters between the local population and the colonial invaders. However, the power imbalance established in colonial times, expressed in the non-reciprocal practice of taking without giving, remains valid until today, with the research and development of new products based on indigenous knowledge input being conducted without the consent of the respective communities, and with highly valuable patents based on traditional knowledge still being held by companies from the Global North. Apparently, most profits still flow in the same one-way direction that they have taken for the last few centuries, though under different political and legal circumstances.

With the politics of the CBD, this one-way road was supposed to shift towards the more equitable sharing of benefits. The attempt to make political reparations for the past brings about new contact zones, enforced by new national political regulations and applications; for instance, in attempts to negotiate ABS agreements, or to negotiate non-disclosure agreements, as was the case in the plant exchange between the Kukula Healers and the cosmetic company Godding & Godding. This evokes and nourishes imagined spaces of hope for indigenous communities that they can economically draw on medicinal plants, and for the state or scientific institutions that they can gain a financial share and/or expand political power. For others, like medicinal plant retailers, it creates frustration over complicated new regulations that cause administrative uncertainty. All of these actors meet in new contact zones. What do these contact zones look like? Which actors are involved in their formation? By which hopes are they nourished? To shed light on these questions, my own position in the field and the reactions towards me as a (white) researcher from the Global North researching in the field of bioprospecting reveal that this field is still ambiguously influenced by past misappropriations. I too ostensibly appropriated indigenous knowledge and was thus facing a constant dilemma with regard to my research questions, intentions and in relation to my research participants.

Bioprospecting Contact Zones:
From Past to Present

Bioprospecting is a field of many different past and present contact zones. The trading and barter of goods has always been a component of human existence and interaction, and from the beginning has played a vital role in the development of civilizations (Mulligan & Stoett 2000: 227). The disclosure of knowledge in these encounters did not always occur voluntarily. Although disclosure was mostly a side effect of the interaction and exchange of goods between people, it was at the same time always determined by power relations, control over resources and notions of unequal exchange. This was particularly salient during colonial times, where colonial invaders were on the quest for resources "that might add to the nation's (or their own) wealth and power either on European soil itself or (…) in the rich and fecund soils of one of Europe's tropical colonies" (Schiebinger 2004: 72).

In her book 'Imperial Eyes. Travel Writing and Transculturation' (1992), Mary Louise Pratt critically engages with colonial travel literature written by the white male subject whose imperial eyes passively looked out and possessed (Pratt 1992: 9). Pratt defines contact zones as the "space in which peoples geographically and historically separated come into contact with each other and establish ongoing relations, usually involving conditions of coercion, radical inequality, and intractable conflict" (Pratt 1992: 6). The word contact "foregrounds the interactive, improvisational dimension of imperial encounters (...) it emphasizes how subjects get constituted in and by their relations to each other" (ibid.). It does not suggest "separateness but co-presence, interaction, interlocking understandings and practices, and often radically asymmetrical relations of power" (ibid.).

With the beginning of the history of 'botanizing' in the age of colonial empire building and exploration, bioprospecting encounters took new directions, where curious travelers and early researchers encroached into as yet unknown land and encountered the local populations there. As a result of these sometimes peaceful, at other times more violent, encounters, they brought medicinal plants and other specimens back home to European universities and/or botanical gardens and "made up the most extensive scientific network in the world" (Mackay 1996: 39) while extending European De Materia Medica" (Ellen & Harris 2000: 5). Taxonomic classification systems were created that are still in use today (such as Carl Linnaeus's 'Systema Naturae' from 1775). The traditional medicine database (TRAMED III), begun in 1994 (cf. Flint 2012), is still the most extensive database in South Africa[1].

---

1   See: www.mrc.ac.za/Tramed3/ (last accessed November 8, 2014).

South African Colonial and Apartheid
Bioprospecting Encounters

Colonial bioprospecting in South Africa started with the arrival of Jan van Riebeck at the Cape of Good Hope on April 6, 1652. Van Riebeck, a young Dutch colonial administrator for the Dutch East India Company (Vereenigde Oostindische Compagnie, VOC), had stopped over at the rugged Cape of Good Hope on his way to the East Indies, Dutch colonial terrain at the time. The Dutch and the later arriving British colonist (who ruled at the the Cape from 1815 until 1915), were first reluctant to leave the safe Cape region. But with the number of settlers from Europe increasing, fertile land soon became scarce and migration towards the center of the country increased. The colonial invaders, among them adventurous travelers and early scientists, soon took notice of the rich and fertile land and high biodiversity of the country. Many plant species were discovered on their intrepid trips into the mysterious and wild interior of this unknown land. On these trips, explorative and exploitative collections of plant species were gathered and documented, first in travelers' diaries and hand written notes, and later in more structured formats such as the early botanical taxonomies. Ethnobotanical information on the Cape's floral diversity can be ascertained from early travelers' accounts, such as those of Willem Adriaan van der Stel, Peter Kolbe, Carl Peter Thurnberg, known as the father of South African botany (Forbes 1986), William John Burchell (van Wyk 2008: 332) and Anders Sparrman (1784). Their accounts include many general references to South African *materia medica*. Other botanists like Karl Wilhelm Ludwig Pappe (1847, 1850) and Andrew Smith (1895) were more focused on medicinal plants in South Africa and laid the foundation for medicinal plant taxonomies.

The exploration – and exploitation – of the 'natural warehouse of the colonies' would not have been possible without the support of knowledgeable indigenous peoples. The chance of discovering merchantable and medicinally valuable plant species grew immeasurably with their help. The legitimacy of simply taking plant species and the knowledge of native people without compensation was drawn from the colonial assumption that South Africa in the 17th century was still a *terra incognita* or *terra nullius* – an empty land. However, although many South African history books only start with the European invasion of the Cape, the Cape region was long before inhabited by the San, also known by the (colonial derogatory) name of 'Bushmen', and the Khoikhoi, also known by the (colonial derogatory) name 'Hottentotts'; the two were later often referred to collectively as Khoisan (Schultze 1928: 211).

Although the original knowledge holders on the plant varieties in South Africa were certainly the San and Khoikhoi, with the invasion of Bantu tribes (ca. 1500–2000 BC) their knowledge later fused to form an inscrutable mix of knowledge(s). For the European settlers, Khoikhoi and San knowledge on the rich plant diversity of the Cape and the wild inaccessible interior of the country was invaluable. Khoikhoi and San people were constantly exploited as servants and knowledgeable guides, but they hardly received any credit or reputation, nor were they regarded as individuals with distinct knowledge(s). They were virtually non-existent to the mainly male travelers and early scientists, who did not even regard themselves as important in their accounts of colonial nature and resources. Nature, in the beginning of colonial times, was virtually dehumanized. Mary Louise Pratt argues that natural history "asserted an urban, lettered, male authority over the whole of the planet; it elaborated a rationalising, extractive, dissociative understanding which overlaid functional, experiential relations among people, plants and animals" (Pratt 1992: 38). She describes the process of dehumanization of colonial flora and fauna:

> The landscape is written as uninhabited, unpossessed, unhistoricised, unoccupied even by the travellers themselves. The activity of describing geography and identifying flora and fauna structures an asocial narrative in which the human presence, European or African, is absolutely marginal, though it was, of course, a constant and essential aspect of the travelling itself (...) Not only is 'European authority and legitimacy uncontested', but indigenous voices are almost never quoted, reproduced or even invented (ibid. 51f).

The dehumanizing and rationalizing approach started with Carl von Linné (Carl Linnaeus, 1707–1778). Linné is known as the father of modern taxonomic systems, with his book 'Systema Naturae' (1775, cf. von Linné & Agnethler 2015) representing the beginning of a systematic approach to nature, the structuring and ordering of the world as part of the European Enlightenment project (cf. Foucault 1966/1994). These taxonomic collections of plants and chemical compositions still exist in databases today.

Apart from mere data collection, interaction and exchange between early travelers and botanists and native inhabitants were part of the encounters right from the beginning. Knowledge could not have been exchanged between native people, perceived and described as "noble savages" or "sad Negros" (Comaroff & Comaroff 1991: 108ff.), and Europeans, primarily Dutch and French settlers, without encounters and relationships between these groups. Augusto Geri (2007) has pointedly claimed that

> South Africa's "ecological knowledge" (Clarke & Fujimura 1992) has always been a complex space where, despite their highly unequal powers, practitioners from all different knowledge traditions have exercised agency – none of the systems has been heretically sealed with respect to culture and practice, and none has remained unchanging or static (Geri 2007: 139).

Against the backdrop of common colonial discourses of hegemonic power relationships between Europeans and the native population, Geri's argument is corroborated by the voices of others such as Peter Kolbe, Anders Sparrman or William John Burchell, early travelers and devoted botanists who to some extent spoke with high regard about some of their native guides and were aware of that fact that they were dependent on local people to explore nature (Beinart 1998: 777). Peter Kolb (1675–1726), who worked at the Cape from 1705 to 1713, was the first to give detailed descriptions of the geography, climate, flora and fauna, and not least of the Hottentots and their language, customs, rituals and habits (Kolb 1922, 1979). Kolb represented the Hottentots as "cultural beings" rather than as "non-existent" (Pratt 1992: 52), and thus resisted the often-endorsed subjugation of the Khoisan, affirming their ways of life as valid and of equal legitimacy as European life. William John Burchell meticulously documented the names of the plants, places and people that he encountered on his long journeys into the center of the country. Short descriptions of roots, bushes, trees and food – like the "heads of flowers, boiled, make a dish which may, in taste and appearance, be compared to spinach" (Burchell 1822: 51f.) – fill his descriptions of the Cape landscape. He also took reference to what "the salves and Hottentots cook, roast, fry and eat" (ibid: 51). A detailed description of the features and appearance of the Hottentott man Stoffel Speelman and his wife Hannah, both of whom accompanied him on many of his journeys, illustrate his curiosity and interest in the native people he encountered (ibid.: 167). Burchell also noticed, with regard to his efforts to rename places and plants, a common habit to dehumanize the environment and make it legitimately accessible for colonial inquiry: "It is certainly bad taste to substitute, in any country, a modern or a foreign name, for one by which a place has been for ages known to its native inhabitant[s]" (Burchell 1822: 202).

The quote from Moreau de Maupertuis (1698–1759) given at the beginning of this chapter demonstrates a similar acknowledgment of the knowledge of the indigenous population. Equally reflective were Anders Sparrman's regular, appreciative references in his 1784 book of his trip to the Cape of Good Hope, the southern polar regions and beyond in the years 1772 to 1776 (Sparrman 178/2010) to Hottentott knowledge and techniques, such as their use of plant and animal products, which he openly acknowledged he had learnt directly from his servants (ibid.). His reference to his Hottentott guides also reads with a feeling of astonishment about their capabilities:

Außerdem, dass der Hottentotte bei dem Geschmiere der Haut sich gütlich zu tun sucht, so ist er auch zuweilen auf Wohlgeruch bedacht, seinen Körper und Kopf vermittelst eines von Kräutern bereiteten Pulvers über und über zu pudern, oder beides in die Salbe einzureiben. Dieser Geruch aber ist zu gleicher Zeit etwas stinkend und gewürzartig, aber riecht eben beinah so wie mit Spezereien vermischte Mohnsaamen. Die Gewächse, welche sie dazu gebrauchen, bestehen aus verschiedenen Gattungen des Duftstrauchs, die in ihrer Sprache Buchu heißt, und zugleich als kräftige Arzneimittel angesehen werden (ibid.: 175).

Buchu (*Agathosma betulina*) is one of the many South African medicinal plants available on the international market today, either as a tea or as an additive in cosmetic products. The plant was first 'officially' recognized by colonial travelers such as Sparrman, but had of course long been in use by the native population. An acknowledgement of this was also articulated in André Brink's novel 'Praying Mantis' (2006), where he describes the knowledge of soap making of the "Bushwoman Anna Vigilante," for which she was famous in the Cape region:

> There is nothing about making soap she [the Bushwoman Anna Vigilante] does not know. First, she will tell you, comes the lye. For this one needs ganna bushes, nothing else. In these parts, they grow luxuriantly, and easily as a big man. These shrubs are burned to provide ash. What is added, is lime. It can be dug out from the ridges in the mountains, but to her taste nothing is as good as burned shell-grit – which means making an arrangement with somebody on his way to the sea (...) (Brink 2006: 71).

This section of Brink's novel illustrates the capabilities of Anna Vigilante, and thus Brink represents another, although much later, voice contrasting the often-repeated discourse of colonial bioprospecting as colonial biopiracy, with exploitation, unrewarded taking and theft as part of the daily agenda in the contact zones of the harsh interior of the country in encounters between Khoikhoi/San and early travelers and researchers/botanists. Meanwhile, early reports of travelers and botanists could also be read in terms of interactive knowledge production between indigenous peoples and the European understanding of 'science', something that was not a clearly defined space in early colonial times (Beinart 1998: 778). These moments of interaction are in contrast with the ongoing "weakness of past writings" on African history, whereby "indigenous and scientific, African and settlers' ideas are often considered separately" (Beinart and McGregor 2003: 3; see also Geri 2007: 139).

The multiplicity of South Africa's biodiversity, the different cultural influences – not only within the country but also from other African countries and the Southeast Asian colonies – formed a conglomerate of knowledge(s) and knowledge practices that influence epistemological knowledge production in South Africa until this day. A simplified dualistic approach of colonialists versus native people would not do justice to this diversity. Those who have written the historical documentation, mostly European scholars, are responsible for these hegemonic, one-sided discourses. Other voices have hardly had a chance to be expressed, at least not in the written documentation of the time. An acknowledgement of the knowledge of the Hottentotts clearly does not substitute for the opinions, feelings or distress of the local population, of which hardly anything can be found in the written accounts of the Europeans. In this context, the idea of benefit sharing was persistently ignored or not even considered by early bioprospectors. The disclosure of knowledge on the part of the native population was generally taken for granted. Under this prerequisite, the "natural warehouse of the colonies" worked on the basis of a non-reciprocal relationship of taking without giving.

This relationship did not change much with the implementation of the Apartheid system from 1948 until 1994. In fact, it became even more cemented with land dispossessions implemented by homeland politics, which began with the Natives Land Act of 1913 and 1936. The Natives Land Act, or Bantu Land Act or Black Land Act (No. 27 of 1913), provided the basis for racial segregation, on which the ideology of "separate development" could build (Zenker 2011: 118). Land was distributed along racial lines, with the black population receiving 10% of South African land in total[2]. Black people were virtually declared landless, and were given only restricted access to certain, often inhabitable, remote and in some cases malaria-infested areas, one of them being the homeland of Gazankulu, located in today's Bushbuckridge Municipality. These conditions became more restricted with the establishment of national parks and protected areas, which strongly enforced the displacement of the black population, limiting their access to these park areas and to the plants in the parks. Protected areas such as Kruger National Park (opened in 1926) were not the unbiased creations of conservation planning, but "reflect the relations of power and privilege which have shaped South African society" (Cock & Fig 2000: 23). This underlines the fact that "biodiversity conversation in South Africa has been, and continues to be, the domain of whites" (Kepe 2009: 873). With the end of the Apartheid regime in 1994, attempts at reconciliation and the reintegration of the former 'independent' Bantustans into the Republic of South Africa increased the number of land claims by dispossessed people (Claasen & Cousins 2009; Zenker 2014), as well as of nature-based political attempts to regain self-determination and achieve the empowerment of local communities.

Historically, indigenous knowledge systems have always been a highly contested terrain between white colonial rulers on the one side and African efforts to sustain their livelihood on the other (Flint 2008). For instance, the Transvaal Crime Ordinance Act of 1904, Ordinance 26, made it illegal for "any person who for the purpose of gain pretends to exercise or use any kind of supernatural power witchcraft sorcery enchantment or conjuration or undertakes to tell fortunes or pretends from his skills or knowledge in any occult science." Under the Apartheid regime, traditional healing practices were prohibited under provision of the Witchcraft Suppression Act No. 3 of 1957, amended in 1970 (based on the Witchcraft Sup-

---

2   An attempt was made to rectify this imbalance with the Communal Land Rights Act in 2004 (Act No. 11 of 2004) (Claassens & Cousins 2008).

pression Act of 1895 of the Cape Colony), which was developed with the intention of suppressing 'malicious' indigenous healing practices, which were incorrectly defined and diminished using the derogatory term 'witchcraft'. In fact, there is no evidence that traditional healers perform witchcraft (Phatlane 2006: 9). Under Apartheid, traditional health practitioners were also prohibited from practicing as a result of the Health Act 1974, which stated that all health practitioners must be registered with the South African Medical and Dental Council in order to practice medicine (Freeman & Motei 1992; Summerton 2006). Depending on the area and the executing local municipalities and tribal authorities, this registration was accomplished, but was more often simply ignored. "White people," it was said, "do not understand our culture and belief, why would we have to register according to their demands" (Pelgrim 2003: 95).

Traditional healing has always been part of the daily lives of black people in South Africa. Without traditional healers, under Apartheid the health situation in the Bantustan would probably have been uncontrollably dire due to the inadequacy of biomedical health personnel and services (McElyea 2011). In spite of their day-to-day importance, and the claim, that witchcraft was more an accusation in Apartheid times, witchcraft accusations against healers continue until today (Niehaus 2005; Ashforth 2005), with witch burnings (Comaroff and Comaroff 1998: 293ff), witchcraft related crime and persecution (Pilgrim 2003), and regular media reports on bewitchment and witchcraft murder in many areas of the country (e.g. Braids 1998; De Waal 2012; see also Alley 2009) appearing in the daily press and in talk on the streets. Research on medicinal plants, which was limited in the final years of the Apartheid regime due to lack of funding as a result of international sanctions, was mostly conducted without the contribution of traditional healers. The few research results on medicinal plants that did come out and which were based on the knowledge of indigenous people, was, however, not regarded as knowledge that belonged to the local population.

With the introduction of new biodiversity and human rights politics in the late 20th century, the relationship between indigenous people, biodiversity and the South African state changed slowly, with continuous efforts and struggles to implement these politics at the national and local level. One of the major challenges was the definition of terms such as 'indigenous', 'indigenous or traditional knowledge/systems' and 'indigenous communities'. These definitions also result in ambiguous politics in current bioprospecting contact zones, where ABS agreements and knowledge protection are also discussed on the basis of vague definitions.

Knowledge Encounters and the Question of 'the Indigenous'

The terms 'indigenous', 'indigeneity', 'indigenous people' or 'indigenous communities' are generally not easy to define, deeply problematic and fragile political and legal terms subject to extensive legal, political and anthropological debates (Banard 2006; Friedman 2008; Kuper 2003; Niezen 2003; Zenker 2011). In the anthropological literature and political debates, the term indigenous[3] was for a long time not used at all. More derogatory terms such as 'primitives', 'savages' and 'natives' were, also as a legacy of colonial rhetoric, used instead. Only in light of post-World War II politics and an increasing recognition of indigenous peoples' rights did the term eventually gain political relevance. In the 1980s, the term 'indigenous' found acknowledgement in the United Nations (UN), with political programs reflecting the new acknowledgement of indigenous peoples and their needs. In 1982, the United Nations Working Group on Indigenous Populations (WGIP) was initiated to "promote and protect fundamental human rights and freedoms of indigenous peoples" (WGIP 1982). The International Labor Organization (ILO) (Convention 169 of 1989) and Declaration on the Rights of Indigenous People (2007) have also increasingly recognized the collective human rights of indigenous and local communities. The United Nations declared the years 1995 to 2004 to be the International Decade of the World's Indigenous Peoples (this was followed by the declaration of a second decade, from 2005 to 2014). UNESCO has defined indigenous as "a group, community or custom that is generally considered to belong to a certain region or country and which cannot be shown to have originated elsewhere" (UNESCO 2002: 1).

In South Africa, a country with a long history of migration and colonial invasion, it is not easy to define who is indigenous and who originates in the country. The San and the Khoikhoi were supposedly the first peoples in South Africa and other sub-Saharan countries. But what about later migrated Bantu groups such as the amaXhosa or Shangaan people? Adam Kuper has in turn provocatively suggested that the much later arrived Dutch settlers should also be considered indigenous (Kuper 2003; see also van Sitter 2012). Given these ambiguities, who is indigenous then? Some scholars assert that the term indigenous should not be used at all because of its "essentialist notions" (Kuper 2003). Others hold that indigenous groups all over the world have divergent claims of identity, including forms of resistance expressed in movements of autochthony and (ethno-)nationalism, claims of (political) confinement in negotiation with or against the nation state (Zenker 2011) or processes of positioning themselves in the global world (Blaser et al. 2010). Irrespective of these claims, the problem, according to Barnard, is the attempt to

---

3   The Latin etymology of 'indigenous' is translated as 'native' or 'born within'. See: Oxford Dictionaries (www.oxforddictionaries.com/definition/english/indigenous).

gather all indigenous people under one umbrella term. Instead, he suggests "a redefined indigeneity according to local requirements for the achievement of legitimate political goals" (Barnard 2006: 9). Saugestad, appealing to a similar philosophy, suggests four main criteria for indigenous peoples: first to come; non-dominance; cultural difference; and the experience of subjugation and self-ascription (Saugestad 2001: 43). Barnard's and Saugestad's approaches seem the most appropriate for the context of my research. Instead of clear definitions, I suggest working on the grounds of indigenous people 1) defining themselves and their distinct cultural identity, and 2) doing so according to the context and the (political/legal) targets pursued by this definition[4].

The Kukula Healers, for instance, define themselves as a community of healers. Each member of this healers' community is at the same time part of other communities (i.e the village or church community). The healers' community consists not only of the regionally dominant group of Shangaan people from Mozambique, but also includes people of Swazi, Tswana and Zulu origin. The healers often spoke of themselves as indigenous people. It was unclear to me, however, whether this was done as a way to claim political autonomy, making use of (learned) rhetoric, or as a conscious claim for an indigenous identity. I would therefore treat the term 'indigenous community' as a concept that enables communities to autonomously negotiate their rights with third parties (Hitchcock & Vinding 2004: 19)[5]. The concept of indigenous knowledge is similarly complex. Graham Dutfield (2003) has defined it as a body of knowledge articulated by a group of people who over generations have lived in close contact with nature. This definition is relatively broad, and implicitly suggests that the knowledge of a farming family in Lower Saxony, Germany, is as much 'indigenous knowledge' as the knowledge of a local cattle farmer in the Kalahari. However, nature and the close connection of indigenous people to their surrounding environments remains key in the definition of indigenous

---

4   Article 33 of the United Nations Declaration on the Rights of Indigenous Peoples (2007) also underlines the importance of self-identification. It says that 1) indigenous peoples have the right to determine their own identity or membership in accordance with their customs and traditions. This does not impair the right of indigenous individuals to obtain citizenship of the States in which they live. And 2) indigenous peoples have the right to determine the structures and to select the membership of their institutions in accordance with their own procedures.

5   The South African Biodiversity Act (2004) defines 'indigenous communities' as "any community of people living or having rights in a distinct geographical area within the Republic of South Africa with leadership structures and a) whose traditional uses of the indigenous biological resources to which a (bioprospecting) permit relates, have initiated or will contribute to or form part of the proposed bioprospecting; or b) whose knowledge of or discoveries about the indigenous biological resources to which an application for a permit relates are to be used for the proposed bioprospecting".

knowledge and indigenous knowledge systems[6], and their analogues traditional knowledge, traditional ecological knowledge and folklore (Anderson 2009; see also Agrawal 2002). The main traits of indigenous knowledge can be summarized as

> oral, undocumented, simple, dependant over the values, norms, and customs of the folk life, production of informal experience through trial and error, accumulation of generation wise intellectual reasoning of day to day life experiences, lost or rediscovered, practical rather than theoretical as well as asymmetrical distributed (Das Gupta 2011: 373; see also Cleveland & Soleri 2002; Ellen and Harris 1996).

Such knowledge is supposed to be practical rather than theoretical and enduring over time (Habsbawn & Ranger 1983). The most vital aspect, however, is that indigenous knowledge, despite prevailing claims of it being unchangeable, fixed and simple, is in fact mutual, not static, permeable, in constant flux and changeable. As Flavier et al. put it, it is "the information base for a society, which facilitates communication and decision-making. Indigenous information systems are dynamic, and are continually influenced by internal creativity and experimentation as well as by contact with external systems" (Flavier et al. 1995: 479). Indigenous knowledge is thus not only changeable and in flux, but it is also influenced by other knowledge systems. Scientific methods, substances and thoughts, for instance, strongly influence traditional healing practices and knowledge, and the other way round. The mutual influence of knowledge systems jettisons the common dualistic approach of indigenous knowledge versus scientific and/or Western knowledge (Verran & Turnbull 1995; Renn 2015). As Lesley Green has proposed

> ...but it is also the case that the idea of knowledge itself needs critical scrutiny, and in this sense, research on Indigenous Knowledge holds the possibility of bringing considerable insight into our understanding of knowledge itself. Achieving this goal, however, demands the study of knowledge, and not just the study of Indigenous Knowledge in relation to, and measured by, science. In other words, there is a need to dispense with the binary of 'Indigenous Knowledge' and 'science' right at the outset — not only because of the uncomfortable history of the duality in the discourse of 'primitive' and 'civilised', but because the notion of 'the indigenous' is not, I believe, a conceptually useful one (Green 2007: 135).

Drawing a strict demarcation in a terrain where the boundaries are actually blurred is not a useful approach. Early anthropologists such as Bronislaw Malinowski (1948), Franz Boas (1911/1938), E. E. Evans-Pritchard (1976) and Claude Levi-Strauss (1966) were already beginning to question this dichotomous approach

---

6   Indigenous knowledge systems, an extension of indigenous knowledge, include systems of classification, a set of empirical observations about the local environment, and a system of self-management that governs resources (Dutfield 2001).

to knowledge. Dualistic thinking at first seems inevitable when comparing the knowledge production in a scientific laboratory to the knowledge production in a traditional healers' community. This dichotomy, however, soon dissolves when further comparisons come into play. Kalahari peasants' knowledge on cattle breeding can hardly be compared to traditional healers' knowledge on medicinal plants in the Eastern Cape, and both again cannot be compared to the knowledge of a neuroscientist in a laboratory in New York or a pharmacologist in a laboratory in Cape Town. The scientist's knowledge is also locally and culturally bound and non-universal, despite the often repeated claims to the contrary (Watson-Verran & Turnball 1995). I therefore concur with Howes and Chambers (1980: 330), who prefer to differentiate indigenous knowledge from scientific knowledge on *methodological*, rather than *substantive*, grounds (cited in Agrawal 1995: 417). There are structural differences between these knowledge systems, but also similarities. The rituals of a scientific experiment, for instance, may be based on intuition and dreams, in contrast to the prevailing idea that science is open, systematic, objective and analytical, as much as traditional healers can use evidence-based methods to prove the efficacy of a medicine by, for example, holding patient files or testing a medicine through trial and error, despite the idea that indigenous knowledge is "closed, non-systematic, holistic, [and] advances on the basis of experience" (Banuri & Apffel-Marglin 1993: 10ff.; see also Howes & Chambers 1980; Agrawal 1995, Sillitoe 2002). Both traditional and scientific knowledge can be conceptualized as *local* knowledge systems:

> Western European Science is a particular standardized form of local knowledge produced by [the] scientific revolution of the seventeenth century. It was then universalized through colonialist and capitalist practices of knowledge production and ownership. During this period traditional knowledge was defined as a product of witchcraft, superstition, and heresy. It was marginalized and its social value was considerably undermined (Vermeylen & Martin & Clift 2008: 202).

Beyond the ascription of knowledge as always being locally formed and constructed, it is nevertheless subject to power structures. Avoiding dualistic approaches does not mean negating existing power structures. It would also be an intellectual challenge to avoid the term 'indigenous' in a field where the main stakeholders use it regularly, for various reasons (perhaps as political affirmation or rhetoric). But indigenous knowledge should not be contrasted to scientific knowledge. Instead, the ontological practices, production and representations of knowledge systems should be analyzed by looking at the interface, or contact zones, *where they meet* and the translation processes *when they merge*. They may nevertheless be distinguished but the focus should be on the interaction between the knowledge systems and the results of this interaction. How do policies dealing with biodiversity and indigenous peoples' (knowledge systems) influence and change other social actors (individuals, organizations, institutions) and the other way round? How do laws and policies create and influence contact zones?

Unresolved Politics: Knowledge and Natural Resources Protection

The interaction between indigenous knowledge, biodiversity and politics was politically envisaged for the first time after World War II, and global policies have continued to develop until today. With the enforcement of the CBD and the TRIPS agreement in the mid-1990s, governments, scientific research institutes, commercial companies, NGOs and indigenous peoples have been in the pursuit of amalgamating both the protection of natural and cultural resources and their commercial use in a neoliberal market system. Laws and policies can be viewed as influential 'actors' (Latour 1996, 2009), which form the field of bioprospecting and interact "with other social agents in processes" that are "dynamic and contingent, and therefore have unpredictable effects" (Shore et al. 2011: 4). They have a huge influence on the conjunctures on the ground, while the people on the ground in turn influence the development and amendment of these policies. Instead of following a top-down analytical approach to policies, *studying through* (Reinhold 1994: 477–479; Shore and Wright: 1997) – "the process of following the source of a policy – its discourses, prescriptions, and programs –through to those affected by the policies" (Wedel et al. 2005: 39–40) – provides a better understanding of the interaction between policies, people and plants. This approach will subsequently be pursued, also as an indicator for the rest of the book.

The Convention on International Trade in Endangered Species of Flora and Fauna (CITES), adopted in 1963, was a first attempt to protect endangered plant and animal species. But CITES neither engaged with human rights issues nor with ABS. The international and binding (for members) treaty of the Convention on Biological Diversity (CBD) of 1993 was the first such treaty to bring biological diversity protection, knowledge protection and human rights together in its three major objectives: 1) the conservation of biological diversity; 2) the sustainable use of its components; and 3) the fair and equitable sharing of the benefits arising from the utilization of genetic resources. With the CBD, the implementation of these goals, as well as the sovereignty over genetic resources, was designated to nation states. The objectives of the CBD were endorsed in article 8(j)[7] on *traditional knowledge, in-*

---

7   Article 8(j) of the CBD on Traditional Knowledge, Innovations and Practices states: Each contracting Party shall, as far as possible and as appropriate: Subject to national legislation, respect, preserve and maintain knowledge, innovations and practices of indigenous and local communities embodying traditional lifestyles relevant for the conservation and sustainable use of biological diversity and promote their application with the approval and involvement of the holders of such knowledge, innovations and practices and encourage the equitable

novations and practices and in the legally non-binding 'Bonn Guidelines on Access to Genetic Resources and Fair and Equitable Sharing of the Benefits Arising out of their Utilization' (2002)[8]. These guidelines aim to assist parties, governments and other stakeholders in establishing legislative, administrative or policy measures on ABS. Eight years later, the Nagoya protocol (2010) on 'Access to Genetic Resources and the Fair and Equitable Sharing of Benefits Arising from their Utilization to the Convention on Biological Diversity' was adopted, which

> aims at sharing the benefits arising from the utilization of genetic resources in a fair and equitable way, including by appropriate access to genetic resources and by appropriate transfer of relevant technologies, taking into account all rights over those resources and to technologies, and by appropriate funding, thereby contributing to the conservation of biological diversity and the sustainable use of its components (Nagoya Protocol 2010:4).

The CBD and the Nagoya Protocol (2010) represent an important step towards overcoming the colonial heritage inherent in the economic and technological power relations that persist around the globe today (Merson 2001: 2001) and fortify the turn towards new global politics and away from the long globally accepted approach to perceiving nature as 'common heritage' (FAO 1983) free to all. These were the first treaties to include mandatory ABS regulations. Member states that signed the treaties (South Africa signed the CBD in 1995) are obliged to put their goals into practice, also as they have become the official stewards of national biodiversity. The Nagoya Protocol officially accredits the bio-cultural community protocol (BCP), for instance, as a tool to enable indigenous communities to strengthen their position as stewards of the biodiversity in which they live and custodians over their knowledge, in particular when confronted by third parties. The treaties may also encourage commercially and/or scientifically interested parties to negotiate with indigenous knowledge holders. A BCP is thought to provide for the sustainable use of biodiversity, empower indigenous knowledge holders and recognize culture and nature as a form of social capital (Coombe 2009: 395). So far, BCPs as a tool only represent the political will to support indigenous peoples in *rights-based* and *dialogic* approaches to their tangible and intangible property. Long-term effects are still to be seen.

The Agreement on Trade Related Aspects of Intellectual Property Rights (TRIPS) of the General Agreement on Tariffs and Trade (GATT), administered by the World

---

sharing of the benefits arising from the utilization of such knowledge innovations and practices.

8   Secretariat of the Convention on Biological Diversity (2002): Bonn Guidelines on Access to Genetic Resources and Fair and Equitable Sharing of the Benefits Arising out of their Utilization, Montreal (https://www.cbd.int/doc/publications/cbd-bonn-gdls-en.pdf).

Trade Organization (WTO) in 1994, then pushed for the economic usurpation of intellectual property by claiming twenty years of protection for individual patents. TRIPS strongly favored private ownership of intellectual property rights and profit-based systems (Massod 1998) and made intellectual property a highly contested economic good in the neoliberal market economy. Intellectual property protection is tentatively aligned to the internationally applied intellectual property rights (IPR) protection system, which includes copyright, patents, trademarks and geographical indications. Such rights are not adaptable to indigenous knowledge, as they demand individual ownership, innovation and applicability to the economic market. Indigenous knowledge, however, is mostly collectively held, sensitive and sacred knowledge embedded in community life and customary law protection systems. Applying this collectively held knowledge to the current IP system is virtually impossible, since intellectual property law does not engage with different 'regimes of value' (Appadurai 1986), but merely with individualized economic value. But denying the relational and historical aspect of knowledge "is to deny people's cultural and inalienable heritage" (Strathern 2000a: 5).

Meanwhile, anything that is not protected under IP law is, according to TRIPS, considered to be in the public domain, and can thus be exploited by anyone without concern for the needs of the original knowledge holders and without sharing any of the revenues (Tedlock 2006: 256). TRIPS thus inflicts private intellectual property rights on the biodiversity and communities of the Global South. "Such development reveals the absolute fragility of distinctions between intellectual and physical property, tangible and intangible resources, nature and culture" (Parry 2002: 679). It exposes the one-dimensional IP law perspective on property. Moreover, the mostly poor indigenous communities of the Global South will hardly be able to finance the expensive patenting process. A patent has to be registered in a national patent office, which does not imply the validity of the patent in other national patent offices. The multiple patent registration process is a costly, legally strenuous one, usually conducted by professional IP lawyers. As a result, affluent corporations or research institutes in the Global North hold most of the past and current patents.

For indigenous communities, this opens up the ambiguous space between disclosure and knowledge protection. Once knowledge is disclosed, communities have to adjust to and rely on intellectual property law to protect their disclosed knowledge and material, irrespective of their own customary laws and knowledge protection systems. If they cannot cope with the complexities and costs of engaging with IP law, they will hardly stand a chance to control their resources once they are in the public domain. The enforcement of IP rights widens the already existing gap in the unequal relationship between North and South that was cemented by the TRIPS agreement.[9] Tony Simpson and Vanessa Jackson purport that such disregard for the ownership of knowledge

> will deepen the North/South rift, with ensuing unfair and unequal exchange; the agreement will facilitate increased occurrence of bio-piracy of biological and genetic resources from indigenous peoples; and communities and cultures may be irreversibly damaged by the forced introduction of foreign concepts of intellectual property law (such as the concepts of exclusive ownership and alienability), and the further erosion of their means of self-determination (Simpson & Jackson 1998: 45).

The CBD, in contrast, even though it is also entirely economically directed, recognizes the collective rights of local communities, a largely contradictory space between TRIPS and the CBD. The CBD provisionally promotes the solution of ABS, but does not, maybe knowingly, provide any measure or scenarios for its concrete application. Without clear objectives, laws and treaties to protect traditional knowledge are unlikely to be effective (Dustfield 2006). The World Intellectual Property Organization (WIPO) also provides no solution for the protection of indigenous knowledge. WIPO does, however, differentiate between *defensive protection*, which aims to stop people outside the community from acquiring intellectual property rights over traditional knowledge (e.g. documentation of traditional knowledge or databases), and *positive protection*, which is the granting of rights that empower communities to promote their traditional knowledge, control its uses and benefit from its commercial exploitation (e.g. national legislation or biocultural protocols)[10].

While the CBD and TRIPS agreements, and with them intellectual property rights, appear to be repressive politics, they have also simultaneously become new tools for indigenous peoples to exert political leverage. The same intellectual property processes that marginalized and disenfranchised communities started to seem like a promising new tool for economic and political leverage, if started a bit earlier (Posey & Dutfield 1996). The Mataatua Declaration, drafted at the First Inter-

---

9   Article 27.3b of the TRIPS agreement on traditional knowledge and biodiversity, which deals with the patentability or non-patentability of plant and animal-based inventions and the protection of plant varieties, was placed under review. A briefing paper discusses the reasons for this review, with some parties arguing that CBD and TRIPS contradict one another, and other parties arguing that they do not. For more information, see: www.wto.org/english/tratop_e/trips_e/ipcw
368_e.pdf (last accessed April 8, 2014). Earlier calls by some developing countries to change article 27.3b were rejected by the US and Europe on the grounds that the WTO cannot be subordinated to other international agreements. This, in effect, confirmed that the WTO is prepared to sacrifice the environment for trade (Shiva 2000: 507).

10   "Traditional Knowledge and Intellectual Property – Background Brief", January 24, 2019 (http://www.wipo.int/pressroom/en/briefs/tk_ip.html).

national Conference on the Cultural and Intellectual Property Rights of Indigenous Peoples, held in New Zealand in 1982, claimed that intellectual property is a right implied in the right of self-determination: "We declare that Indigenous Peoples of the world have the right to self-determination, and in exercise of that right must be recognized as the exclusive owners of their cultural and intellectual property" (ibid.: 205). The United Nations Draft Declaration on the Rights of Indigenous People likewise asserted in 1993 that "Indigenous peoples are entitled to the recognition of the full ownership, control, and protection of their cultural and intellectual property" (ibid.: 186). This is asserted and legitimized by the urge to overcome the historical asymmetry between Western and indigenous societies that was symbolized by the practice of perceiving indigenous knowledge as freely available goods of common heritage in the public domain (Brown 2005). Goods that have not been removed from the public domain under state auspices cannot be subject to limitations (Brush 1999: 540). While this measure was intended to prevent uncontrolled biopiracy, it also might result in conflicts between nation states that view themselves as owners of natural resources, corporations that call for free access to these resources, and indigenous communities that start declaring themselves owners and custodians over their tangible and intangible resources. Legal scholars Chandar and Sundar (2004) have commented:

> Native peoples once stood for the commons... But in the advent of an awareness of the valuable genetic and knowledge resources within native communities and lesser developed nations, the advocates for the public domain – and, in turn, propertization – have flipped. Now, corporations declare the trees and the shaman's lore to be public domain, while indigenous peoples demand property rights in the resources (Chander & Sundar 2004: 1335).

Apart from protecting knowledge by means of the common IP system, *secrecy* and *customary law* were and still are the best modes of protecting (sacred and spiritual) knowledge. The incentive of prospective benefits, as proposed by the CBD does, however, motivate indigenous knowledge holders to disclose their knowledge in the hope of participating in economic benefits; a hope that so far has not often materialized in the South African context. Even the widely discussed benefit sharing agreement in the *Hoodia Gordonii* case did not yield much financial revenue for the San community (Wynberg et al. 2009), which indicates an often repeated position of "informed consent, yes, direct benefits, no" (Hayden 2007: 739) and shows the reality behind the objectives of political agendas.

The alternative to a one size fits all solution of knowledge protection may be divergent *sui generis* modes of protection. The Traditional Knowledge Protection Bill released by the South African government in 2013 is one attempt to tackle the difficult question of how to protect traditional knowledge, and how to properly anchor it in the constitution. The bill does not include the protection of traditional knowledge on medicinal plants, but concerns arts and folklore. In addition, these modes of protection do not facilitate guidance for indigenous knowledge protection per se. IP lawyers, legal scholars and activists are in the pursuit of appropriate solutions that integrate indigenous communities directly (De Beer et al. 2014), with a trust model for indigenous communities (Cocciaro et al. 2014) being just one of them. However, to date, the only realistic way of ensuring property protection for indigenous people might indeed be to either keep the knowledge secret or, alternatively, to adapt to the current patent system. Darrell Posey claims "global trends that substitute economic and utilitarian models [e.g. TRIPS] for the holistic concept of the 'sacred balance' need to be reversed" (Posey 2002a: 3). Instead of a reversal, I would rather suggest gaining a better understanding of knowledge practices, production, protection and the relationship between these and customary law, the surrounding environment and the larger community. This would add insights to future models of indigenous knowledge protection beyond the scope of prevailing common IP law protection[11].

South Africa, with its diverse history, culture and biology/ecology was forced to adjust to the political demands of the CBD and TRIPS agreements, both of which came into being contemporaneously with the vast political changes that South Africa faced with the end of the Apartheid regime in 1994.

New Contact Zones: South African Biodiversity and Indigenous Politics

Post-Apartheid South Africa, after an extended period of economic isolation and embargo during the years of the Apartheid regime (1948–1994), came to realize the economic and socio-cultural value of natural resources and associated (indigenous) knowledge, and reacted – after having rewritten and promulgated the new democratic constitution – to international and national political developments with novel policies and forms of legal advocacy pertaining to the protection of biodiversity[12] and indigenous knowledge (systems). This was also part of the nation building process, which was linked to the notion of an 'African Renaissance', as proclaimed by Thabo Mbeki[13] in 1998, which involved the revitalization of African values, culture,

---

11   In April 2013, the South African government released a draft version of the 'Protection of Traditional Knowledge Bill' to nationally delineate the protection of traditional knowledge. However, knowledge on traditional medicine was not included in the bill.

12   According to the CBD, biological diversity is "the variability among living organisms from all sources, including, 'inter alia', terrestrial, marine, and other aquatic ecosystems, and the ecological complexes of which they are part: this includes diversity within species, between species and of ecosystems."

13   Thabo Mbeki was the second post-Apartheid president from 1999–2008, after Nelson Mandela.

science and economic power in the global market (Diop 1996; Makgoba 1999). Mbeki emphasized that "the colonizers sought to enslave the African mind and to destroy the African soul," and that therefore "the beginning of our rebirth as a continent must be our own rediscovery of our soul" (Mbeki 1998). In post-Apartheid South Africa, indigenous knowledge and biodiversity were considered vital for the rediscovery of African identity and cultural heritage. This emotional rediscovery tone was well aligned to the economic expectations bound to natural and cultural resources. Traditional medicinal plants and associated knowledge were persistently viewed as economic leverage with high revenues from trading and commercializing the plant material as scientifically verified commodities.

The link between state, science, market, local knowledge and *muthi* took on a new relevance in bioprospecting in the African Renaissance. This was a link that was also promoted in other political forums as a tool for innovation, such as by the World Intellectual Property Organization stating that together with modern technology [it] is [the role of] the pharmaceutical or other sectors to increase the rate of innovation (WIPO 2006; see also African Bioscience Initiative and NEPAD 2001). The political attempt to bring democracy, economy and current politics into practice was also part of the process of 'healing the nation' of the legacy of colonialism and Apartheid (Lund 2003). The Anglican Church Bishop Desmond Tutu claimed, "Our land needs healing. We have all been traumatized by Apartheid. We are wounded people, all of us" (Tutu, quoted in Frost 1998: 24).

Indigenous knowledge systems in general and traditional healers in particular play an important role in this healing process (Thornton 2009: 19; Lund 2003; Wreford 2008: 60–61), since traditional healers, more than any other group, represent South African indigenous knowledge and value systems. It has often been said that 80% of all Africans[14] and at least 60% of all South Africans regularly consult traditional healers. Healers were resurrected as new political agents in post-Apartheid South Africa, adopting an aggressive position in the political debates around cultural identity and heritage. To politically enforce the African Renaissance and the healing process of the nation, the African National Congress (ANC) government, after bringing into force the new democratic constitution in 1996, released in the subsequent years a number of policies designed for the development and support of indigenous peoples and their knowledge systems. Subsequently, the ANC government released policies that engaged with indigenous knowledge systems, tra-

---

14   This figure of 80% is one that is often repeated, especially by the WHO, but with virtually no evidence base. South African General Household Surveys of 2011 (http://beta2.statssa. gov.za/publications/P0318/P03182011.pdf) and 2014 (www.statssa.gov.za/publications/ P0318/P03182014.pdf) have shown that this number is vastly overrated. The black population first consults public hospitals, and there is a low rate of consultation of traditional healers. A similar result was found in the MRC South African Demographic and Health Survey (www.mrc.ac.za/bod/sadhs.htm).

ditional healing and intellectual property[15]. The promulgation of the Biodiversity Act (2004), the Indigenous Knowledge Systems (IKS 2004), the Bioprospecting and Access and Benefit Sharing Agreement (2008) and the Traditional Health Practitioners Act (2004, amended 2007) indicate the effort of the government to constitutionally promote indigenous knowledge systems and the implementation of ABS agreements. The inclusion of 'indigenous matters' into the legislation expresses not only the integration of rights of the thus far excluded, but also evoke a number of questions. What are these policies aiming at? Under whose authority are they produced? What values and whose interests are promoted and supported by these policies? And "what new subjects and relations of power do such policies produce" (Ball 1990: 154)?

Policies Endorsing Indigenous Heritage

Indigenous knowledge systems found anchorage in the country's constitution with the South African Indigenous Knowledge Systems (IKS) Policy (No. 10 of 2004). It was adopted by the South African Cabinet in 2004, "thus laying in place the first important milestone in our efforts to recognize, affirm, develop, promote and protect Indigenous Knowledge Systems in South Africa" (IKS Policy 2004: 1), wrote Musibudi Mangena, Minister of Science and Technology, in the introduction. The policy was developed by eleven ministries under the lead of the Department of Science and Technology (DST) as

> an enabling framework to stimulate and strengthen the contribution of indigenous knowledge to social and economic development in South Africa to balance out the profound negative effects on the development of South Africa's economy and society, resulting in the distortion of the social, cultural and economic development of the vast majority of its people (ibid.).

This excerpt from the policy alludes to the objectives of the African Renaissance, with its focus on economic development and growth impacting the social development of the country. The policy also encouraged "the affirmation of African cultural values in the face of globalisation, a clear imperative given to the need to promote a positive African identity" (ibid.). Additional concerns that framed the policy were biopiracy, benefit sharing and the recognition of knowledge holders (Green 2008: 132). It was thus set in place to better understand the historical and cultural context and the value of indigenous communities, to ensure the contribution of indigenous knowledge to the economy, to eradicate poverty and fortify innovation

---

15   The Intellectual Property (IKS) Laws Amendment Bill (2010) and the Draft Protection of Traditional Knowledge Bill (2013) deal with intellectual property in particular.

and economic growth (IKS Policy 2004). Against this background, the South African government also attempted to align to the demands of the WIPO, the CBD and the UNESCO Convention for the Safeguarding of Intangible Cultural Heritage (2003)[16].

But why is the IKS policy promoted by the Department of Science and Technology? asked Lesley Green (2008) provocatively. According to Green, the approach of the government to accredit the IKS policy under the lead of the DST "was a shot across the bows of universalist approaches to the sciences" (ibid.: 49). This positioning would not lead to an extended dialogue between science and indigenous knowledge, but rather to an assimilation of indigenous knowledge into science (Green 2007: 130). In her view, it contradicts the original motivation of the policy to promote African values and identity. "Would not the Department of Arts and Culture (DAC) be the more appropriate overseeing department?" she asked during an informal conversation that we had at the University of Cape Town in March 2009. The scientific approach was emphasized in the IKS policy by promoting "the interface with other knowledge systems, for example indigenous knowledge is used together with modern biotechnology in the pharmaceutical and other sectors to increase the rate of innovation" (IKS Policy 2004: 9). In this sense, indigenous knowledge serves as a support system for (scientific) innovation. It is obviously not viewed as innovative in its own right, but instead serves as a source for *scientific* innovation.

This was also realized through a number of scientific institutions and programs that were founded to conform to the objectives of the IKS Policy, with the IKS Lead Program and the National Indigenous Knowledge Systems Office (NIKSO) being two of them. NIKSO was installed in 2006 to engage not only with traditional healing, but with a range of other knowledge systems (e.g. indigenous farming methods, indigenous mathematical knowledge, arts and crafts, and indigenous games). The IKS Lead Program of the Medical Research Council (MRC) was implemented in 2001 and the laboratory opened in 2004/5. It aims to bring together science and the indigenous knowledge (systems) of traditional healers to support indigenous people and their knowledge systems and generate scientific innovation relevant for the global market.

This recognition of traditional knowledge holders was further stipulated in the Traditional Health Practitioners (THP) Act (2004, amended 2007 by the Department

---

16   The Convention for the Safeguarding of Intangible Cultural Heritage was adopted by the UNESCO General Conference in October 2003 to safeguard the uses, representations, expressions, knowledge and techniques that communities, groups and in some cases individuals recognize as an integral part of their cultural heritage. See: www.unescor.org/new/en/santiago/intangible-heritage/convention-intangible-cultural-heritage/ (last accessed October 5, 2014).

of Health), which seeks to integrate traditional healing and traditional health practitioners into the legislation. It is estimated that about 350,000 practicing traditional health practitioners (Flint 2012: 260) work in the primary health care sector.
Their knowledge systems are immeasurable in terms of daily health care delivery
for local populations. The THP Act therefore focuses on traditional health practitioners, their professionalization and their obligatory registration[17] "to ensure the
efficacy, safety and quality of traditional health care services" (THP Act 2007: 5), including the establishment of the Interim Traditional Health Practitioners Council.
The Act also included provisions for the registration, training and practices of traditional health practitioners, and the protection of the interests of members of the
public who use the services of traditional health practitioners. The THP Council,
founded as a result of the Act, appointed by the Minister of Health, consists of nine
categories of traditional healer and each category of traditional health practitioner
– diviner, herbalist and traditional birth attendant – as well as 'non-traditional
members' such as a member of the Department of Health, a lawyer, a pharmacist
and a member of the Health Professions Council. All traditional healers in South
Africa ought to be registered at the Council. Healers are then entitled to prescribe medical certificates and sick notes. After the prohibition of traditional healers
during the Apartheid regime, the THP Act was an important step towards their official recognition. The endeavor to 'professionalize' traditional health practitioners
takes cognizance of the importance of traditional healing as cultural heritage, but
at the same time attempts to formalize a profession this is difficult to formalize.
How, for instance, can practices such as trance or the evocation of ancestors be
measured and regulated?

In interviews with traditional healers, I noticed two positions regarding the
Act. One group fully endorsed the efforts to regulate the profession, while the other
group rejected and/or ignored the new power assumed by the state over traditional healing. Nceba Gqaleni, Chairperson of the DST's African Traditional Medicine
Bioprospecting and Product Development Platform and Professor at the University
of KwaZulu-Natal, claimed that traditional healing systems must be self-regulated
by traditional healers, and should not be subject to state regulation and control,
as this can be viewed as a new secularization process. "What happens," questioned Gqaleni, "when the ancestors say something other than the law?" According
to Gqaleni's firm conviction, traditional healing should not be regulated; the different healing traditions, the huge differences between traditional healing contexts

---

17   The Act stipulates that "a person who is not registered as a traditional health practitioner
or as a student in terms of this Act is guilty for an offence if he or she (...) treats or offers to
treat, or prescribes treatment or any cure for, cancer, HIV and AIDS or any prescribed terminal
disease." Anyone who does so is liable to "a fine or to imprisonment for a period not exceeding
12 months or to both a fine and such imprisonment" (Thornton 2009: 20).

in rural and urban contexts on the one hand, and the diverse rules that regulate traditional healing on the other, are too complex to put them into one regulatory framework (Interview with Gqaleni, January 2010, Durban).

Aside from the IKS policy and the THP Act, the national Department of Health (DoH) has demonstrated significant commitment by including traditional medicine as one of the objectives of the National Drug Policy (1996). The policy recognizes the potential role and benefits of available remedies from African traditional medicine for the National Health System. The DoH has established a Traditional Medicine Directorate, headed by Dr. Mayeng. Its main objective is the coordination of the development of traditional medicines, including formulation and implementation. Supplementary South African regulatory frameworks such as the Traditional Medicines Draft Policy (2008) and the Medicines Control Council (MCC), the latter of which regulates the performance of clinical trials and the registration of medicines, including traditional medicine. All publicly available plant medicines should be registered under the MCC, even those sold at street markets and the big *muthi* markets. Registration is a long process, as it includes pre-clinical and clinical trials to be conducted before registration; a long and cost-intensive process unaffordable for most traditional healers. This rule is, therefore, barely applied; the informal traditional medicine plant market is far too complex and uncontrollable. Nevertheless, the value inherent in medicinal plants means that there are not only calls for more control, but hopes have also been ignited by the potential – untapped – economic value of plants.

Economic Incentives: In Muthi We Hope

It is not only indigenous knowledge systems that are considered important in the new post-Apartheid South Africa; medicinal plants, due to their potential economic importance, can also no longer be ignored. As said earlier, the commercialization and trading of medicinal plant material has always been an economically profitable business. Today, however, it is a multi-million dollar business. Herbal medicines produce an estimated global value of US$ 65 billion (WHO 2001). In the year 2000, the global value of plant-based pharmaceuticals was calculated at around US$ 500 billion (Mander et al. 2006: 169), with the numbers continuously increasing. While developing countries provide most of the world's natural resources, they receive little of the incoming profits in return; a recurrent discrepancy between resource rich but economically poor and economically rich but resource poor countries (The Crucible Group 1994). A survey from South Africa on the national market estimated that 35,000 to 70,000 tons of plant materials are consumed per year, with a market value of US$ 75 to 150 million (Mander & Le Breton 2006: 4). This sum comprises raw and semi-proceeded plant material utilized for daily medicinal health care and body hygiene by the black South African population, who are dependent on medicinal plants for their primary health care provision.

To date, of the more than 30,000 species of higher plants in South Africa, 3000 are commonly known and used as medicines (van Wyk & Gericke 2000). About 350 of these species are traded as medicinal plants (van Wyk et al. 2009), with Devil's Claw (*Harpagophytum procumbens (Burch.)*), Umckaloabo (*Pelargomium sidoides*), Hoodia (*Hoodia gordonii*), Buchu (*Agathosma betulina*), Aloe ferox (*Aloe ferox Mill.*), Rooibos tea (*Aspalathus linearis*) and Honeybush tea (*Cyclopia genistoides*) being the most common. The immense quantity of (partially wild) harvested plant material on the market poses an enormous threat to the already threatened national biodiversity. Mixtures of commonly known barks of the Pepper Bark tree (*Warburgia salutaris*) and the Red Stinkwood tree (*Prunus africana*), bulbs of African potato or bundles of *Imphepho* (*Helichrysum odoratissimum*) – South African ritual incense – are sold in large quantities in markets and informal shops along the roadsides of former homeland villages and city townships. The daily need for plant material as well as the growing global interest in medicinal plants also leads to an increase of wild harvesting by so-called '*muthi* hunters', for local use (Cunningham 1988), for the large and small *muthi* markets in Johannesburg and Durban, and for the (international) food, pharmaceutical and cosmetic industries. *Muthi* markets are of such importance that the pharmaceutical industry in Johannesburg even perceived them to be in direct competition with the pharmaceutical market. The battle between the pharmaceutical industry and the *muthi* markets went so far that the pharmaceutical industry in Johannesburg considered trying to enforce the closure of the government-owned Faraday Muthi Market (Interview with Faraday Muthi Market liaison manager, January 2010, Johannesburg).

Figure 2 Muthi Market in Durban

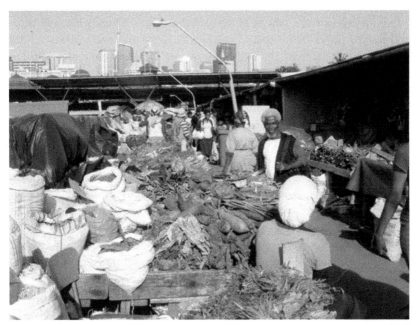

© B. Rutert.

Many local plant collectors live from supplying the national and international market with medicinal plants. As a consequence, some plant species are close to extinction. To prevent wild (over) harvesting, some local governments have enacted a ban on collecting specific plant species such as *Pelargonium sidoides* in the Eastern Cape[18]. Instead, it has been proposed that medicinal plants be bred on plantation sites to supply the markets. Twasa, the traditional healer in Mboyti, Eastern Cape, told me "that Nature Conservation," the governmental environmental protection organization, had come to his village to debate

> with the chief that they [the healers] cannot collect medicine, they must go and plant it up there [on top of a small hill in the village]. Nature [Conservation] is going to plant them somewhere here, because they are preventing the inyangas from taking the plants and the roots of the forest. They must go to a special place where they are allowed to fetch these medicines. But then Nature disappeared and never came back to do that (Interview in Mboyti, October 2009).

---

18   www.environment.gov.za/sites/default/files/gazetted_notices/biodiversitymanage-ment_pelargonium_sidoidesplan.pdf (last accessed November 25, 2015).

Mboyti lies in the Maputaland-Pondoland-Albany Biodiversity Hotspot and covers a wealth of rare plant species endemic to the area[19]. Twasa also claimed that it is not the *inyangas* who take all of the medicine from the forests but poor people collecting plants for 10 Rand (ca. 1 Euro) a bag for the *muthi* markets and the pharmaceutical industry. The wild harvesting of *muthi* hunters was regarded as an enormous threat to the environment and to the practices of the healers. Nevertheless, the hope for 'green diamonds' is not an illusory one, given that around 25% of all available synthetic biomedicine is based on natural resources (Mander and Breton 2006). Probably the most prominent example is acetylsalicylic acid, popularly known as aspirin. It originally derives from the bark of the willow tree and was used by the ancient Greeks against headaches and was eventually extracted by a French chemist in 1853 (Jeffreys 2008). The economic value of aspirin (and equivalent products) is immeasurable. Acetylsalicylic acid was discovered long before the CBD was adopted, and the discovery was not based on indigenous knowledge. Umckaloabo, by contrast, a phytomedicine made of the plant *Pelagonium sidoides*, originates from the knowledge of communities in the Eastern Cape and Lesotho. Its wide medicinal use/exploitation unleashed a huge debate over the misappropriation of medicinal plants and the breaching of patent law (see also chapter VI). Economically, Umckaloabo is a successful product with an estimated value exceeding Euro 80 million per year on the Germany market alone (van Wyk 2011: 824) and demand is continuing to increase on the global market.

The general success rate for research and development (R&D) in natural remedies processes is claimed to be one in 10,000 compound screenings ending in a successful drug (Reid et al. 1993). Indeed, the costs of the R&D process often stretch beyond the income generated by a product. For that reason, only a small number of big companies are able to develop pharmaceuticals based on biological or genetic resources. Parts of the R&D process are outsourced to smaller companies or institutes like the IKS Lead Program. The rescreening of already existing libraries or the screening of natural samples directly collected in nature is a common and successful practice. Plants used as medicines have to pass laborious safety and efficacy tests and clinical trials before entering the formal market (Gibson 2011). Others, like Rooibos tea, fall under the law of less strict rules for congestible goods. The rich biodiversity of South Africa might contain many more as yet undiscovered 'green diamonds' (Wynberg et al. 2009) inherent in (medicinal) plants. New biotechnologies and advances in medicinal botany have also added to an increase in ethnopharmaceutical research (Martin & Vermeulen 2006) and the hope to medicinally

---

19   South Africa hosts hosts 10% of the world's higher plant species (van Wyk & Gericke 2000) in three so-called biodiversity hotspots: the Cape Floristic region in the Western Cape, the Succulent Karoo region in the interior of the country, and the Maputaland-Pondoland-Albany region along the cost from Eastern Cape Province to Mozambique.

and economically revolutionize the pharmaceutical market with valuable new products. The probability of finding new valuable chemical compounds in medicinal plants is relatively high in South Africa's rich biodiversity.

Ethnography in Bioprospecting Contact Zones

The historical and current political and economic situation that emerges from bioprospecting in South Africa is obviously a convoluted mixture, reaching from the past into the present. I only came to realize how much past influences reach until today after I, as a researcher, went through some rough, mostly irritating, sometimes overtly hostile, encounters with my interlocutors. I regard these situations as encounters in current bioprospecting contact zones; zones of interaction loaded with past power imbalances and resulting mistrust that, most probably, had nothing to do with me as a private person, but with me as a researcher in a field that has for a long time been determined by imbalanced power and a newly arising African consciousness, propagated by the African Renaissance and subsequent indigenous policies. Drawing a line between the personal and the professional was difficult here. At first, I was unaware that "bioprospecting is a [political] minefield" (Informal conversation with Anne Hutchings, Empangeni, January 2009). It took me considerable time to adjust to the political diplomacy and cultural sensitivity that the field required. An ostensibly protective attitude and some rough encounters with healers and other interview partners made me aware of just how much the field of bioprospecting is still influenced by the past, and that my research was challenged not only by my own lack of experience. I began to understand reluctance and secrecy as an important category in the context of my data, and understood that the field is highly influenced by past colonial and Apartheid politics. But I also noticed how much the interactions between my interview partners and me depended on the geographical region and institutional context. Conducting research in the Eastern Cape under the name of the IKS Lead Program seemed to present many obstacles, while research conducted in Bushbuckridge in the name of Natural Justice rather seemed to be met with open doors. This could partly be due to my lack of experience in the first research phase at the IKS Lead Program and my greater experience in the second research phase; but I am inclined to believe that it is not irrelevant that I was associated with the IKS Lead Program as an institution that "wants to have something" (knowledge and plants), while Natural Justice is an organization that "wants to give something" (knowledge and expertise).

Case studies of three different sites will describe my position as a researcher (from the Global North) in the field of bioprospecting. My first encounter with traditional healers of mostly isiXhosa-speaking background started with a focus group discussion that my German PhD colleague Peter and I conducted at the IKS

Lead Program's headquarters in February 2009. During the FGD, the healers disregarded my interview questions and almost aggressively refused to give permission for audio-recording or the taking of notes. The next opaque encounter happened in Mzansi, a small village in Eastern Cape Province, where one healer nearly hit me with a stick and yelled in furious anger, "You white people are not going to take our knowledge away!" (Fieldnotes, February 2009). In an informal conservation at the annual Indigenous Plant Use Forum (IPUF) conference at Stellenbosch University in July 2009, a professor of biology at Johannesburg University roughly asserted, when I approached him to get advice regarding the problems of approaching traditional healers for interviews, "Go back home. You will never get the information you are looking for. They [traditional healers] will never give you any information" (Fieldnotes, July 2009). "My own experience with traditional healers had been challenging," he continued. "It is not easy to approach them, even for me as a South African." At the same conference, a PhD student of pharmacology confided to me, "This [bioprospecting] is a dangerous field, you must be very careful. If you ask too many questions, they might even kill you" (Fieldnotes, June 2009). At the IKS Lead Program laboratory, one of the PhD researchers took me aside, asked me how my research was going, and after I told him that it was generally difficult to get information, he nodded knowingly. "If I may advise you, don't talk openly to anyone here, only use email or the phone if you have questions" (Fieldnotes, August 2009).

All of these warnings, threats and words of advice made me think about the backdrop to these words. Why did the professor recommend that I "go back home"? Who are the people who would possibly kill for the sake of medicinal plants and knowledge? Why did the healer think that I wanted to take her knowledge away, even though I never asked her or her fellow healers for any specific knowledge? Why was the researcher at the IKS laboratory being so cautious when he advised me not to talk openly? And what was my role in all of this? The reasons behind these views might have been manifold, ranging from the after-effects of colonial biopiracy and Apartheid racial politics, which are still deeply inscribed in people's minds; to the increasing recognition of knowledge as valuable currency in the global knowledge economy and as a significant socio-cultural good of cultural heritage; to medicinal plants being a contested good for scientists and companies seeking innovative patents and products; to my position as a researcher investigating in a field that is economically, politically, socio-culturally and emotionally highly contested.

In light of these short remarks, it is fair to say that bioprospecting is a highly politicized and competitive field. The new value of knowledge in the global knowledge economy makes knowledge holders increasingly aware of the value of their resources. Even though the motivation for protective attitudes might have been different for each stakeholder, it is based on the protection of this newly ascribed value. For a researcher, this situation is like searching for the safe route through a minefield, a situation that can be emotionally strenuous and yet nevertheless valuable for the data collection and analysis process.

Emotions in the Field. Are They Re-Narratable?

Are personal emotions experienced in a such a politicized field as bioprospecting and such a deeply intuitive realm as traditional healing re-narratable? I am sitting in my flat in Berlin, cold, dark winter weather outside, the washing machine rumbling noisily in the background. It has been a year since I was last in South Africa for a holiday, and two and a half years since I conducted my last month of fieldwork. Almost despairingly, I am trying to grasp how I felt during my fieldwork, and how my interlocutors might have felt. Reiterating emotions and making scientific use of them seems impossible while listening to the noise of the washing machine and staring at the first snowflakes falling past my window.

In the villages of the Eastern Cape and Mpumalanga Province, I listened to the barking of dogs, the monotonous clucking of roaming chickens, to Kwaito or Shangaan electro music from faraway music boxes, or to the enthusiastic singing of the Sunday morning service at the neighboring Zion Christian Church. While *there*, I learned movements, inhaled smells, thought new thoughts and felt emotions different to the emotions here. I shared joy, laughter, anger, fear and excitement in resonance with the context. Local adaptation entails emotional adaptation. Yet I remained a middle class, educated white woman from Germany, who, until the beginning of the PhD project, had never experienced ancestors and spirits, or the regular slaughtering of chickens, goats and cows. After many months, such things eventually became familiar to me. When back in Germany, I had difficulties in reconnecting to the world at home. Gradually, however, these emotions vanished the more time passed with me 'just sitting in front of the computer'. In that sense, reiterating emotions from the field is like writing about falling in love for the first time. It is easy to remember the intensity, the desire for closeness, the longing and the suffering when the relationship breaks down. But feeling the emotions as such is hardly possible. Emotions are alive in the present. They exist intensely in the moment, but they do have an expiry date. Emotions are writeable as memories, but the written word will never represent the embodied emotions of the lived moment. In this sense, "fieldwork is an emotional encounter as well as an intellectual exercise" (Sore 1999: 28, cited in Spencer & Davis 2010: 6). The differentiation between writing about emotions *in* the field and emotions *about* the field is vital here. In particular, encounters that made a huge emotional impact, such as with entities like the ancestors, are not easy to recount.

"What counts as data?" asked Tanya Luhrman (2010) in a chapter of Davis & Spencer's book 'Emotions in the Field. A Psychology and Anthropology of Fieldwork Experience' (2010). She describes how her own experiences with magic and the supernatural influenced her position in the field. She draws the conclusion that our own proclivity and experiences affect the way we chose the field in which we work, the guiding interests in the field and the outcomes of the writing: "If you have heard the mermaids singing, you are more likely to ask people about mermaids in different ways than if you have not" (Luhrman 2010: 233). Luhrman's experience lays out an ambiguous intersubjective encounter between a human being (herself) and a non-human being (supernatural power). "Because Being is never limited to human being, the field of intersubjectivity includes persons, ancestors, spirits, collective representations, and material things" (Jackson 1998: 9).

Integrating interactions of emotional meaning into ethnographic analysis argues against the long maintained idea that emotions have no epistemological value. It has been said that subjectivity only has a corrosive effect on research and undermines the process of knowledge production in general (Davis & Spencer 2010; Stodulka 2014). I intend to show, however, that *radical empiricism* (James 1976; Davies & Spencer 2010, Jackson 1989), an approach to the field that does not cut between object and subject, person and person(s), person and method (inter-methodology), and between person and materiality/environment (inter-materiality), is the most suitable methodological approach to engage with emotions evoked by human (healer) and 'half-human' (ancestor) actors. Radical empiricism focuses on the relations *between* people, things, concepts, the environment and the self and is also informed by psychological perspectives (Jackson 1989, 1998). Radical empiricism looks at fieldwork as a relational and intersubjective process (Spencer 2010: 3; Jackson 2007), "and takes into account the researcher's own position in an intersubjective relationship with persons, ancestors, spirits, collective representations and material things (Jackson 1998). As an atheist, who was raised in a protestant household and educated in the academy, all entities and beings beyond 'the familiar' initially went unrecognized in my fieldwork. I was ontologically unaware of the ancestors and unknowingly underestimated their power and thus did not integrate them into my anthropological knowledge production. They simply did not exist for me. I probably fell victim to what Bourdieu (2000) called "scholastic fallacies," the assumption that identity and knowledge are stable and intrinsic properties of persons and groups and that human interactions are primarily motivated by abstract ideas and rational calculations (Jackson 2007: 149). Only with time and a "shift in cultural anthropological methodology from participant observation toward the observation of participation" (Tedlock 1991: 69) did I begin to make "a transition from objectifying methodology to intersubjective methodology" (Tedlock 200:471). This also corroborates the approach of actor-network theory, which in a similar manner does not deal with object-subject divisions but looks at the relational aspect of the interaction of human and non-human actors.

The ancestors, though neither totally human nor non-human, belong to the network of all human and non-human actors in the field of bioprospecting and do have a significant influence; this was not only the case for my own access to data, but also in terms of the political debate on intellectual property rights and knowledge protection. I therefore suggest rephrasing Luhrman's quote above to the following, which applies to my own fieldwork: If you have heard the ancestors speak, you are more likely to ask healers about ancestors in different ways than if you have not. I will show that 'getting to know the ancestors' challenged the research process significantly, in a way that 'getting to know pharmaceutical biochemistry' was unable to do. While a laboratory could be observed from a distant point of view, the ancestors are an intangible and invisible entity that one can only experience and never observe. The following case studies cannot recreate the respective emotional experiences to the fullest. At first naïve and unaware of the politically charged field of bioprospecting, and of the lived world and interests of traditional healers, I went through intense key emotional episodes (Berger 2010) where I "plunged into the life of the natives" (Malinowski 1922: 22). In all contexts, these key emotional episodes were always relational encounters that happened in particular bioprospecting contact zones. Kirsten Hastrup used the term "raw moments" to describe

> thresholds of knowledge, and lived narratives (...) being highly charged with emotions. The raw moments are different from diagnostic events, as we usually talk about them in anthropology, because they are intensely emotional and related to the feelings of the fieldworker rather than the analytical habitus. The raw moments strip us bare of conceptual prejudice and deliver us to pure sensation (Hastrup 2010: 204).

While Hastrup experienced a raw moment in the arctic landscape by envisioning a *huldumadur*, "a man of the hidden people," a vision that is impossible to have without experiencing the landscape (ibid.), I experienced the key emotional episodes during my fieldwork more as inter-relational turning points, dependent upon my interlocutors, politics, the ancestors and the perception of knowledge and medicinal plants. They were based on many different emotions: fear and distress, lack of time, my position as a white researcher in a politically – and racially – charged field, talking past each other (Jackson 2007: 158ff.), but also my growing confidence, commitment and experience, as well as the trust of my research participants in me. Clearly, these encounters contributed to gaining a better understanding of and access to the field. In the second research phase, the experiences of the first phase helped me to gain easier access to the field and its people.

In describing these key emotional episodes and raw moments, I do not only want to reveal my own, naïve, inexperienced and vulnerable role in a highly ambiguous field, but also to show how the trajectory from participant observation to the observation of participation changed my access to the field. This trajectory happened in a field that is strongly shaped by past contact zones reaching into the bioprospecting contact zones I encountered in the present. My own emotions and reactions, as well as the emotions and reactions of my interlocutors, were hence not only situational affects, but were also based on past and present political and economic contexts. I therefore refer to the experiences I made as *emotional contact zones*, an assemblage of deep emotional immersion, an "emotional apprenticeship" (Shreshta 2010). I will start with an encounter at the IKS Lead Program and continue with two situations in the Eastern Cape. To show how emotions and access to the field changed over the twenty months of fieldwork, I will conclude with a situation involving the ancestors that occurred during my second research phase.

Focus Group Discussion at the IKS Lead Program: Politics or Personal Liability?

I arrived in Cape Town on January 5, 2009, a research proposal, a tape recorder and the contact details of Dr. Mastabisa, Director of the IKS Lead Program, in my luggage. Upon arrival, my German colleague Peter was coincidently also in Cape Town for his own research project on Masculinity and HIV/AIDS. After I had settled in at the IKS laboratory, my main research site for the year, a staff member, Mirranda, helped me to organize a focus group discussion with traditional healers from nearby townships. I intended to investigate the healers' perceptions on knowledge and knowledge protection. Peter was also interested in interviewing the healers on men's health, and we agreed, after consultation with Mirranda, to conduct the focus group discussion together. A week later, Mirranda had organized a minibus to pick up the healers. The healers, six female and one male, arrived at 10 in the morning at the IKS Lead Program's head office, chatting and singing. We welcomed them and gathered in the small meeting room of the IKS office. Biscuits and coffee were served and we introduced ourselves. The ancestors were greeted with a prayer. Because most of the healers spoke only isiXhosa, Mirranda translated from isiXhosa to English. After the introduction, Peter and I ask for permission to audio record the interviews, but the healers unanimously refused any kind of recording. It was my first focus group discussion in South Africa and I was surprised by the fierce refusal. I put the turned off tape recorder in front of me on the table. This was regarded as insulting, as I would learn later.

Peter began with his questions on men's health and a lively discussion ensued and continued until we switched and I introduced my own research subject. Curiously, the atmosphere among the healers immediately turned icy. They abruptly asked me not to take any notes at all. I was infuriated. Peter had taken notes, why should I not? Had I offended the healers unknowingly? I continued to ask my questions on knowledge and intellectual property rights. Reluctantly, the healers answered. The main spokesperson summed up: there is a big gap between the knowledge and ancestral wisdom of the healers and the knowledge of the IKS Lead Program. And the government will not be able to protect knowledge, wisdom and dreams by means of a policy [the THP Act]. The government basically cannot protect our knowledge, the healers claimed. And then, suddenly, the atmosphere became even more closed off, and the main spokesperson, a tall and insistent woman, started nagging: "You pose very offensive questions." She continued, "Why do all these white people come to take away our knowledge? What are we getting out of it in the end? We will never get anything out of it!"

Although I was capable of rationalizing this response, in the moment I felt insulted. I found her questions reasonable, yet I was unable to answer appropriately. First and foremost, I was in South Africa for my PhD. But, I tried to explain, I might write a book that may represent the voices of the people. After releasing her anger, the atmosphere became even icier, and after twenty minutes I gave up and ended the interview. Had I asked the wrong questions? Formulating comprehensible questions on property took me almost the entire first research phase. I learned that property was an abstract concept for most traditional healers. And I actually had too little experience with the political explosiveness of the subject. I could easily and unknowingly have dropped a brick.

Either I, or me in the position as an IKS associate and researcher from the Global North, seemed to have aroused negative emotions in my interview partners. Aside from the fact that I was a white researcher wanting to know something about traditional healing and knowledge, which arguably was a controversial position, the hostility of the healers was disturbing. I must have crossed a number of ethical boundaries I was unaware of. And probably, conducting research under the auspices of the IKS Lead Program made the situation even more complicated. Peter was a researcher independent of the IKS, while I was an IKS associate. I obviously had a doubly threatening role in this scenario: I was a researcher from the Global North, who by means of my research subject could potentially be interested in the healers' knowledge, and I was associated with a research institute that was also interested in their knowledge. In the focus group discussion, I heard criticism posed against the IKS, and against the government's attempt to 'professionalize' traditional healing (see also Laplante 2015). The healers basically mistrusted the governmental IKS Lead Program. And yet they cooperated with it; I saw some of these healers at other activities of the IKS Lead Program. The institutional mistrust seemed ambivalently torn between politics of interests and the desire to participate in educational courses, knowledge sharing and possibly the honor of partaking in a governmental program.

When I later asked Mirranda what had gone wrong, she avoided me and simply claimed that I had not been allowed to interview the healers; the focus group discussion had been meant only for Peter. I would need ethical clearance from the MRC ethical research committee before I could conduct interviews. Later, I learned that this was an MRC approved informed consent form that both my participants and I would have to fill in and agree upon at the start, a common practice since the Biodiversity Act 2004. Probably the IKS director simply had forgotten to tell me before? Research participants would have to agree by signing the informed consent form, which declared that the information exchanged would be "confidential and that there shall be no reckless publications that may jeopardize the creation of intellectual property that could result from the information supplied" (Informed consent document, MRC South Africa). From then onwards, I adhered to this procedure when I conducted research in the name of the IKS Lead Program. I offered information on the project, in particular when I conducted interviews with traditional healers, where I briefly introduced the purpose of the study, my expectations of the study and the possibility for participants to withdraw from the study whenever they wished. But still, even when informed consent procedures were scrupulously followed, further challenges emerged.

"Experiencing the Ancestors": Immersion in the Field

The first to introduce me to the ancestors was my landlady Annelie in Cape Town. Annelie is a white Afrikaans-speaking woman with a Bachelor degree in Philosophy and Theology, who had been working in the media as a "corporate princess," as she called herself, for many years before, having been called by the ancestors, she started her apprenticeship as a *sangoma*. It is the ancestors who choose a traditional healer-to-be (*thwasa*). In fact, it is the ancestors who are the inner voices, forces and powers that make a diviner (a traditional healer who is capable of evoking the ancestors). For my landlady, her calling manifested as a physical and mental burnout and recurrent meetings with a black woman in her neighborhood, who after some time insisted that she should train as a healer. Annelie knew that "Africa is going to be my doctor," and soon after she started her apprenticeship in the Eastern Cape Annelie's story is unusual, but not totally unheard of in the new post-Apartheid South Africa. More and more white people are crossing the imaginary and real segregation boundaries between black and white citizens to train as traditional healers, and thus immerse themselves in black community life (cf. Bührmann 1984; Hall 1995; Wreford 2009). Traditional healing still remains mostly outside of the experience of many white South Africans, but is nevertheless fully part of South African life and consciousness (Thornton 2009: 17). At the beginning, I was suspicious about white people becoming African traditional healers, and about the concept of the ancestors. Why immerse oneself in something so unfamiliar? I aimed to study *muthi*, indigenous knowledge systems, access and benefit sharing schemes and concepts of knowledge protection. My mind was totally inclined towards allegedly objective, rational thinking.

In the end, my own personal encounters with the ancestors finally confounded my inner belief system and enabled another, more procedural access to the field. In the following sections, I will describe how a string of misfortune and negative

experiences – of theft, accidents and inner turmoil in my bioprospecting encounters – and my being supposedly healed of it, eventually brought me closer to the
realm of healing and the healers in the second research phase, when I eventually
even extended my role to a triple role as an ethnographer

Being Jeopardized in Mzansi, Eastern Cape

Mzansi is a conglomerate of houses along a sloping hill just off the N2, not far
from Butterworth, in the former homeland of Transkei, Eastern Cape Province.
Mirranda had joined me as a translator and traditional healer to interview traditional healers about their perceptions on knowledge as property. After five days of
interviewing healers in Transkei villages not far from Mthatha, she suggested we
visit her friend Mamjoli. I could stay there for some days and learn more about medicinal plants, she said. She knew Mamjoli from her training in the Eastern Cape.
Upon our arrival at Mamjoli's house, about twenty young girls from the village sang
and danced to welcome us. Mamjoli, happy to see her old friend again, greeted us
with joy. After our joint journey had been overshadowed by financial struggles, I
saw Mirranda relaxing for the first time, being among her peers. At the IKS Lead
Program, she came across as constantly tense in her attempt to cope with her own
triple role of being an IKS staff member, a traditional healer and a student of anthropology. She joined the dancing girls with laughter and sparkling eyes. A bit
later, we went into Mamjoli's small *indumba* to greet the ancestors. "Otherwise they
will feel neglected," said Mamjoli. She told the ancestors that I would stay with her
for a couple of days to learn about *muthi* and traditional healing.

The next day, when Mirranda left Mzansi to go back to Cape Town by bus, we
again greeted the ancestors to bid farewell to Mirranda and offer her blessings for
her long journey. Mamjoli burnt *Imphepho*, the aromatic plant used to evoke the
ancestors. We agreed that I would stay with Mamjoli for five more days to visit
a number of other healers and participate in medicinal plant collection. The next
day, after we had gone to run some errands at the local *muthi* shop, a small, dusty
shop on a side road in Butterworth, we started by interviewing an old healer in a
small village between Butterworth and Mthatha, the next big city. When Mamjoli demanded that I pay 250 Rand for the interview, I was irritated, as I found this
quite an overrated sum. I did not want to cause trouble or exploit my interlocutors,
however. I paid but felt exploited myself. I tried to explain that I am not the rich
person that she might think. But how to explain that, when I am the one who had a
car and fancy technical devices like a tape recorder, a computer and a camera? Was
250 Rand per interview possibly the price I had to pay for the time and information
my interview partners were willing to give me? I felt split over the antagonism of
inner resistance to pay such an overrated price and the willingness to accept the
price I seemingly had to pay as an anthropologist who would build her career on

the information she received from people who, in the long-run, would remain economically less privileged than me. Although these are thoughts that probably every Western anthropologist has encountered when researching in countries in the Global South, I was additionally working in a field with a long history of biopiracy.

On the fifth day, after a few more financial tensions over buying beer, food and paying interview costs, we went for plant collection. "On Sundays the other healers will be free," said Mamjoli. "Nowadays, it is too dangerous for women to collect plants alone," she insisted. "People get robbed and mugged in the forest." We picked up some of her friends, three female healers and one herbalist, to collect *muthi* at a river about one hour from Mzansi. "Plants grow much better along rivers," explained Mamjoli. We strolled along the river, the healers dug for roots, scratched moss off stones and took bark off trees. Mamjoli, although seemingly in a good mood, did not say much but muttered every now and then about "all the work we have to do on a Sunday." I, on the other hand, thought it was a relaxed excursion, and I learnt basic rules of plant collection, such as "offering a silver coin to the ancestors before removing a plant" or "not to ring bark a tree or else it will die."

After two hours of picking and chatting, we went back to one of the healers' houses. The healers went into the *indumba* to present the collected plant material to the ancestors. The gathered plant material was then shared among the healers along hierarchical distribution rules, with Mamjoli getting the largest share as a leading figure among the healers of Mzansi. After this, the day continued with us drinking beer, eating roasted maize and dancing with occasional outbursts of ancestral spirits expressed in sudden dance and trance episodes. It felt like a joyful Sunday afternoon. The ancestors were part of many of the healers' activities. They served as guardian angels for journeys, as the receivers of interview costs, as guides in plant collection, as moral influence in approving the harvest, and as voices and supporters in singing and dancing. They were an essential part of the healers' lives. Although I got to know the ancestors during the day, I still looked at them from an observant and distant position.

Figure 3 Plant collection close to Mzansi, Eastern Cape

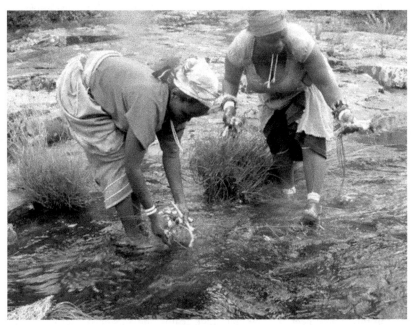

© B. Rutert.

In the evening, back at Mamjoli's place, I prepared my luggage to leave Mzansi to return back to Cape Town the next day. I struggled to figure out an appropriate price for accommodation and translation. But before I could come to a conclusion, Mamjoli suddenly entered the room, smacked down a piece of paper in front of me, and turned around, saying briskly, "I am coming back." She then left to lock the gate of her compound. The piece of paper calculated in clear letters and numbers the amount of 2000 Rand (200 Euro). She had summed up 250 Rand for accommodation per night, 500 Rand for the plant collection and 500 Rand for the translation of interviews. Given that I had already paid for food, beer and the interviews, this seemed like an unreasonable sum of money. The next morning, I offered her the 1200 Rand I had still in cash. She freaked out, ripped my bag with my computer and camera off my shoulder, and threatened to hit me with a stick. She wanted to force me to go to Butterworth to withdraw more cash. "You white people," she yelled loudly, "you are not going to take all our knowledge away!" Eventually, I convinced her to give me my bag back and to open the compound gate. I left immediately without farewell. After ten hours of driving, I reached the Western Cape to spend the night in a backpackers hostel. Only then did I feel my inner tension. A note in my field diary says:

Wilderness beach Backpackers, place of transition. Back from the world of the amaXhosa, straight into the white fancy world of beach town Wilderness, once the holiday resort of the Afrikaner Apartheid regime elite, P.W. Botha's[20] former beach villa not far from here. I didn't know how different these "two worlds" are and how much they are still existent in South Africa. How much must this twofold world profoundly influences the country, and in particular bioprospecting? For now, I am glad to be back here. What happened? Did I "fall victim" to my own lack of experience and imprecise communication structures or of centuries old structures of inequality and abuse? How could I have done better, without knowing anything about the lives of traditional healers? Well, I should take it as a lesson learnt. How does this continuous switching between the "two worlds" work for Mirranda? She felt like a different person in "her world." Can these "two worlds" ever speak to each other? (Wilderness Beach Backpackers, April 1, 2009).

The dichotomy between these "two worlds" (Buhrman1984) was nourished by many racially pointed comments that I heard during the course of the research from both sides, such as "You white people, you are not going to take our knowledge away!" or "Don't spent too much time in black communities, they have powers that we [white] people don't know." Although I personally refrained from expressing any racist notions myself, I hardly stood a chance to escape them in South Africa. Whatever the reason might have been for Mamjoli's rage against me, this encounter taught me a number of crucial lessons. First, I was a researcher from the Global North with money and a mission, after all; a fact that did not matter to me as someone who was not born under the Apartheid system, but that obviously mattered to those who had been born in the system. To the healers, my mission may not have looked very different to the missions that other affluent researchers had: to take something away without appropriately compensating for it or fairly redistributing the ensuing benefits. I constantly had to reflect on my position as a 'potential biopirate' and remained insecure about how to fairly redistribute or compensate for the value of the information I received. Often I was told "this is what the ancestors want," as legitimation for the (in my eyes) overpriced interview costs. While I initially considered this to be a manipulative way to get more cash, I also slowly learned more about the ancestors in the everyday world of traditional healers and their crucial influence in the field of traditional healing.

---

20   Peter Wilhelm (PW) Botha served as both Prime Minister (1978–1989) and State President (1984–1989) of South Africa. He was known by the name Die Groot Krokodil (The Big Crocodile) for his rigid and cruel Apartheid politics.

There Is Another Side of the Coin: Getting Healed in Mboyti

The ancestors slowly became more than a distant category for me. Gradually, they began to influence my attitudes and thus the data collection process. This influence was not only threatening, as it was in Mzansi, but also had a (maybe imagined) healing effect. After my laptop with the data of five months of research and my purse had been stolen, and after I had been involved in two serious car accidents in Eastern Cape Province (in one of which a young man had died), I temporarily lost my inner balance. Instead of taking a break, I decided to deal with this string of unfortunate situations "the African way." The leaflets of traditional healers often proposed that they could treat everything, including misfortune. Although I did not believe in these healing methods, I nevertheless thought that it would be a valuable experience, also for the understanding of traditional healing and its practices, to search for treatment with a healer. I decided to consult Twasa, a healer in the small coastal Eastern Cape village of Mboyti. I had interviewed Twasa a couple of months before and regarded him to be an honest person.

To reach the coastal village of Mboyti, it took a three-hours drive through the uninhabited, endlessly green Magwa tea plantations and Magwa Forest. Magwa Forest is the largest indigenous coastal forest in South Africa. It belongs to the Pondoland Centre of Endemism, which is part of the three South African biodiversity hotspots, the Maputaland-Pondoland-Albany Biodiversity Hotspot, stretching from Mozambique to the Eastern Cape. In this richly biodiverse area, Twasa had explained the last time I met him, "One can even meet a leopard from time to time. When you see the leopard while you collect medicinal plants, you must stop collecting plants and go straight back home." When I passed the winding gravel road through the forest down to Mboyti, I could easily imagine a leopard slipping out of the deep bush, crossing the road to immediately be swallowed back into the green. Mboyti has been made accessible for tourism, with electricity and running water reaching the fancy Mboyti River Lodge at the entrance to the village. But beyond the lodge, such facilities abruptly stop, and life in Mboyti comes and goes with daylight. Twasa, who lived close to the sea, had never left Mboyti further than Lusikisiki, the buzzing trading town.

After I arrived, greeted the family and settled in, I explained to Twasa about the string of misfortunes that I had recently experienced. Dava Rasta, who had agreed to join me, translated from English to isiXhosa. Twasa listened carefully. Then, after some minutes of silence, he said, "I am going to help you." He left the hut and for the rest of the afternoon disappeared to prepare a *muthi* mixture. I observed him while he sat in the entrance to his *indumba*, cautiously burning roots and mixing the ashes (in isiXhosa charred medicine is called *Insizi*)[21] with an oily liquid and some salt like crystal white powder in a mortar. His movements were calm, quiet, tender. He seemed to juggle with the ingredients, immersed and concentrated in his movements. I was curious about the ingredients, but I felt that I should not disturb the tender movements and the harmonious interplay between him and the *muthi*. Instead, he asked me to sit in the round hut opposite the *indumba* and wait until I was called. The huge round hut was part of the healer's homestead, which had five huts in total. It was a meeting point, sleeping room and place for ceremonies all in one. Attached to the wall, I saw feathered chicken scalps and a huge snakeskin, relics of past ceremonies and medicine hunting. Time moved slowly. After about an hour, Twasa asked me to come over to the *indumba*.

Gently, Twasa advised me to sit down on a small wooden stool placed on a goatskin. The light had become gloomy in the meantime; it was by now late afternoon. The last sunrays shimmered through the small half broken window, interfering with the dusty cobwebs that crossed the window frame. Slowly, Twasa started to unwrap a thin razor blade. The small wrapping paper slowly glided down to the goatskin. Still I did not know what would happen, but I figured that I had to trust the healer. Not an easy task, when articles spoke about high levels of toxicity through herbal medicines (Steenkamp et al. 2006). With precision, he pointed at the hairline on my scalp and with a quick movement scratched two little cuts into the skin. A fierce moment of pain rang through my body. Next to him stood an empty Coca-Cola bottle. I could see a black, shiny, oily paste – obviously the one he had mixed earlier – on top of the lid. With his fingertips he rubbed a bit of the black paste into the tiny wounds. A burning sensation ran through my veins. He continued, making similar little cuts at my temples, under the collarbone, on my shoulders, my chest, above and under the navel and further down on each side of my knees. Little trickles of blood oozed out of the small wounds. I wished I could ask questions, but again his gaze told me to keep quiet. Finally, he closed my eyes with one hand and indicated for me to leave the small *indumba*. I felt dizzy. Later, Twasa explained that I might feel bad for two days, but after that I would recover and would have no further trouble. I stayed another two days, felt tense and tight for some time, but then became very calm. I paid 500 Rand (50 euro) for his services and finally left Mboyti.

After the treatment, my inner and outer situation improved. I had no further accidents or other forms of disruption. While this might have been mere coincidence, I nevertheless started to have another feeling for the practice of traditional healers that, until then, I had only had the chance to observe, but not to sense physically and emotionally. Interestingly, Twasa had nothing to do with the IKS Lead

---

21   Burning poisonous plants takes the poisonous effect away. This is a method that is not only practiced by healers but also in scientific laboratories.

Program; I had met him through contacts of my landlady Annelie. Our time together was marked by peaceful interaction and respect. The tensions experienced in
connection with the IKS did not play a role at all in Mboyti.

One and a half years after the first research phase, I returned to South Africa for
my second research phase in Bushbuckridge Municipality, where I would conduct
six months of research. The longer I stayed, the more I also became involved in
helping to organize the activities of the healers. This soon brought me into the
position of not only being a participant observer, but an active participant. With
growing trust and an at first seemingly insignificant private 'raw moment', I slowly
immersed myself into a third role: that of healer's apprentice. In outlining this role,
I will reflect on the question of whether 'going native' is a threat or a benefit for the
data generating process. I will also show that, although I seemingly 'went native',
I was still never quite 'native enough'.

On Being 'Called' and Taking on a Triple Role in the Field

During the second research phase, I had just spent two months in Hluvukane/Share
when in January 2012 heavy rains flooded the sandy, dusty lowlands of Bushbuckridge Municipality. Roads and bridges were flushed away by rapidly rising rivers,
and the house I lived in with Rodney's family had not a single dry spot after five
days of incessant rain. We had to shuffle ankle-deep water out of the living room
every two hours. On the sixth day, the rain stopped, and I decided to escape to a
backpackers hostel 60 km away in the hilly Drakensberg Escarpment. Although I
lived with Rodney's family, I suddenly felt isolated and lonely. Being alone in the
field is always a challenge, even though the healers were unbelievably kind and
hospitable.

At the cozy Graskop backpackers hostel, I went for a run to ease my feelings. I
had learned from traditional healers that I had to ask the ancestors for help when in
a bad situation. Although I still did not fully understand the ancestors, I intuitively
followed the healers' advice and asked the ancestors for help. On the way back to
the hostel, I passed a housing area with wealthy looking houses, which may have
been owned by white people. When almost back at the hostel, I saw an old string
with red and white beads and a copper bracelet lying by the roadside, covered with
grass and dirt. Such beads and bracelets are usually insignia of traditional healers.
Red and white are the sacred colors of *sangomahood*. Why were they lying here, in a
seemingly white suburb of an old mining town in the Drakensberg Escarpment? I
assumed that no traditional healer would find his/her way to this area of town, and
if so, why would he/she lose such valuable items? Carefully, I retrieved the string of
beads and the bracelet from the grass. When back at the hostel, the cleaning lady
of the house, a small (black) woman with a witty sense of humor, observed me as I
was washing the dirt off the beads, and asked me where I had found them. After I

told her, and said how unusual I thought it to be, she said, "This means good luck for you," and then, a little later, "Maybe this is your calling?"

The next day I went back to Hluvukane, beads and bracelet in my pocket. It took me a couple of days before I dared to ask Rodney what he thought about the items. He actually did not say much, but soon afterwards he started including me in his work as a healer. During the previous two months, we had conducted interviews together or organized activities of the Kukula Healers. But soon after I told him about the beads, he started to integrate me into his practice. I became his de facto healer's apprentice, without ever officially becoming one. He asked me to help him with his patients. I prepared *futhas* (steam bath with *muthi*), I made fire, boiled water, heated up big stones in the fire and helped the patients to wash with *muthi* mixtures. Meanwhile, Rodney prepared the *muthi* mixtures and treated the patients.

Later, the finding of the beads and the bracelet would be interpreted as a 'calling' by various healers in Bushbuckridge and elsewhere. But I did not take notice of it, as I could not see myself in the role of a South African traditional healer. But I did notice a sort of 'initiation', a coming into being with the healers with whom I worked, as if I had traversed the role of a stranger and researcher and had become more one of them. With this new role, I suddenly had a 'triple role' in the second research phase: I was an ethnographer in the pursuit of data and I conducted participant observation on the lives of the Kukula Healers; due to my close cooperation with the NGO Natural Justice, and the cooperation between the healers and the K2C committee, I started being an assistant in the activities of the Kukula Healers Association and a mediator and translator between the different 'languages' of NGOs and healers; and finally, I was the helping hand in Rodney's healing practice, wherein I learned about the preparation and use of medicinal plants.

Against this background, I can say with assurance that I never fully 'went native'. The triple role allowed me to be engaged in the healers' lives and activities, but it also always brought me back to other activities, like the work of NGOs and my own research agenda. Although I had the feeling of deep immersion in the field, I remained what I was: an anthropologist from Germany, who had encountered the contested values of plants and knowledge in bioprospecting contact zones. These contact zones were also emotionally loaded; for the healers, for whom knowledge is part of their identity, and for me, who was confronted with an at first unexpected situation of disdain. Only my own deeper immersion – by getting to know the ancestors and consequently the field of traditional healing – was what enabled me to gain a deeper understanding of bioprospecting as a field influenced by the past reaching into the present.

Conclusion and Outlook

Bioprospecting is an ambivalent field. It is motivated by economic and scientific incentives and unleashes contestations over contextually framed values attached to medicinal plants and associated (indigenous) knowledge. In colonial times, this contestation was already well established, when travelers and scientists insisted on staking their claim to the resources collected in this *terra incognita* or *terra nullius*. This claim was clearly instigated by the power of the colonizers, but was nevertheless acknowledged by some of the invading travelers and researchers themselves as not always justified. With the increasing political manifestation of colonial power, policies came into force aimed at undermining indigenous knowledge systems and their knowledge holders, here traditional healers. This was only reversed with the end of the Apartheid regime in 1994 and subsequent policies that aimed at empowering knowledge systems and protecting the degrading biodiversity. Traditional healers and their knowledge were then viewed as an important component of the cultural heritage of the country and they were seen as custodians of biodiversity related knowledge.

This new political configuration had an influence on a new form of protection of knowledge and the contestation of resources, which I, as a researcher from the Global North, encountered in manifold ways. These encounters showed that the contestation is not only resentful and averse; rather, such encounters are complex and dependent on the relationality of the involved actors. Deep immersion in cultural spaces may affect the protective attitude of knowledge holders. Long-term stays (like the one during my second fieldwork stay in Bushbuckridge) create trust and access to the knowledge systems, while short-term research stays (such as in the Eastern Cape) can be hindered by mistrust and resentfulness. As a friend, I was allowed to access knowledge and inaccessible spaces, such as the healing practices of my research assistant and healing teacher Rodney Sibuyi. But as a researcher from the Global North, conducting investigations in the name of both international (Freie Universität Berlin) and national (IKS Lead Program) research institutes, I was regarded as someone who wanted to take something away without fairly sharing the benefits, a resistance that had been learned from past experiences.

My perceptions here may be biased by the fact that Mirranda initiated all of the contacts with healers, which I had in connection with the IKS lead Program. Hence the mistrust on the part of the healers might have had its roots in a mistrust that Mirranda held against me, and which she transported, and translated, to her fellow healers. The disdain might have been a personal feeling. But it might also have been caused by 'institutional friction'. Bioprospecting contact zones are not only political and economic spaces, but are also influenced by emotions attached to tangible (plants) and intangible (knowledge) property. These emotional values attached to property strongly influence the contested field. Emotions are more likely to be shared when friendship, trust and understanding is involved. This was the case in my relationships with Twasa and Rodney, both of which were framed by mutual trust and support.

While this chapter reflected on past and present bioprospecting contact zones and my own position in these contact zones, the next chapter deals with the relationality of plants and knowledge in traditional healers communities. How are medicinal plants and associated knowledge embedded in healers' communities? How are knowledge and plants shared and protected and what does this say about potential concepts of (indigenous) knowledge protection and access and benefit sharing agreements?

Chapter IV
"Our Knowledge Belongs to Our Ancestors":
Topographies of Knowledge and the Question of Property

> Knowledge involves creativity, effort, pro-
> duction (...)
> Marilyn Strathern (1999: 20)

Introduction

The previous chapter illustrated how the value of traditional medicinal plants and indigenous knowledge has changed over time. Both have been subject to power relations, political and legal alterations and economic interests on the one hand, and negotiation processes in contact zones on the other. In today's global political (knowledge) economy, plants and knowledge have become highly contested and protected. The prevailing North-South power imbalance that characterizes this knowledge economy was also evident in my own ethnographic research, when during my encounters with local knowledge holders I was often viewed with suspicion as a 'representative' of the Global North.

Today, the (knowledge) economy that valorizes (indigenous) knowledge drawn from natural resources, mainly according to its economic value, has a strong influence on the value that indigenous people attribute to their own resources. Irrespective of economic influence, however, indigenous people also have their own system of meaning for their knowledge, expressed in a distinct system of pooling, sharing, transferring and protecting knowledge and medicinal plants. This system functions within a community of healers, and is also embedded in additional relationships, such as those with the ancestors, patients, tribal authorities, local municipalities, the family and village communities, as well as the surrounding environment with its biodiversity. This chapter is therefore concerned with the question of how exactly knowledge – and with it the plants from which this knowledge derives – are embedded, managed, protected and valorized in traditional healers communities and the larger communal context. Sharing and protection are subject to specific rules and customary laws. How are these rules and laws constituted? What values are ascribed to this knowledge – as intangible property – and to the respective plants – as tangible property?

To reflect on these questions, this chapter follows a trajectory that begins with 'just plants in nature' – material matter that grows in a specific environment, and produces oxygen and nutritive substances that influence the environment, animals and human beings alike (cf. Ingold 2002, 2011) – through to the knowledge derived from these plants, knowledge that has been developed and refined through human intervention over the course of centuries. Over time, a huge corpus of knowledge is established through trial and error, where the healing properties of plants are detected and tested. Knowledge here is understood as (intangible) property, and as such implies a series of rights and restrictions, rules and obligations. Among healers, it is often claimed that knowledge of medicinal plants derives from the ancestors. Knowledge in this context is thus always subject to rights-based negotiations among groups of people – such as living healers and patients – as well as with other entities such as the ancestors. It is defined by the value that people give to this property and to the relationships that are connected to the property. Benda-Beckmann et al. assert that "property in the most general sense concerns the ways in which the relationships between society's members with respect to valuables are given form and significance" (Benda-Beckmann et al. 2007: 14). The relationship between plants, living healers, patients and the ancestors thus denotes a "bundle of rights" (Hann 1998: 8), whereby "property always belongs to someone who then owns the right to something, but not the thing itself" (ibid.: 4).

To understand these relations that assemble around knowledge, the following questions will be examined: Who holds the rights to knowledge and plants in the relationship between the healer, the healer's community, the patient and the ancestors? How are these rights to knowledge and medicinal plants negotiated? What practices and rules are adhered to in order to keep knowledge stable and yet adaptable to outside factors? The system of knowledge sharing, transference and protection follows similar rules in most South African (black) healers' communities. I will jump back and forth from interviews and participant observations conducted with traditional healers in the Eastern Cape, KwaThema/Johannesburg and Bushbuckridge Municipality. While this may not do justice to the complexities of each socio-cultural context and the depth of the life worlds of the healers, the focus is more on the relations between the different actors in the production of meaning and the value of knowledge. Depicting this web of relations will enable a deeper understanding of property relations in healers' communities, which may then help to point out the challenges and frictions that arise when knowledge and plants traverse into a biochemical laboratory and then into mainly economically oriented access and benefit sharing negotiations.

Topographies of Muthi and Knolwedge

At the very beginning, a plant grows, as yet undiscovered, in a specific environment. It may contain medicinal properties or it may not. A plant's medicinal value may be discovered over the course of centuries through observations; for instance, of animals eating the plant, or of trial and error experiments performed by healers and lay people, which are added to by the knowledge of the ancestors. The accumulated knowledge about one plant may then lead to a variety of treatments for different ailments. *Sutherlandia*, for instance, was discovered as being valuable in boosting the immune system as well as against depression; *Imphepho*, the plant used to invoke communication with the ancestors, is also used to treat coughs, fever and insomnia (van Wyk et al. 2009). Along the trajectory of a plant, from being discovered in nature to being regularly used in treatments by traditional healers, the ancestors play a significant role. Without the ancestors, much knowledge would basically never have come into existence. Healers regard the ancestors as the originators of all knowledge. However, at the very beginning, a plant is still just a plant in nature.

From Being (Just) a Plant in Nature to Being a Plant in Use

Common shrubs like *Sutherlandia* and *Imphepho* grow in specific environments, which constitute an assemblage of climate, altitude and/or soil. Some plants prefer the aridity of the semi-desert of Karoo or the humidity of the Western Cape; others only grow along swampy riverbeds or prefer the cool darkness of dense forests. Most plants, however, have in common the fact that they produce chlorophyll, oxygen and minerals, and require minerals, water and soil in turn. They grow in a web of relations to their surrounding environment, at first independent of human influence (leaving aside the general influences of environmental pollution) and indispensable for the surrounding environment[1]. They are plants in nature, sometimes growing en masse, sometimes isolated from most other plants. Until the moment of discovery by a healer or other persons, a plant is but one of many that contribute to an area's biodiversity.

At some stage, selected plants will be eaten by animals and/or human beings, and will serve as nutriment or medicine. Once the plant has been collected and its nutritive and/or healing properties detected, it enters into a human–non-human

---

1   Some scholars have gone as far as to think of plants (or forests) as thinking entities. Eduardo Kohn's book 'How Forests Think. Towards an Anthropology Beyond the Human' (2013), for instance, is written in the tradition of the "ontological turn" (cf. Candea 2010). By following Philippe Descola (2013) and Eduardo Viveiros de Castro (1998), Kohn questions the dualistic human–non-human approach, seeing instead more interrelatedness between the two.

relationship whereby knowledge may be generated through trial and error. Healers may learn about the healing potential of plants by observing animals that eat certain plants for self-treatment. "Especially goats," one healer said. "They are very clever and one can learn a lot by observing them" (Informal conversation, Mtambalala, Eastern Cape, October 2010). Through such observations, many plants have been discovered by humans in their quest for survival and health maintenance.

Sutherlandia frutescens, for instance, is such a plant. It is a shy but commonly known plant that grows all over the Western Cape. Unlike many Aloe varieties or the even more prominent Protea, one of South Africa's landmark plants, *Sutherlandia*, with its powerful red blossoms, prefers to grow among other plants. It has long been known for its great immune boosting and healing powers. Grandparents, parents and healers alike have used it over many generations and have built up a corpus of knowledge around the plant and its generalist healing capacities, which today has even spurred heated debate and ongoing research into its potential to strengthen the weakened immune systems of HIV/AIDS patients[2]. Yet when seen along the roadsides of the Western Cape, this unassuming plant would not seem to have such strong healing power nor such a significant impact on today's pharmaphyto landscape. It is basically just a green shrub with red flowers.

Another example is *Imphepho* (bot.: Helichrysum odoratissmum; Afr.: Kooigoed; Engl.: Everlasting) (cf. van Wyk et al. 2009: 168). It is a light green shrub with soft round silvery leaves and yellow flower heads, which when they blossom in spring and summer produce a pungent fragrance. *Imphepho* grows in many parts of South Africa: the Western Cape variety with its large round leaves grows on Table Mountain in Cape Town and along the dusty roadsides; the variety that grows in the Eastern Cape and parts of KwaZulu-Natal, Mpumalanga and Limpopo Provinces is ground creeping and has smaller leaves. Although quite unimposing in looks, *Imphepho* – both in nature but especially when triturated, dried or burnt – has a strikingly strong, spicy smell, which is also known as "the air of the spirits" (Dugmore & van Wyk 2008). It is commonly used by traditional healers in ceremonies and rituals to evoke the ancestors, in celebrations and in the treatment of patients. It is said that the smoke crosses the barriers of the mind and thus invokes a better connection and communication with spirits and ancestors. The plant thus connects human beings with semi-human beings (the ancestors).

Imphepho, like *Sutherlandia*, was discovered over the course of human interaction with nature. Both plants convey the fact that *muthi* is not *muthi* right from the beginning. Through observation, trial and error, and experience, plants in nature progressively transform into *muthi*. It is a long process that progresses continuously, with changes in cross-generational knowledge. Knowledge on a specific *muthi*

---

2   For media articles and other related information on research into *Sutherlandia frutescens* use by HIV/AIDS patients, see: www.sutherlandia.org.

only becomes subject to political, economic and legal enquiry when it enters the public domain as a commodity, which then also prompts and intensifies the question of ownership and intellectual property, which, until then, had been a matter of local customary laws and regulations. Customary laws are, as will be shown later in this chapter, also politically, economically and legally structured, but they have different implications than common intellectual property law. The examples of *Imphepho* and *Sutherlandia* also show that *muthi* is multifaceted. One plant in a specific environment is not equivalent to the same plant in another environment. Even two plants of the same type growing next to each other may not have the same healing value. Furthermore, as a healer in Beaufort West taught me, plantation site plants generally have weaker healing property than the same plants growing independently in nature (Informal conversation with Antoinette Pinhaar, Beaufort West, March 2009).

Knowledge about plants is, consequently, context dependent. With the changing environment, a plant's attached knowledge and healing value also change. *Imphepho*, for instance, is used a great deal in healing ceremonies in the Eastern Cape and KwaThema, but very little in the Bushbuckridge area, due to the simple fact that the plant does not grow much in Bushbuckridge. Similarly, *Sutherlandia* is well known in the Western Cape, but known little or not at all in Bushbuckridge. Knowledge thus develops contextually, depending on the environment. In the context of traditional healing, however, all knowledge about medicinal plants is known to have the same origin: the ancestors.

The Origin of Knowledge:
"It All Comes from the Ancestors"

The beliefs and practices of traditional healers in Southern Africa have been well described over the years (cf. Berglund 1976; Junod [1912]/1962; Sundkler 1948: 220–37; Hammond-Tooke 1985, 1989, 2002; Hirst 1990, 1998; Ngubane 1977, 1981; Du Toit 1980; Cumes 2004; Wreford 2008; Janzen 1992; Thornton 2009), especially by anthropologists and psychoanalysts who themselves trained as healers or at least spent considerable lengths of time with healers (Buhrmann 1986; Hirst 1997; Stoller & Olkes 1987; van Binsbergen 1991; Wreford 2008). In these accounts, however, the production of knowledge on medicinal plants and the process of knowledge transference are scarcely looked at (Thornton 2009: 25). Generally, traditional healing knowledge is said to be ancient knowledge that extends across time, cultures and languages and derives from pre-colonial African systems of belief (ibid.: 17). The knowledge of a traditional healer, who has knowledge of a specific treatment and a plant that s/he uses, is bound to a long genealogy of past knowledge, embodied in the ancestors, transferred by cultural rules and protected by customary laws, which protect the mostly secret and partially sacred knowledge.

The knowledge that healers acquire (through their training, for instance) is subject to an exchange system between the trainee healer (*thwasa*), the healer trainer (Xh./Zl.: *magobela*) and the ancestors. Every traditional healer is connected to a long line of deceased members, a specific lineage and/or clan of ancestors. These lineages are organized into specific healing schools (Zl.: pl. *izimpande* / sing. *impande*; Engl.: roots). These schools have hierarchical structures, with the healer elders serving as leaders, teachers and trainers. With the graduation ceremony (*goduswa*), an apprentice is not only initiated as a healer but also as a member of an exclusive *impande*. The members of the *impande* consist of living beings as well as of ancestral spirits[3]. There are many words to denote these ancestral spirits: *amathongo* (Zl./Xh. pl. / sing. *ithongo*) is the general term for all departed spirits (Ngubane 1977: 50), while *amadlozi* (Zl./Xh. pl. / sing. *idlozi*) are ancestral spirits responsible for protecting or disciplining descendants (ibid.)[4].

While everyone has a line of ancestors in his/her life, traditional healers have the special gift of being able to communicate with them and channel information through the medium of dreams and divining bones (Cumes 2003, 2013: 59). Bantu-speaking Africa has a long tradition of healing cults (Janzen 1992; Devisch 1993) that work with different ancestral spirits. In South Africa, two different groups of ancestral spirits are known: the possession and trance mediums of Nguni groups. Nguni is a collective ethnic name that includes Xhosa, Zulu and Swazi. These ancestral spirits are commonly more explicit and overt among the Nguni than in the other groups of Venda, Tsonga or Sotho (Hammond Tooke 1998), which use more 'objective' systems such as interpreting the 'throwing of the bones'[5]. Other ancestral spirits, such as forest, water and mountain spirits, as well as alien spirits such as the *ndau* spirit (an emotional spirit that may cause significant harm when a healer has not been trained thoroughly), add to the landscape of ancestral spirits that require special attention and integration into a healer's training. Many healers work with many different ancestral spirits, and train in different traditions, as the

---

3   During interviews, the terms 'spirits' and 'ancestors' were used interchangeably, and the difference is also not clearly delineated in the literature. John Janzen, for instance, uses both terms interchangeably (Janzen 1992: 37ff.). It is therefore difficult to describe them as different categories.

4   During my fieldwork, several healers, for different reasons and on various occasions, said to me: "You have *amadlozi*," implying that I have ancestral spirits, and that I could be trained to make use of their healing capacities.

5   This contradicts what John Janzen has said, namely that "among the Xhosa, undramatic, meditative and counseling techniques are used between healers and their clients. The spirits who are called on are usually ancestors, or vague evil or nature spirits. Among Zulu diviners, mechanistic bone-throwing techniques prevail. The Swazi, however, although the same holds true for parts of their work, have recourse regularly to far more demonstrative possession trance behavior as they are visited by a series of increasingly powerful nature and alien spirits (i.e. ndau spirit)" (Janzen 1992: 37).

following short excerpt from an interview with one Kukula Healers member, Lion Thethe, whom we met at his friend's homestead (Orliandah Ngomana, a traditional healer who had trained in the *ndau* tradition, among others), outlines.

BR: Is this an indumba [pointing to a small hut]?

LT: Yes, this is one. There are others. She [Orliandah Ngomana] has three indumbas for her different ancestors, from the mother, from the father. Once you have one, there are others, they will come. And they don't want to be together. So this indumba is for her mother. So this only is a mark so far, because it is so expensive to build a house, so you go to this mark. It depends on how many ancestors you have. This woman, she got ancestors from her family, where she comes from, and from the mother and from where the mother belongs and also from the people called Ndau. They are needy people. So previously, in Africa, they [the Ndau] used to go to anothertribe, and eh, we were not welcoming these people and it happened that they would be killed. And that spirit will become part of the family, it will follow until today. (...)

BR: And is she trained in the ndau spirit?

LT: Yes, she is working with it. She was in Beira [Mozambique] to train.

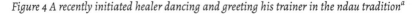

Figure 4 A recently initiated healer dancing and greeting his trainer in the ndau tradition[a]

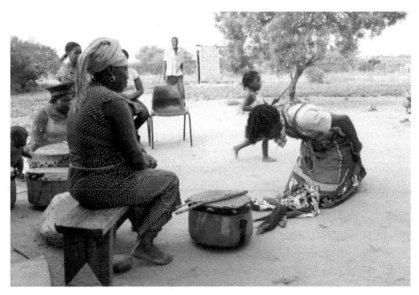

© B. Rutert

Dreaming Plants: Ancestors and the Production of Knowledge

In any of the abovementioned traditions, the role of the ancestral spirits in the process of knowledge transference (during the training and beyond), sharing and protection, as well as the influence of the ancestors on the collection and use of plants
in the treatment of patients, is immeasurable and indispensable. Subsequently,
this role will be laid out based on the interviews that I conducted with traditional
healers in the Eastern Cape in March 2009. The first interview was conducted with
Ntate Ndeni, a 62-year-old male healer who lived in a village 10 kilometers south
of Mthatha, the main city in King Sabata Dalindyebo Local Municipality, Transkei,
Eastern Cape Province. Ntate Ndeni had been working as a director at the Department of Justice long before he started his training as a healer. He continued
working in his well-paid job for the two-year training period, but finally quit to

a   The Ndau people are originally a sub-group of the Tsonga people from Mozambique. In
      spiritual terms (cf. van Warmelo 1934), the ndau spirit is particularly common and strong
      among the Tsonga because they had been incorporated during the Nguni-Ndau wars in
      Mozambique. The *ndau* spirit would enter the body of those who killed a Ndau person, or
      would be inherited by the descendants of those slain. The spirits would then cause suffer-
      ing, as the deceased had not received a proper burial or funerary rites. Appeasement would
      occur through the training as a healer (cf. Keene 2013).

concentrate fully on his *sangomahood* and, according to him, never regretted this decision: "It is such a freedom to work as a *sangoma*," he said. "You can walk barefoot whenever you want, no one restricts you." As he was relatively fluent in English, Mirranda's role as a translator was rather limited during the interview. Instead, she contributed to the conversation in her own capacity as a healer.

> **BR:** Where does your knowledge about plants come from?
>
> **NN:** My father was an herbalist, so I grew up with knowledge about botanic plants. He taught me. And some of them I dream of. [The dreams] tell me that they [the plants] will be at such and such a place, perhaps in the forest in such and such a place, so usually, they [the dreams] would direct me, because I always pray to the spiritual ancestors. So they come to direct you, until you get it [the plant].
>
> **BR:** Ah, so you dream about the plants?
>
> **NN:** Yes, I do dream about the plants. More specifically, if somebody is seriously ill, I go to them [the ancestors] and I pray to them. Ask them: I have this problem, what advice would you give me?
>
> **BR:** So, you concentrate on dreams? Can you go to sleep and ask for dreams? [Mirranda and Ntate Ndeni giggle.]
>
> **NN:** No, it is not possible. Usually they [the dreams] come on their own. Perhaps at times there is a problem approaching you and they will come and give you advice. It needs a lot of concentration and dedication in a certain mood. Then you get what you need. It is a bit taxing on your body, because you need to concentrate, and it needs a lot of time. They [the ancestors] may visit you the following day or any other day. Our belief is that our ancestors are not looking for me alone, we are a big family and all our brothers and sisters are being cared for by our ancestors. That is what we believe, even if the answer might not come today or tomorrow.

This short excerpt from a one hour-long interview depicts the strong connections between the healer, plants and the ancestors. Ntate Ndeni had always been interested in medicinal plants. His father had taught him about their healing power. He had grown up with this knowledge, which he continuously extended and manifested through his connections with the ancestors. Once he was trained, he relied on insights received from them, mostly through dreams, about a plant's position in nature or about which plant to use for a specific illness. The ancestors are 'guides' to find the right plants and they support Ntate Ndeni in treating patients. As such, the ancestors, via the healer, care for the whole community. Accordingly, ancestral knowledge is multi-generational, collectively held knowledge bundled in the person of the healer, which contributes to the community's health. The healer is the one who brings the past (ancestors) to the present (community). Medicinal plants function as a bridge between the healer, patients and the ancestors. The plants, such as *Imphepho*, open up the pathway for communication with the ancestors and serve as medicine for patients. Often, a healer will prescribe different *muthi* to patients, depending on the illness or other, more socially oriented concerns. A plant or plant mixture may serve as spiritual medicine to cleanse the patient's body or the patient's house or invoke a connection to the patient's ancestors. A plant or plant mixture may also serve as medicine to treat a specific illness. Plants are strongly connected to the healer's inner visions and dreams, which are infused by the ancestors. The healer, plants, ancestors and patients, as well as the surrounding community and environment, thus form an inseparable unit.

On the same day that we spoke to Ntate Ndeni, we conducted another interview with Andaleti Nkomo, a 64-year-old female healer and herbalist. She lived with her adult daughter in a small homestead consisting of two small round huts. She invited us into one of the huts where she had separated off a corner with blankets in order to consult patients undisturbed. For the interview, we sat on a small bench in the large hut, right in front of the *indumba*.

> **BR:** Where did you get the information from about the plants?
>
> **AN:** I am a sangoma, so I always have dreams about the plants. Sometimes I dream that someone [is] coming with a problem and then I see her going to the forest, collecting certain plants and then that person will come and I will go and collect that plant and will treat the patient with that plant.
>
> **BR:** And what kind of plants are these?
>
> **AN:** I have got a plant Nciciponga. So sometimes when people are talking bad to you, I will use this plant to stop people talking bad about that person. You have to wash yourself and then they stop talking about you.
>
> **BR:** Who taught you about that?
>
> **AN:** My trainer never told me anything. But your trainer depends on you and what you dream about, what your ancestors tell you. So then the trainer will help you on that. So it's all from the ancestors.
>
> **BR:** Was your father or mother already a healer, or someone in your family?
>
> **AN:** Oh, my father's sister, my aunt, was a healer. It is in the family. Sometimes those who passed away become your ancestors and they will help you with dreams about a plant. So you will know the name of the plant and what the plant is for.

Andaleti Nkomo, like Ntate Ndeni, also reported that she obtained all of her knowledge on plants from her ancestors. Her trainer had helped her to interpret her dreams and correctly use the plants she had dreamt of. When consulting patients, she also asked the ancestors for advice on illnesses, the respective medicinal plants and where to find them.

The role of the ancestors was often stressed in the Eastern Cape[6]. In Andaleti Nkomo's case, it was her aunt who had been a traditional healer. The gift of healing is often inherited within the family. Hence knowledge is not only learned in the training situation of a specific *impande*, but also has – or can have – its origin in the family. Some healers have a calling, however, without any preexisting familial knowledge. Nevertheless, they do have ancestors, who appear in dreams or as inner voices and deliver knowledge to them.

Figure 5 Andaleti Nkomo with itshoba (the sangoma stick) and muthi

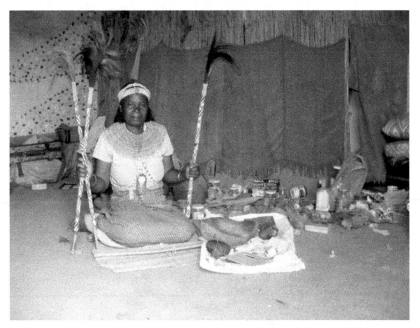

© B. Rutert.

The notion of healing as an inherited gift within the family also came up in other interviews with healers. The next day, Mirranda and I conducted an interview with Ntate Fuyani, a 58-year-old healer who lived in a small village north-west of Mthatha. His interest in medicinal plants had started at a young age, when he had learned a lot about plants from his grandfather, who had also been a healer. As a young man, Ntate Fuyani used his knowledge to seduce girls.

6   *Izimpande* were hardly mentioned in the Eastern Cape. This was probably due to my lack of knowledge about the context of traditional healing during the first research phase. I simply did not know about *izimpande* and hence never asked about them. Curiously, my interview partners also never mentioned them; instead, family members were said to have played a crucial role with respect to traditional healing.

With a naughty smile he said, "You have to put this specific plant on their door-step and you will see, they come to you. Yes, it works." In his early 30s, he finally started training as a healer. He learned about the healer who would become his trainer in his dreams:

> **BR:** From where do you get your knowledge?
> **NF:** I dreamt about my trainer and then I went there. I decided to accept it [the calling] in 1989. Then I trained for eight years.
> **BR:** That is long. And what did you learn in the training?
> **NF:** I was trained to know different plants and their use. I was trained to foresee things before they happen. And I was trained to consult [clients] and to respect [patients and the ancestors]. You must know how to consult.
> **BR:** And how are you actually consulting, how are you healing?
> **NF:** So, there are two different ways. First, maybe someone who has lost some-thing, then you must know: where is it, who took it? And then sometimes a client is ill, so you must be able to find out what happened.
> **BR:** And how do you find out?
> **NF:** The ancestors help me. There are several ways to deal with the ancestors. Sometimes you hear them speaking from nowhere and you can interpret and translate what they see, but the client will not hear or see. But to talk to them you must pray and burn Imphepho. Pray. But if they don't want to talk to you, you must tell the client, ah, ah, I can't see anything. So try someone else. You must be very honest.
> **BR:** And plants, to whom do they belong?
> **NF:** Plants are for everybody. But it depends what you want to use the plant for. And your ancestors will tell you what the plant is for. Then you collect the plant. But it belongs to everybody.
> **BR:** Is the position as a sangoma very accepted?
> **NF:** Everything I have is from my practice. The house up there, even the cows. I paid for lobola [brideprice]. Some clients pay with money, some pay with chick-ens. I don't mind. I take everything.
> **BR:** But still, I don't quite understand how consultation works.
> **NF:** It happens like as we are sitting here. The patient starts telling me or showing me something and at the same time the ancestors tell me what the problem of the client is. They are showing me something, your problems. There is something happening that helps me. It can happen any time of the day. So, anytime, the ancestors can show you something, where to go, what to do.

When I asked my interview partners to describe the ancestors, they answered in terms similar to what Vera Bührmann found in her research in South Africa, name-ly that "they mostly referred to daydreams, intuition and inner voices" (1984: 50ff.).

Ntate Fuyani, for instance, explained that inner voices (the ancestors) advise him when he consults patients. The ancestors, as well as the trainer, are the first entities involved in the transference of knowledge to a healer apprentice, such as that about plants and their application. Traditional healers, in their capacity to communicate with the ancestors, are thus capable of getting in touch with a form of knowledge that other people are not capable of perceiving. Accordingly, they are carriers of an immeasurable sum of knowledge on environmental, biodiversity, healing and spiritual affairs, and are therefore able to sustain the spiritual life of their communities and beyond. Although not many healers take written records of their knowledge, mostly because many of them are illiterate, their repertoire of knowledge on local biodiversity and healing needs is vast. Furthermore, undergoing the training gives a special quality and value to their knowledge. It is exclusive, inert knowledge that serves the community and beyond. The quality and quantity of their knowledge makes traditional healers important carriers of the traditions of the community. With time and experience, a healer increases his/her knowledge on treatment methods and the use of *muthi*. He or she will extend this knowledge throughout his/her lifetime, through ceremonies, consultations and ongoing communication with other healers as well as the ancestors. Over time, a healer will develop skills in particular treatments and applications of *muthi* that will make him/her a specialist in treating certain physical and psychological conditions. Then patients will travel from faraway places like Johannesburg or Cape Town to remote areas to consult a specialized healer who is known for his/her specific healing virtues.

The Healer as an 'African Intellectual'

The allocation of knowledge as well as specialization are thus embedded in a lifelong – essentially intellectual – learning process. Knowledge therein is never a fixed, terminal entity, but subject to transformation and change, as every new knowledge holder adds a personal component to the knowledge, which is composed of a particular moment in time, adaptation to the environment, personal discoveries and inventions, as well as collectively accumulated wisdom. Traditional healers view themselves as "members of [a] profession with a distinct intellectual tradition" (Thornton 2009: 17). Due to the body of knowledge and intellectual capacity that healers build up over the many years of training, as well as after the training, traditional healing has been referred to as "African science" (Ashforth 2005: 147ff.). Healers do not only provide the fundamental basis for communal healing, but also strengthen and support cultural identity and heritage through their system of knowledge sharing and transference, and convey an exclusive form of knowledge authority in their communities (cf. Ngubane 1977). In this sense, traditional healers can be referred to as the intellectuals of their communities and as the preservers of cultural heritage.

The following excerpt from an interview with 62-year-old Ntate Manyeni highlights the intellectual capacities of traditional healers and herbalists. Ntate Manyeni lived with his family in a house far off the N2. The living room was equipped with a fancy couch, still covered with the plastic cover that it had been delivered with. His *indumba*, which he proudly showed us after the interview, was stuffed with many different types of *muthi*. The most interesting aspect of this interview was the fact that, in contrast to most of his fellow healers and herbalists, Ntate Manyeni had documented most of his knowledge on medicinal plants from South Africa and beyond in an archive of handwritten notebooks. The pile of notebooks that he showed us was only a small part of his library, he said.

BR: How did you become a healer?
NM: I was interested in this plant and I went to an herbalist and so I started being interested in plants. I went all over [Africa] and I learned through sharing knowledge. I was first interested in plants and then I started dreaming around plants and even went as far as Zimbabwe to learn about plants. I like using plants. You always need to inform yourself about plants.
BR: You are an herbalist. What is the difference between a sangoma and a herbalist?
NM: Ahh, everybody dreams. Everybody has got ancestors. So only because you are dreaming, you do not have to be a sangoma. Even you have ancestors, because you also dream. The learning about plants comes one by one. You treat one patient and then you know and another patient comes and you learn more. It is important to know the names of the plants, because in these days they [chemists] are also selling plants. So it is important that you know the plants from the forests, you know the plants and the names, so if you go to the chemist, they cannot rob you, because I know the plants from the forest. There are lots of people who want money today (...). I have all these books with all the information. I go all over the country and write all the information I get. So whenever a client has a problem, I go to the books and look for the information. I keep [a] record. Even those people who work in the chemist, they don't know about the plants. They just buy the plants, for instance from KwaZulu-Natal or wherever. If you tell that person [the chemist] to fetch that plant, he does not know that plant. You see, they are just making business, making money. (...)

Ntate Manyeni was notable for his accumulation of 'cross-border' knowledge. He presented an exceptionally rich written account of knowledge that is generally accumulated only in non-written form by traditional healers. As the professor of biology whom I spoke to at a conference in Stellenbosch in June 2009 said to me, "When we are not able to document this knowledge, it will simply die with the dying of the healer." I would add that it is not only the knowledge that would be lost, but also the social relations of past and present that will die with the passing of a healer, a person who habitually grants the continuation of life. Accordingly, the ancestors (and/or spirits) play a significant role in the inter-relational encounters between plants, knowledge, trainees, trainers, the training process and the everyday practices of a traditional healer. They not only guide the training and healing process of a healer, but also teach the healer about medicinal plants and how to use them in his/her healing practice.

The ancestors are thus responsible for the transfer of knowledge from the past to the present. This knowledge carries spiritual and emotional value in terms of inherent cultural identity and the long genealogy of knowledge holders of past generations. To carefully preserve this valuable knowledge, trainee healers have to go through a thorough preparation phase, where they learn to connect themselves to the ancestors and learn the rules and regulations of knowledge transference and protection. This process is called *ukuthwasa*. In the context of this book, *ukuthwasa* is relevant as it is the first moment in a healer's life when he/she accesses an exclusive mode of (spiritual) knowledge production, transference and protection.

Knowledge Transference:
Knowledge, Plants and Ancestors

Trainee healers are often taken by surprise when they receive their 'calling'. Some, like Ntate Ndeni, were working in ordinary jobs as administrators, farmers or fruit vendors. Since traditional healers are part of the everyday life of local (black) communities, most trainee healers had had prior contact with healers and traditional healing, but very few had really thought of becoming a traditional healer themselves. Many initially refused to accept the calling, and followed it only after a long period of resistance. The training is extremely hard and demands perseverance and abstinence from 'normal life', often for many years. Once engaged in the process, the trainee healer learns, among other things, the rules of knowledge accumulation, transference and protection and how to make use of medicinal plants. The following section concerns the trainee healer's entrance into the realm of healing and its knowledge transference system: the process of *ukuthwasa*.

The Coming of Sangomahood:
Ukuthwasa and Knowledge Transference

Ukuthwasa is originally a Bantu term meaning, "to become visible, appear (of moon and stars); to commence (of the seasons)" (Hammond Tooke 1998: 10). It is also referred to as "the sickness of the calling" (Berglund 1976; Buhrmann 1984; Hirst 1990; van Binsbergen 1991), a calling that leads to a person being initiated into the diviner's role (*(uku)thwasa kwegqirha*) (Hirst 1990: 90). *Ukuthwasa* refers to the process of becoming a diviner (Xh.: *igqirha*; Zl.: *isangoma*) and learning the system of divination (Thornton 2009: 24). In the beginning stages of this process, most diviners who are called by the ancestors are troubled by numerous symptoms (Xh.: *inkathazo*). The process and state come with characteristic signs, including dreams (Xh.: *amathongo, amaphupha*) and visions (Xh.: *imibono*), psychic experiences, pains, madness and possibly leaving the homestead to live in the forest (Hirst 1990). Often, before trainee healers follows their calling (Xh.: *ukubiswa*), long episodes of misfortune, mental or psychological disease, and/or the constant occurrence of death and illness within their circle of friends and family members constitute part of the situation that makes them realize their fate (Berglund 1976; Buhrmann 1984; Hammond-Tooke 1989; Hirst 1990; Reis 1999; van Binsbergen 1991; Wreford 2005).

Many healers told me that before they had commenced their healer training, they had experienced several unexplainable physical and mental problems. One female healer in the Eastern Cape said that she did not menstruate for many years and was unable to get pregnant. This instantly changed once she accepted her calling. Gogo Mule in KwaThema told me that she had been a TV actress for soap operas. But then some unexplainable diseases and deaths occurred in her family. She knew that she had the calling, but she refused to follow it until the moment when she realized that if she continued to deny it, she would destroy her entire family. Mama Rose, an associate of the Kukula Healers, claimed that she had suddenly become blind for many months and no doctor could help her. Only the advice of a *sangoma* to follow the calling relieved her and she eventually regained her eyesight once she started training. Rodney Sibuyi had been obese and had had severe pains in his legs before he accepted the calling and started his four year long training, which slimmed him down significantly and improved his general physical appearance. Often, trainee healers would deny their calling for a long time, because the training is demanding and requires enormous emotional and financial commitment.

Ukuthwasa begins with a diagnostic consultation, called a *vumisa* (Xh.), with a healer. During the *vumisa*, it is determined whether the ill person should begin *ukuthwasa* or whether the illness has other roots (Buhrmann 1984: 36). Once the *ngoma* (Ndembu) "cult of affliction" – which Victor Turner defined as "the interpretation of misfortune in terms of domination by a specific non-human agent and the attempt to come to terms with the misfortune by having the afflicted individual, under the guidance of a 'doctor' of that mode, join the cult association venerating that specific agent" (Turner 1967: 15–16) – is finally accepted, the apprentice's *rite de passage* (van Gennep [1960]/1990) or graduation (Thornton 2009: 18) begins. *Ngoma*, the art and philosophy of healing the self and others, which is a therapeutic institution that transforms sufferers into healers (Janzen 1992) in the "quest for fruition" for mental and physical well being (van Dijk & Reis & Spierenburg 2000), is a tradition that varies significantly in Bantu-speaking Africa (Janzen 1992; Thornton 2009)[7]. Aside from being "a way of articulating and commenting on processes of transition or transformation," *ngoma* also produces "a certain type of power and authority which is based on claims to a specific association and communication with the spirit world (...) expressed and effected in rhythm (drumming, singing, dancing)" (van Dijk, Reis & Spierenburg 2000: 7). In most traditions, the training involves procedural characteristics that were similar across my research areas in the Eastern Cape and Bushbuckridge Municipality, but which included different techniques and practices. Throwing the bones (*tinhlolo*), for instance, is not taught in the Eastern Cape, but is an essential part of the tradition of the Shangaan people who inhabit the Gazankulu area. Commonly, the 'afflicted' person will move into the household of their healer trainer to live with his/her family and contribute to household duties such as cleaning, cooking and collecting water and wood, usually for the entire duration of the training, sometimes many years. This often includes long periods of distance from spouses and children, abstinence from sexual activities, the restriction of eating habits (e.g. no sugar, eggs and milk) and immersion in a close but very hierarchical mentor relationship, expressed, for instance, in the act of the trainee kneeling down in front of the trainer while communicating. The training's basic intention is to allow the trainee to let go of his/her individual person and transform into a medium guided by the ancestral spirits. The trainer supports the trainee to open up the path for deep communication with the ancestral spirits, though it is emphasized that connecting to the spirits is a process left solely to the *thwasa*.

The actual 'treatment' of the afflicted begins with a number of rituals, such as inner and outer cleansing with *muthi*, receiving small razorblade cuttings into which *muthi* is rubbed, and wearing the white or red beads and typical *thwasa* clothing (simple white or red cloths)[8]. This is followed by an intense dance and drumming session, while the *thwasa* sits under a blanket to slowly glide into a form of trance and expel the names of his/her ancestral spirits from deep in the subcon-

---

7   It was beyond the scope of this research to look into the details of each individual healing tradition. To truly understand the different traditions, I would presumably have had to become engaged as a *thwasa*, or at least do research on a long-term basis on traditional healing only, as other anthropologists have done (see Ashforth 2005; Stoller & Olkes 1986; Wreford 2009). Instead, I was a short-term observer of the private and professional lives of an array of different healers in different traditions.

8   In the Nguni tradition of the Xhosa, the *thwasa* wears white clothes and is often painted with white chalk throughout the entire training period (see figure 6). White is the color of purity and symbolizes the state of withdrawal and abstinence from normal life. In the Tsonga/Shangaan tradition, which is closer to the Swazi tradition and is influenced by the emotional *ndau* spirit, *thwasas* wear red.

scious[9]. For the remainder of the training, the *thwasa* attends *inthlombes* (ceremonies) and learns the *xhentsa* (ritualized dancing), which wakes up the spirit of the *thwasa* (Thornton 2009: 28)[10]. All of these ritual practices are intended to deeply connect the *thwasa* with the ancestral spirits. Once they are evoked, the process continues throughout the entire training, with the slaughtering of animals (chickens and goats) and purification rituals such as purging, steam baths with *muthi* (*futha*), and washing with and drinking herbal mixtures and smoke (Buhrmann 1984: 41–42).

Getting to know *muthi* is one of the most crucial parts of the training. The ox, which is slaughtered in the final *goduswa* ceremony to initiate the apprentice into full *sangomahood*, is sprinkled with *muthi*. The tail of the slaughtered ox is retained and serves as the upper end of the *sangoma* stick (*itshoba*), which is wrapped in beads. *Muthi* is fixed between the stick and the beads. Other practices and techniques involve particular *muthi*, for the most part *ubulawu*, so-called dream medicine, a plant or plant mixture that, when dissolved in water, opens the path to dreaming and connection to the ancestors. To prepare *ubulawu*, a huge bucket of *ubulawu muthi* is mixed with water and stirred with a wooden blender. The froth that develops on top of the liquid is consumed before sleep, or before ceremonies and rituals. *Ubulawu*, which has an earthy, wooden and slightly sour taste, is associated with the clan of the *thwasa*'s teacher and offers a direct way to the clan ancestors (Berglund 1976: 223). It also enables the *thwasa* 'to see' (Xh.: *umhlahlo*). 'Seeing' is a central characteristic of a healer (Wreford 2005: 113). Learning to see is also a principal aspect of the training. 'Finding the *imphilo*' (Xh.) means finding a secret or hidden object. This exercise evokes and manifests the initiate to see illnesses and other

---

9   In her book 'In Two Worlds' (1984), Vera Buhrmann, a psychotherapist and psychoanalyst, examined the meaning of the ancestors in South Africa and correlated them to what C.G. Jung called the subconscious.

10   I attended a number of *inthlombe* in the Eastern Cape, Johannesburg and, to a lesser extent, Bushbuckridge. *Inthlombes* are spiritually intense, socially dense gatherings of community members and healers. These events vary considerably in nature and complexity (Bührmann 1984: 56). An *inthlombe* can last between many hours to many days. It includes dancing, ritualized praying to the ancestors, singing, drumming and the slaughtering of animals. In one *inthlombe* that I attended, the participants whirled a chicken around their heads before the animal was finally slaughtered. Until today, I find it difficult to write about these events, where enormous spiritual energies were released by the dancing *sangomas* and attending community members. Writing about this spiritual energy would demand a more poetic approach, as the spiritual is not legible and hence eludes easy description. "There are things one cannot put into words, only feel them in one's body," a healer said to Vera Buhrmann (1984: 56). When I attended an *inthlombe*, I often experienced severe headaches and migraine attacks, either during or afterwards. I assume that my bodily response was based on a mixture of anxiety of the unknown and discomfort over being spiritually (and linguistically) excluded from a space that I only had the chance to observe.

conditions in a patient. It exacerbates the ability to identify problems and locate the causative illness in and outside the body. It is basically an act of deep intuitive seeing.

Figure 6 A thwasa in front of a bucket of ubulawu, Eastern Cape

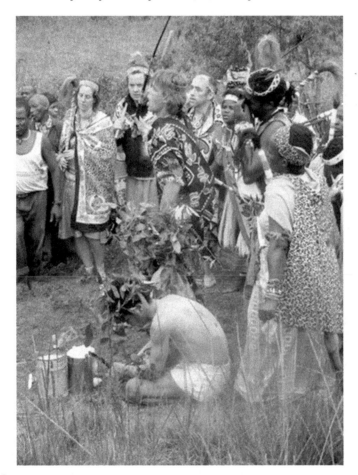

The ancestors guide the entire training period and support the apprentice to regain health and strengthen his/her healing capacities. They also help the *thwasa* to find the right animal for the *sangoma*'s drum, which is made of the skin of a goat, cow or any other animal, and finally to dream about the ox to be slaughtered in the *goduswa*. Ancestors often expel themselves out of the *thwasa* with noisy, roaring sounds. The *thwasa* becomes totally overwhelmed and occupied by this explosive force, leading to shivering, sweating and trance-like conditions. These ancestral encounters happen during the night and the day, and those at the healer's homestead must support the possessed *thwasa* to release the ancestors by beating drums. When more than two *thwasas* are living at one time in a healer's household, nights and days are filled with roaring séances and with tiredness after the intense emotional discharge. This can be a physically and psychologically exhausting process. The *thwasa* has to regularly participate in ceremonies in the larger community, where he/she dances, serves food and prepares *muthi*. Community members support the *thwasa*'s process, for instance by supporting the obligatory *xhentsa* dancing with drumming, hand clapping and singing. A hierarchically structured greeting of the ancestors, the healer trainer, other elders and the community precedes the dancing. Greeting the ancestors entails the *thwasa* kneeling down on the floor while leaning on two sticks (*isthoba*), reciting the names of ancestors (parents and grandparents) and burning *Imphepho*. The training is not only emotionally strenuous but also economically demanding. It includes the trainee paying to stay at the trainer's homestead, and for the many smaller and larger ceremonies on the way to graduation. The graduation ceremony itself is probably the most expensive part, as the *thwasa* has to pay for the graduation ox (which can cost 8000 Rand, ca. 470 Euro, or more), for a number of goats and chickens, for *muthi*, for the ingredients of *umqomboti* (homebrewed beer), and other beverages such as beer, cold drinks and tea (cf. Wreford 2009).

Ritualizing Muthi: Finding the Imphilelo and Finalizing Ukuthwasa

The following descriptions stem from KwaThema, a township east of Johannesburg, where I, together with my landlady Annelie, spent four days in March 2012 to visit Gogo Mule. Annelie had finalized her own healer training, which she had started in Mtambalal in the Eastern Cape, with Gogo Mule in 2010. She had come to train with Gogo Mule for two reasons. First, Gogo Mule was, in addition to Zulu, fluent in English and Afrikaans, and was thus capable of training white *amathwasa*. Second, she had no issues with training gay people in what is otherwise an extremely unfriendly and homophobic environment. In KwaThema, for instance, 24-year-old Noxolo Nogwaza was killed in 2011 after an inhumane and horrific corrective rape for being a lesbian[11]. At my landlady's homecoming ceremony in Cape Town, where she was ritually reintegrated back into her family after having been part of her trainer's family for the duration of the long training period in KwaThema, half of

---

11   See David Smith (2011): www.theguardian.com/world/2011/may/03/south-africa-homophob
ic-attacks and Clare Carter (2013): www.nytimes.com/interactive/2013/07/26/opinion/26corr
ective-rape.html?_r=0.

the healers and *amathwasa* who participated in "bringing Jacobus home"[12] to Cape Town were gay men and women. Indeed, in South African healing traditions, it is said that same-sex partners can get married if they are traditional healers, because a male ancestor of the one healer may want to marry the female ancestor of the other healer, being referred to as the "ancestral wife" or "ancestral husband" (cf. Nkabinde 2008; Morgan & Wieringa 2005). For Gogo Mule, this was a reasonable explanation. According to her, she only fulfilled her duty as a "role model, counsellor, therapist, guide" (Janzen 1992: 170). "I only do what I need to do. A *thwasa* is a sick child that needs help," she explained.

Below, I will briefly recount two situations that took place during the four days that I spent with Gogo Mule. The first describes how the current *thwasa* at Gogo Mule's house was engaged in finding the *imphilelo*. Finding the *imphilelo* is an important exercise to consolidate the intuitive power of finding, seeing (*umhlahlo*) and knowing illness in a patient. The second is a brief description of a final initiation ceremony (*goduswa*). Describing these situations will help to better picture and contextualize *muthi* and knowledge in the training process and to show how much they are bound to social and ancestral relations. Finding the *imphilelo* and the homecoming ceremony are practiced both in the Eastern Cape region and in the Bushbuckridge region, but with different practices and *muthi*.

The freshly polished and waxed backyard seemed to vibrate under the noisy drumming beat out on old, rusty truck wheels strung with cow- and goatskins, and which resonated heavily on the freshly cleaned concrete floors and walls of Johannesburg's townships. "The floor has to be clean," said Gogo Mule, "for the ancestors and spirits to feel welcomed and at home." In her early years, Gogo Mule had been a soap opera actress and stage diva. Later, in her mid 40s, she received the calling after she had experienced an extended phase of suffering, bad luck and deaths in her family. At first she refused to follow the calling; it was much more convenient to stay where she was, on stage and in front of the camera. But after yet more severe accidents and deaths had occurred in her family, she finally accepted her fate. Today, she trains *amathwasa* and graduates *izsangoma*.

During a particular time when she did not have any *amathwasana* (as she called them), she thought of herself as having been bewitched by someone who was jealous of her success as a trainer. She thought about consulting the *magobela* of her *impande* in Swaziland, which she eventually did. After performing cleansing rituals with different *muthi*, a new *thwasa* eventually arrived to train with her, which not only strengthened her power as a healer but also her financial situation. When we visited her in spring 2012, the weather in Johannesburg was still warm, though the nights were cold, and during the day the concrete floors radiated heat. The weekend had begun with the cleaning of the house and backyard and the visit of some

---

12   Annelie's ancestral spirit expelled itself during the initiating ritual as Jacobus.

friends, among them a lesbian couple that Gogo Mule had recently wedded. Both women were trained healers. In midst of the visiting people, the cleaning of the house and cooking for dinner, the current *thwasa* (aged 28), started having a few ancestral fits after she had drunk *ubulawu*. It was time for her to find the *imphilelo*, the hidden secret (cf. Wreford 2008:114f.). Roaring and whining sounds came from the *indumba* in the rear corner of the backyard. In the meantime, some neighborhood children and Gogo Mule's adoptive son Pitso, whose parents had died of AIDS, prepared the drums. They started drumming, and with the increasing noise of the rusty truck wheel drums, the *thwasa* was slowly propelled into a trance-like dance. Gogo Mule burned *Imphepho*. The *thwasa* danced energetically, then knelt down in front of the *Imphepho* to greet the ancestors, then danced again and then knelt down in front of Gogo Mule, rubbing her hands, accompanied by the weeping and sighing sounds and repetitive shaking of the head typical of the *ndau* spirit, in which Gogo Mule trains her *amathwasa* (including my landlady Annelie). She answered the *thwasa*'s greeting by clapping her hands, greeting her and saying:

> **Gogo Mule:** We have hidden something for you. Go and find it.
> **Thwasa:** What is it?
> **Gogo Mule:** It is a thing I gave to you.
> **Thwasa:** Where is it?
> **Gogo Mule:** It is inside.
> **Thwasa:** Where inside?
> **Gogo Mule:** Go and find it. [The thwasa runs and comes back to kneel down in front of Gogo Mule.]
> **Thwasa:** I did not see it. Where can I find it?
> **Gogo Mule:** It is inside. Go and find it.

This exchange continued a couple of times. Finally, the *thwasa* came back with a yellow-green snuffbox that had been hidden under the pillows of one of the two beds in the house. She knelt down in front of Gogo Mule and the rest of the present audience supported her with *siyavuma* (their agreement). The community was satisfied with the *thwasa*'s performance, and so was Gogo Mule. This would not be the last time that the *thwasa* would have to find the *imphilelo*, as it is a regular exercise in the training. In addition to finding the *imphilelo*, the *thwasa* stays in a very close bonding relationship with her/his trainer. Daily rituals and activities, which include individual communication with the ancestors, collecting *muthi* in the field or bush, preparing the *muthi* by cutting it into pieces and grinding and pulverizing it, consulting patients together with the healer trainer and learning how to tell a patient's fortune by reading the bones, preparing the *futha* (steam bath) with *muthi*, drinking *ubulawu* and sharing dreams with the trainer, in addition to daily household chores such as collecting wood and water (in the rural areas) and cleaning the house, constitute a large part of the training. The trainer–*thwasa* relationship is hierarchical, full-time and therapeutic. It can also lead to tensions and conflicts, though these are mostly regarded as a normal part of the process (cf. Wreford 2009).

After the *thwasa* had found the *imphilelo*, we left Gogo Mule's house to join the *goduswa* of another *thwasa* at Gogo Gonegwani's house. Gogo Gonegwani is a close friend of Gogo Mule and also a healer. The *goduswa* ceremony separates the ancestors of the trainer and those of the *thwasa* to enable the *thwasa* to work independently, but as a member of the same *impande*. The graduating *thwasa* was a 64-year-old woman who had hardly been able to sustain the training due to her physical weakness and severe leg pains. Nevertheless, she managed to train for three months with Gogo Gonegwani, who explained that three months were enough for the old lady; she only had to be connected to her ancestors. She received the cuttings rubbed with *muthi*, slaughtered chickens and a goat for the ancestors, and had chosen the ox for the *goduswa* ceremony, which had already been ritually slaughtered, cooked and served to the community. Feeding the guests is one of the most important aspects of the ceremony. The *goduswa* ceremony also entailed the burning of *Imphepho* while the *thwasa* danced her *gida* and aspects of finding the *imphilelo*. This time, the *imphilelo* was a freshly flayed goatskin that was cut into two connecting loops, which the *thwasa* wore around her upper body; the contact of the goatskin on her own skin symbolized contact and communion with the ancestors. In the appropriate way of asking questions while kneeling in front of her *magobela*, and running back and forth to find the *imphilelo*, she eventually found it hidden in the *indumba*. Together with her *itshoba* (cow-tail *sangoma* stick), it was hidden in a bowl covered by a colorful piece of cloth. After the goatskin was slung twice around her body, she danced the *gida*, the final dance that marked her transition to the status of being a fully graduated *sangoma*. Due to her age and health issues, her dancing was limited, and she could hardly bend down to greet the ancestors.

Gogo Gonegwani greeted the *thwasa* compassionately, supported by the drumming and hand clapping of the community. After she finished dancing, the newly graduated *sangoma* sat down on the straw mat, where her husband quietly and humbly welcomed her back. Intimacy is strictly forbidden during the training period, and hence the spouses were glad to be together again. Gogo Gonegwani finalized the ceremony with some words to the community and the reunited couple. She thanked the ancestors for supporting the process, and thanked the community for having stayed so long. "It shows," she said, "that the spirit of this *thwasana* is very high. Normally, people would leave much earlier after having eaten."

Healer, Plant and Ancestors: An Inseparable Unit

Searching for the *imphilelo*, drinking *ubulawu*, burning *Imphepho* and integrating *muthi* into the training all aims to connect the trainee healer – with the help of medicinal plants – to the ancestors. Dream medicine, for instance, enhances dream intensity that then leads to inner visions about animals (e.g. choosing the cow for the final ceremony) or plants (where and when to find plants for specific treatments). Integrating *muthi* into the training thus has a deeply transformative component. It connects living beings with the dead and evokes deep intuition and communication in the trainee healer. It supports the *rite de passage* that is determined by the manifestation of contact with the ancestral spirits (Ngubane 1976: 278). It is also a process of purification. Purity means to wash away the pollution (*umnyama*) of birth and other polluting factors, and to substitute it with the highest possible capability of clairvoyance. The graduation ceremony is the point where the trainee has the strongest clairvoyant power and is hence strongly connected with the ancestral spirits. *Muthi* also serves as a means of clarification and purification (cf. Hutchings 2007). The coming healer washes and takes *futha* with *muthi*, drinks and vomits *muthi* mixtures for inner cleansing. Without *muthi*, connection with the ancestors would not be established, and different *muthi* have different influences. *Muthi* is not only indispensable for *rites de passage* and other rituals and ceremonies performed after initiation, such as when *Imphepho* is used in Xhosa, Zulu and Swazi traditions for its cleansing capacity and to "clear the air for the spirits" (Dugmore & van Wyk 2008). It also helps to treat physical and psychological conditions like back pain, headache, bad luck or bewitchment[13]. The use of *muthi* is taught during the healer training and is manifested and extended through a lifelong learning process, which is ultimately transferred to a new *thwasa* who then, as a healer, transfers the knowledge to the next thwasa.

The knowledge is transferred as a bundle of information that is assembled in the healer, to the *thwasa*. This bundle – or the many bundles – of knowledge are not constituted of individually held pieces of knowledge. Rather, they are a conglomerate of different knowledge(s) accumulated in a healer over years of knowledge transference and sharing, which takes place not only during the training but also in their everyday interactions with other healers, for instance in ceremonies or simply while meeting at home. The process of knowledge accumulation and production is thoroughly guided and controlled by the ancestral spirits. Without the ancestors, this knowledge transference would not be possible. *Muthi* and the ancestors are basically omnipresent and interlinked in traditional healing. Learning to heal me-

---

13   Bryant (1966) wrote an extensive account of medicinal plants and their use in 'Zulu medicine', and Hewat (1970) did the same for 'Bantu tribes'. Both accounts are, however, written in a colonial language that does not give much credit to the experience of the knowledge holders themselves. Today, making such an encyclopedic documentation of plants and knowledge would hardly be possible without prior informed consent and making an access and benefit sharing agreement, as stipulated by the Biodiversity Act of 2004.

ans learning to control and make use of both. And it entails learning to protect the spiritual value of healing knowledge and associated plant knowledge.

Protecting the Value of Knowledge and Muthi

Against this background, the knowledge of traditional healers, and to a certain degree material objects (such as a plant mixture carried as a talisman in a small bottle around the neck), can be regarded as "inalienable possessions" (Annette Weiner 1992), a term that refers back to Marcel Mauss's "objects immeuble" (1954), objects with inalienable wealth that cannot be detached from their origins. Inalienable possessions must be analyzed differently to alienable possessions (possessions that have little or no cultural meaning), which are bound to different economies. When traced back, inalienable possessions originate from a higher order, i.e. a god, higher spirit, the ancestors or any other entity regarded as higher than human beings. Mark Osteen explains that "what makes [a] possession inalienable, I conclude, must be neither time nor the drive for power but an immaterial aura of connection to other humans and to something greater than [an] individual human" (Osteen 2002: 244).

Indeed, "What makes a possession inalienable is its exclusive and cumulative identity with a particular series of owners through time. Its history is authenticated by fictive or true genealogies, origin myths, by sacred ancestors, and gods" (Weiner 1992: 33). Inalienable possessions are imbued with affective qualities that are expressions of the value that an object has when its owner keeps it and inherited along a family line or descent group. An inalienable possession, according to Weiner (1985: 210),

> acts as a vehicle for bringing past time into the present, so that the histories of ancestors become an intimate part of who one is in the present, so that the histories of ancestors, titles, or mythological events become an intimate part of that person's identity. To lose this claim to the past is to lose part of who one is in the present. In its inalienability, the object must be seen as more than an economic resource and more than an affirmation of social relations.

The *hau* described by Marcel Mauss (1957) and the *taongoa* described by Annette Wiener (1992) illustrate that inalienable objects or possessions are involved in a circuit of giving and receiving, which represents the circle of life and death. Giving away something of the inherent power of an inalienable object or possession means giving away something of life. It is actually a life threatening action and hence demands social rules to maintain trust and social order. On the other hand, not giving it away but rather keeping hold of it would entail not continuing with the order of life. Exchange and sharing is therefore a way of achieving social integration. It is "the glue that holds society together" (Graeber 2001: 27).

The exchange of knowledge between a healer trainer, a *thwasa* and the ancestors can be regarded as a gift practice that is caught between the "inalienability of sacred objects" – those gifts from the gods, heirlooms and kinship markers inextricably linked with tribal or social identities – and "the alienability of commercial objects" – things freely exchanged for profit (Godelier 1999: 94). "Gifts are thus double-voiced, speaking now in the voice of ancestors or divine beings, and now in the neutral tones of mere merchandise" (Osteen 2002: 8). This double voice puts knowledge in an ambiguous position: on the one hand, it is an inalienable possession that derives from the ancestors and has a sacred notion; on the other hand, it is embedded in the everyday economy of the healer and the community. The healer–patient relationship entails sometimes high, at other times lower, payments; the training is highly cost intensive and most of the money flows to the trainer, as he/she provides knowledge and practices as well as food and accommodation. Being a healer is therefore, in addition to an invaluable service to the community, also an income generating business (cf. Dietzel 2013: 63ff.). The inalienability of knowledge creates an aura, and a spiritual, inalienable value, that demands highly secured protection. This protection space is taught and learned in the *impande*, a healer's school or clan that holds the ownership over specific inalienable possessions.

The ownership of healing knowledge is bound to a number of social relations within the *impande* and beyond. In interviews in the Eastern Cape and in Bushbuckridge, healers repeatedly claimed that "knowledge belongs to the ancestors." But the situation is more complex. Knowledge derives from the ancestors, who have their origin in the family line of the individual healer as well as in an *impande*. As mentioned earlier, the gift of healing is often inherited within a family. In the training, the healer is then connected to the ancestral spirits of the *impande*. The knowledge that was acquired during the training may only be shared with members of the same *impande*. Each *impande* is characterized by specific knowledge of medicinal plants, healing practices and rituals, as well as ethical and moral values and norms of behavior, expressed in customary laws. The knowledge is exclusively acquired during the training under the auspices of the ancestors of the "new family" (Thornton 2009: 27) of the trainee healer. It is subject to strict rules of adherence, transference and protection.

Members of the Kukula Healers in Bushbuckridge Municipality all claimed to belong to an *impande* – either to the *Dlamini* or to the *Nkomo le Lwandle* (the latter means 'cow from the sea') – while the term *impande* was much less frequently mentioned in the Eastern Cape, sometimes not at all. These two names – *Dlamini* and *Nkomo le Lwandle* – refer back to the original ancestors of the clan. I asked an associate of the Kukula Healers, Mama Rose, to explain the origin of these names. Together with her husband David, she offered the following brief account:

Many centuries ago a man disappeared from his hometown close to Barberton, a small town close to the border of Swaziland, to Komatipoort, a border post to Mozambique. From there he traveled to the coast not far from Maputo. His family thought that he had died, for he did not return for a long time. But what happened instead was that the man went into the sea and when he came out of the sea years later, he happened to have learned the arts of healing. He returned to South Africa as a healer and was the first to heal and train the next generation of healers. He happened to have two sons, whom he also trained as healers. These two brothers first healed and trained together but later split into two separate conflicting healing schools, named Nkomo le Lwandle (the cow from the sea) and Dlamini, in which different forms of knowledge played a role. These two schools again split into different sub-groups, of which one was called Majoye and the other Vondo[14].

According to the above account, an *impande* is said to have an original founder. The founder of this *impande* belongs to a specific clan, which can be traced back along patrilineal lines to a "common clan founder in the male line who gave his name to the clan" (Hammond Tooke 1989: 60–61)[15]. In the above case, the clan founders were the brothers Nkomo Le Lwandle and Dlamini. In other areas and ethnic groups, the clan founders have different names and origins. Knowledge may be shared with members of the same impande, or, exceptionally – and ideally in consultation with the ancestors – with healers of other *izimpande*. This is a rule that seems open to individual modification. One healer in Bushbuckridge, for instance, said: "I don't mind sharing my knowledge, but I have some knowledge I will not share with anyone. It is my own secret" (Thembi Ndlovu, January 2012).

In case a healer wants to secure a certain "healing terrain," he/she may not want to share his/her knowledge with others as this will give him/her an advantage in

---

14   This story was told by Mama Rose personally and is subject to her own views and specifica-
      tions. Origin stories are orally transferred, which often give them a mystical and poetic qual-
      ity. The extent to which they are 'true' is largely difficult to determine. Niehaus, in his book
      'Witchcraft, Power and Politics: Exploring the Occult in the South African Lowveld' (2001),
      recounts the story differently. According to his account, the first Tsonga healers were the
      woman Nkomo We Lwandle and the man Dunga Manzi (Stirring Water, see also Dunga-
      manzi/Stirring Waters, Johannesburg Art Gallery 2007), who were trained by Nzonzo, the
      water serpent. Nzono would capture people underwater, and their release would only occur
      after the slaughtering of an ox. After being released, Nkomo We Lwandle and Dunga Manzi
      emerged as powerful healers (Niehaus 2001: 24).

15   Generally, the linage systems of ethnic groups of bantu origin have a patrilineal, exogamous
      descendent line (the great-great-grandfather, see Wreford 2008: 49), which constitutes large
      categories of people who have a common clan name and believe themselves to be descended
      from a common clan founder. As such a founder lived far back in the distant (sometimes
      mythical) past, it is quite impossible to demonstrate conclusively a relationship to him or to
      fellow clan members (Hammond Tocke 2002, 1985, 1978; Ngubane 1977).

a competitive field. Or he/she may only share selected parts of his/her repertoire of knowledge with a befriended healer or family members. However, it also seemed to be the generally accepted consensus that if knowledge is shared beyond the boundaries of the *impande*, or at least outside of the healer community, "the ancestors may kill you." This warning was made repeatedly in interviews with healers in Cape Town, KwaThema, the Eastern Cape and Bushbuckridge. Furthermore, knowledge that is shared beyond the boundaries of the healing profession will lose its potency. The fear of losing patronage over knowledge may thus be a reason for the strict boundaries and secrecy attached to it (cf. Bhat & Jacobs 1995). As Adam Ashforth has stated, "African science is secret knowledge. This secrecy is the essential core" that nevertheless also "broadens the field of imagination in which potential powers of *muthi* and the people who deploy it play out" (Ashforth 2005: 147). The aspect of being persecuted for witchcraft plays a further, essential role in keeping knowledge secret. When knowledge remains secret, it and its users are protected against outside use and/or abuse, and thus the community is strengthened. Secrecy and selective disclosure only within the boundaries of the *impande* are one of the strongest means of knowledge protection.

George Simmel was the first to sociologically engage with the term secrecy. In his book 'The Sociology of Secrecy and of Secret Societies' (1906), Simmel defined the "role of secrecy as a means for the manipulation and control of a central variable in social organization: information" (Hazelrigg 1969: 323). The secret is the ultimate sociological form of regulation of the flow and distribution of information (ibid.: 324). Secret societies are intentional units characterized by the fact that reciprocal relations among its members are governed by the protective function of secrecy (ibid.: 326; see also Bok 1983: 45 ff.). The *izimpande* may be referred to as secret societies in this sense, since they uphold specific transference rules and boundaries to protect knowledge. These rules and regulations protect the aura of the inalienable possession and therewith protect the 'unspoiled' continuation of the cycle of life and death, past and present. Every trespass of the rules is avenged by the moral and ethical power of the ancestors themselves, sometimes even with death (see, for instance, the story of Gogo Mule; see also Ashforth 2000).

Figure 7 below illustrates the flows of traditional healers' knowledge. It shows how knowledge should ideally remain within the boundaries of a healer's *impande*, though it may be shared with healers of other *izimpande*, and only under very specific circumstances with those beyond the boundaries of the *izimpande*. Customary laws help to uphold specific cultural rules and regulations that protect knowledge as an inalienable possession, which, when transferred by the ancestors, has the mediating character of bridging the past to the present. At the same time, this system is open to modification and changes. As seen in figure 7, knowledge may be shared with other healers, and, if correctly compiled and agreed upon by the ancestors[16], even beyond the boundaries of the *impande*, though this demands new rules of pooling, sharing and protection.

Figure 7 Knowledge exchange within single impande, transmission to healers in other izimpande, and only beyond the izimpande under very restricted circumstances

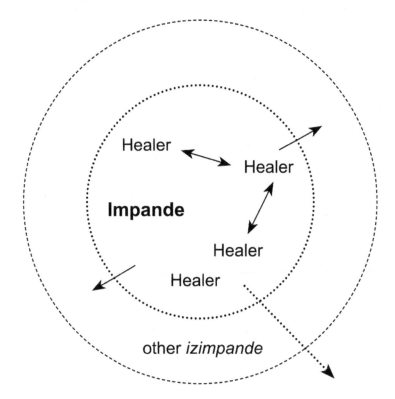

© B. Rutert.

It can occur that moral and ethical rules are disregarded, irrespective of the implications. Hence the system of knowledge protection might be disrupted by intrinsic and extrinsic factors, such as knowledge disclosure enforced by outside parties, or brought about by the seductive hope of participation in the broader knowledge economy. However, to maintain moral and ethical order, customary laws offer a helpful structure. Healer training is thus not only a *rite de passage* into *sangomahood*, but also a transference of the rules of the appropriate protection of the inalienable

---

16   I was never able to fully understand how this ancestral consent actually occurs, as it was always a private process between the healer and the ancestor(s).

objects of a healers' community, and thus also of the community at large. Traditional healers are responsible for the well being of their community. They uphold rules and regulations that protect their own knowledge, the environment and/or medicinal plants, as well as the community. By protecting knowledge, they also protect parts of the social order of their communities, which entails communication with the dead, who – as much as the living – belong to the structure of *ubuntu* (elaborated on below). Customary laws are supportive in protecting this moral and social order. The following section depicts customary laws that enable the protection of knowledge as well as medicinal plants in the environment, and which, to a certain extent, uphold the moral and social order in communities. Customary laws are therefore not only knowledge protection schemes, but social order protection schemes.

Customary Laws: Protecting Knowledge, the Environment and Moral Order

Early anthropologists analyzed customary laws in terms of closed, bounded communities with fixed systems of law and governance (see Schapera 1938; Allot 1970; Gluckmann 1955, 1956; Comaroff & Roberts 1981). Looking at customary laws in South African traditional healers' communities today, however, though some of these laws do maintain certain 'traditional' or fixed moral and ethical standards in the lives of healers and their communities, in general they can be seen as dynamic and, to an extent, intertwined with and contextualized within national law and a constantly changing society.

On my very first day in the Bushbuckridge area, Rodney Sibuyi explained during a side conversation "the customary laws are ethical and moral laws. Respect for the elders, for instance, must be sustained at all times." Customary law is "'living law': law as lived in day-to-day life and [the] norms and values it draws on" (Ehrlich 1936: PAGE; see also Bennett 1995; D Enelbronner-Kolff 2001). Such law must also be differentiated from 'official customary law' as it pertains to local 'native' courts and administration (Oomen 2005). While healers attempt to uphold customary law, at the same time they also have to adjust to official customary law, which, for instance, restricts the unlimited collection of medicinal plants on common land, a law enforced by local tribal authorities (though it must be added that 'living law' and 'official customary law' are often intertwined).

The lived customary laws of traditional healers are an intrinsic part of knowledge systems and, at the same time, an extrinsic regulatory system that protects the sensitive balance of all knowledge, people and environmental relations. These laws have and still go through ongoing changes, from the pre-colonial past until today, which makes their content highly flexible (Gluckman 1969). According to Abrell et al., "[c]ustomary laws are the principles, values, rules, codes of conduct, or established practices that guide the social practices of indigenous communities, including the use and management of natural resources" (Abrell et al. 2009: 7). Customary laws, which are "usually unwritten and mutable, malleable and not drawn to specialization" (Bennett 2004: 2), regulate everyday life in local communities. They are a field of diverse actions, including figures of authority (Oomen 2005) or other local institutions such as traditional healers. As Abrell et al.'s definition suggests, customary law also comprises more than people. In the context of traditional healing, customary law regulates and protects relationships between patients, the community, other healers, the environment, as well as sexual behavior and rules and customs with regard to birth, death and food. Customary law in this sense is concerned with the moral and ethical norms of communities and with maintaining cultural as well as natural resources.

Probably the best-known and most general customary law in the (South) African indigenous context is the moral and ethical principle of *ubuntu*. The term *ubuntu* derives from the Zulu proverb *umuntu ngumuntu nga bantu*, which can be translated as "a person is a person through other people," in which the root word *-ntu* means person or human. Desmond Tutu (1999) summarized the underlying principle of *ubuntu* as follows:

> Ubuntu [is] the essence of being human. Ubuntu speaks particularly about the fact that you can't exist as a human being in isolation. It speaks about our interconnectedness. You can't be human all by yourself, and when you have this quality – Ubuntu – you are known for your generosity. We think of ourselves far too frequently as just individuals, separated from one another, whereas you are connected and what you do affects the whole World. When you do well, it spreads out; it is for the whole of humanity[17].

Ubuntu, the relationality of people, is the principal of 'harmony' and the 'heart of Africanness' that was vigorously promoted in the efforts to unleash the African Renaissance (Ashforth 2005: 86; Bennett & Patrick 2011). In this web of human existence and societies, where everyday life is threatened by uncertainty, relationships to others help one to feel physically, psychologically and spiritually more secure (Manda 2008: 126). *Ubuntu* is a general notion in many African societies[18]. While customary laws such as *ubuntu* have long existed, since the colonial conquest they "have been treated as inferior, scarcely deserving recognition as true laws" (Bennett 2011: 30). With the inclusion of the concept of *ubuntu* into the South African constitution, the perception of customary law as inferior to common law slowly reversed

---

17   Robert Thornton has commented critically that *ubuntu* remains only vaguely defined and is
      often "honored more in the breach than the practice" (Thornoton 2009: 19).
18   *Ubuntu* is a term used in Xhosa and Zulu; the term *botho* is used in Sotho, *bunhu* in Tsonga
      and *vhuntu* in Venda. The word can be found in many other African languages and cultural
      contexts, for example as *unnhu* in Shona, *utu* in Swahili and *umundu* in Kikuyu (see Broodryk
      2002; Ramose 2002; Nkonko Kamwangalu 1993).

(ibid.: 31). The customary laws built around traditional marriage, for instance, were included into the constitution as legally equal to state marital law.

To better understand customary law in the context of traditional healers and their communities and environment, I conducted several interviews with healers in Bushbuckridge on the subject. In December 2011, for instance, I conducted an interview with Adah Mabunda, the second executive officer of the Kukula Healers, to discuss customary laws regarding the protection of knowledge and the environment. Before Adah began the interview, she first invited me to take a look at her *indumba*. It occupied the central hut of the homestead, where she lived with her husband and her youngest daughter. It was an organized and tidy place with a highly polished concrete floor. Her *sangoma* attire (ducks[19], *itshoba*, beads and a brown wig) was neatly arranged in a wardrobe on the right side of the round hut. One duck with the membership emblem of a traditional healers' organization in Johannesburg was attached to the wall. Adah had been a member of the organization for a long time and was, at the time of our interview, a member of both this organization and the Kukula Healers. The tidy *indumba* was also a representation of her for her important strong ethical and moral values.

> The most important thing for a healer is the right attitude, such as not drinking alcohol while you are treating a patient. Because when you give the patient muthi, you can overdose and intoxicate the patient. And then people will say, 'Ah, this one, she is a witch [because she kills people]'. Therefore, you also need to train properly, to teach the coming healer to use the muthi correctly. And you must stay true to the customary laws, e.g. when you have a female thwasa, you as a female healer always have to sleep with the thwasa in the indumba to prevent her from having male visitors. Also, at night, a Tokoloshe [a small naughty dwarf that scares people], might come and scare the thwasa. It is better for them not to be alone. When you have a male thwasa, my husband sleeps with the guy in one hut for similar reasons. Also, as a healer, you are not allowed to start a relationship with your patients. But somehow things changed a lot; today healers have relationships with patients and also with thwasas.

Aside from moral guidelines dealing with sexuality, Adah also recounted some rules regarding medicinal plants and the protection of the environment.

> It is very important that you ask the ancestors before you collect this and that plant [a rule I also heard from healers in the Eastern Cape]. Some plants you can only collect at sunrise, then you take the plant that shows in the direction of where the sun comes from and then you take another plant and combine them for a muthi

---

19   A duck is the cloth that is wrapped around a healer's waist. It is the official attire, and often comes with a printed figure of an animal (such as a lion, snake or rooster), which represents the association's guiding animal.

mixture. After you remove the roots, you must put soil. If you leave it open, it will dry out. Also, the roots grow faster when covered. We are using roots a lot. We also use barks, but not much. That's what we were taught. Roots are strong. It depends on the disease you want to treat. Some roots you cook, some you only put in water, like a decoction. Some plants you can even use as a poison. To know all these things and to treat the knowledge responsibly, a person is supposed to train for at least two years, not only one year or a few months, like people like to do today.

Adah's perspectives on customary law were confirmed in many interviews with members of the Kukula Healers. The laws they referred to were mostly related to sexual behavior, food, and birth or death. For instance: "When a husband or wife dies, you must stay and eat alone, separate from the rest of the community, and you must sexually abstain for a year"; "After an abortion, immediate sex is prohibited"; "When you have a newborn, you are not allowed to touch them after sexual intercourse because their navel wounds will burst and the child will die"; "When you had sex before marriage, you must clean your house with goat blood." While these are general laws that are supposed to be followed in every household, others are more related to the attitude of healers: "Having sexual intercourse with an apprentice during apprenticeship is strictly forbidden"; "It is not allowed to have sexual intercourse in the *indumba*"; "When you had sex in the *indumba*, you are not allowed to consult patients for the week." Sexuality and its fluids have a disturbing influence on a healer's practice, as the healer might be in danger of losing his/her purity, and hence power, when the rules are not guarded closely and proper cleansing instructions followed. Purity is an important condition that must be upheld by both healers and their communities (Douglas 1966; Green 1997; Hammod-Tooke 1989; Ngubane 1977).

The source of pollution is often associated with birth on the one hand and death on the other (Ngubane 1976: 1). The environment, for instance, with its polluting factors such as bad spirits, can have a negative influence, particularly on weaker members of society such as newborn children or the bereaved. They need to be protected, and in case pollution occurs, to be cleansed by a healer. A healer's characteristic trait is the ability to purify patients of harmful substances and dangerous spirits (Reis 2000: 62). The position of a healer is to balance out the (moral) order where there "has been disorder in relation to the position of people vis-á-vis other people, the environment, the ancestors and other mystical forces that produce pollution" (ibid.). Producing and maintaining good health means "the harmonious working and coordination of the healers' universe and thus also of the health of his patient/community" (ibid.; see also Ashforth 2005: 154ff.). Medicinal plants contribute to the process of cleansing and purification, at least when used as *umithi wokwelapha* (Zl.) (Engl.: medicine for healing) (Ngubane 1977: 22), also referred to as *umuthi omhlope* (white *muthi*, Ashforth 2005: 133). Anne Hutchings reported that medicinal plants such as *umSuzwane* (Xh.) (Engl.: Lemon Bush) are used specifically in burial rites, for instance: "A mixture of leaves and roots is used to clean tools and hands before and after the funeral," and "the plant is used when coming from the mortuary to remove bad spirits" (Hutchings 2007: 200ff.). *Imphepho*, African incense, is also used in cleansing rites to purify the body before sleep (ibid.). *Muthi* is basically used in every event that may cause pollution, since it instills protection.

In addition, customary laws regulate access and exposure to nature and the environment, and enforce the relational aspect of traditional healing. For example, customary law requires a healer "to ask the ancestors for permission to harvest plants and thank them after having collected plants" and a healer also "has to cover roots with soil after being collected and should never ring-bark a tree." A tree, when ring-barked, tends to die. Roots, when not covered with soil, dry out, causing the plant or tree to die. Showing gratitude to the ancestors before and after plant collection leads to a respectful attitude towards the plants and the ancestors. It connects nature, the ancestors and the healer in a relational interplay and thus connects past with present and nature with culture.

It was difficult for me to determine whether these laws are strictly upheld each time a healer collects plants. In the interviews and informal conversations with members of the Kukula Healers, it was said that they collect most plants in the close vicinity of their homesteads, generally on communal land. Collecting plants is also often done as a side activity while fulfilling other duties such as bringing the cattle to the commons or fetching water at the river or the local water pump. At a meeting at Rodney's house, I once observed a number of healers ripping leaves off a bush. The leaves, one healer explained, "help protect against snakes: put them at the entrance of your house and the snakes will never come into the house." The collection of the leaves took place, however, without any spiritual preparation that I could observe. Furthermore, when I observed Rodney collecting plant material, it was usually in his backyard or the nearby bush, where he collected the plants and either used them immediately or dried them for later use. He did not seem to pay much attention to any particular preparatory rules, though he did often go into his *indumba*, especially in the early morning hours, to connect with his ancestors and thank them for the plant materials that he had harvested.

Customary laws are thus obviously guidelines, susceptible to situational adaptation and change. They may be reinterpreted or overlooked, and can be subject to personal modification, adjusted to a healer's everyday needs and/or personal proclivities. Every healer executes them in different ways. On the other hand, such laws are also general rules and are a sign of the credibility and self-determination of the healers as moral authorities in the community and as knowledgeable stewards of the environment.

Property in Relation: Property, Environment and Community

So far, I have shown that traditional healing and the transference of knowledge entails a close relationship between the healer, the ancestral spirits and medicinal plants. The following account of Rodney and an interview with Charles Mthethwa, one of the executive committee members of the Kukula Healers, illustrates that these relations are also deeply interwoven with community life and the surrounding environment. The abovementioned customary laws already hint to the fact that traditional knowledge and medicinal plants are fully integrated into the everyday life of the community at large, as well as into the economic life and survival of the healers, a situation that creates a complex web of property relations.

The ownership of medicinal plants depends on access to land, which, especially in the Bushbuckridge area, is often restricted by private ownership. When access to land is denied, access to plants is denied as well. When access is allowed, the collected plant material (an alienable possession) belongs to the healer, who has no obligation to share it with other healers unless the material was gathered collectively. Ownership is therefore dependent on political constraints and obligations, and is at the same time largely open to change and situational adaptation. I observed the Kukula Healers, for instance, discussing access to communal land and medicinal plants growing on the land with the local chief; part of the discussion was also about confining property relations with regard to *muthi* hunters[20]. Access to land enables access to plants, and having such access creates contestation with regard to the property. It creates a network of relations in which some are allowed in and some are not.

In the abovementioned discussion between the Kukula Healers and the local chief, the healers, *muthi* hunters, the larger community and the communal land were all involved in a contestation over land and plants. In other cases, healers attempted to gain access to privately owned nature and game reserves, such as the Mariepskop Nature Reserve. The plants growing on private land belong to the landowner, but rights of ownership may change when access is allowed. When a healer collects plants on private land, he/she is thus allowed to take it home without any restrictions, and hence gains ownership over the plant material.

The ownership of knowledge as an inalienable possession is less tangible, and thus there is a different quality and complexity to the process of sharing and protection, which reaches, as mentioned earlier, back into the past through the involvement of ancestral spirits. The network of relations bound to an *impande*, however, only starts to be permeable when a third party becomes interested in the knowledge. At other times, a healer is entitled to use the knowledge that he/she owns

---

20   For a situation where so-called *muthi* hunters were caught for illegally harvesting medicinal plants on communal land, see chapter VII.

freely and to generate income from it without any further obligations to share it with others. He/she basically owns the knowledge, but has a social obligation to adhere to customary laws. The following examples illustrate the deep connection between healers, plants, the community, as well as income.

Rodney Sibuyi

Rodney Sibuyi (46, Shangaan, CEO of the Kukula Healers) had lived in Share, a very small settlement of about 100 houses not far from Hluvukane, for most of his life. After he had married in his mid-30s, he moved to Thulamahashe, the next biggest city approximately 20 kilometers west of Share, and began his training as a healer in his late 30s. The four year long training healed him from his obesity and heavy legs, and from a certain 'unhealthy' lifestyle: "I loved women too much," he confessed, as he described his early life before commencing training. After completing the training, he moved back to Thulamahashe to live with his wife, who had been waiting for him for the four years that he had been away, though the marriage soon came to an end. "I had changed too much in the training," Rodney reasoned.

He continued to live in the house in Thulamahashe, but soon became restless. He felt that he should move back to Share, to the property where his grandfather had lived. Rodney's grandfather, who had migrated from Mozambique to South Africa in the 1940s, had been a traditional healer and Rodney believed that his healing capacity was inherited from his grandfather. His grandfather told him in dreams that he belonged to Share and that he should build his *indumba* on his property, near the place where Rodney had been born and next to both his father's homestead as well as most of his family (approximately half of the houses in Share belong to a member of Rodney's extended family). Thus his decision to move back to Share was a decision to go back to his roots. He did not make the complete move straight away, however, and for some time he commuted back and forth between Thulamahashe and his new home in Share. One day in January 2012, when a sudden diabetic shock struck him, he believed that his ancestors had become angry with him because he still had not shifted his *indumba* from Thulamahashe to Share. He finally did so around March 2012.

With the move, Rodney's family situation also changed. After his divorce from his wife in Thulamahashe, he negotiated with the family of another woman over the conditions for marriage. Once he and the woman's father had reached an agreement, the marriage went ahead. Rodney was 44 years old at that time and his wife 40 years. The *lobola* (the brideprice a husband pays to his wife's parents), had at the time of my stay with him still not been paid, but, he explained, "it will come." Eventually his wife got pregnant and they had a daughter, and a year later another child followed, this time a boy.

Aside from his concerns about finding the perfect position for his *indumba*, Rodney also began developing plans for how to make more money, because he and his large family – which consisted of six additional children who lived with their mothers (former women with whom he had had relationships) – could not live off the income generated by his healing practice alone. Goat breeding and running a guesthouse and a *shebeen*, a small local pub, were among his plans, and during my time in Share he established a *shebeen* that he called Hlayavasia. "Hlayavasia Accommodation" indicated the road sign on the gravel road leading from Hluvukane to Thulamahashe, pointing to a not yet existing guesthouse. As he explained, "Hlayavasia was the name of my grandfather. He lived here. You will see, next time when you come, there will be rondavels [Westernised versions of African-style huts] for guests. I will have my own guesthouse here on my land." Indeed, Rodney held a permission to occupy (PTO) an approximately one hectare large plot of land, delivered by the Chief Mnisi tribal authorities[21].

The community of Share soon took notice of the new *shebeen* and children were sent to fetch beer and unemployed men sat on upturned beer crates in front of it from morning until evening, dinking Castle milk stout beer with UHT milk. The *shebeen* also offered airtime (credit units for cell phones), cigarettes, maize crisps, soap and other small daily items. Rodney considered extending the *shebeen* to include a stall directly alongside the gravel road to Thulamahashe. The foundations, a small wall of self-made bricks, already marked the small plot of land. All that remained was to complete the building, stock up the shop and employ a person to run it. Pakistani shop owners ran most of the shops in the area. Rodney's little shop, once it had been established, would be one of the few exceptions.

Rodney's father, an old, agile and stern character, lived with his new wife in the next homestead. Together, Rodney, his father and other family members owned about thirty cows, a sign of their wealth. In addition, Rodney owned about ten goats and a number of chickens. Furthermore, he still owned the house in Thulamahashe, which he rented out for 3000 Rand a month. Rodney's income was thus based on multiple sources – the *shebeen*, the rent from his Thulamahashe house, and other irregular sources such as his work as a healer and his cooperation with Natural Justice – all of which allowed him to generate enough money to support his large family. And while Rodney managed his businesses and developed his plans, his 42-year-old wife quietly organized the household. She hardly ever spoke a word. She cared for their two children, did all the sweeping, cooking and washing, and occasionally visited her family on the other side of the village.

Rodney's everyday life wisdom and capacities as a leader – and healer – were apparent in the daily routine that the two of us developed after some time of getting

---

21   Land in the area falls under the supervision of the chief, who allocates PTOs to the people. A PTO is not a title of ownership, but rather the allowance to live on a particular piece of land.

used to each other. One of his core sentences was "I am a leader. As a leader, you have to put everything on the table, you have to be transparent, don't hide anything. Then things will come right." Furthermore, my personal security in the area seemed very much connected to Rodney's reputation as a leader and healer. When I said to people that I was living with the family of Rodney Sibuyi, I often heard in reply, "Sibuyi? Ahh, Sibuyi is a strong man. Send my regards." His power significantly influenced the Kukula Healers. He had strong opinions and a very strong mind that pursued things and activities 'intellectually'. His cow and goat breeding activities, his successful management of the *shebeen* (which grew over the years to include a jukebox, a pool table and a machine electricity units), his huge family network and his position as CEO of the Kukula Healers all made him what could be termed a social entrepreneur and a visionary, a man who believed in his ideas. He often told me, "You must always have plan. Every day, when you wake up, you must follow this plan. Otherwise you get nowhere." He managed everything in parallel and on the go. His phone rang all the time. He organized and managed, made promises and plans, and represented the Kukula Healers, both at the local level and at the national and international levels through workshops and conferences.

Aside from his business and leadership qualities, Rodney often reflected, mostly in the car going to or from an interview, on what it means to be a good healer: "As a healer, you always have to be clean. You must be clean in your mind. You must have things clean in your family." In his own healing practice, however, he did not always adhere to these rules. Against the customary law that you should not drink while treating a patient, he often showed up to a consultation with a bottle of beer. He also never wore his *sangoma* attire, preferring to wear a boiler suit or a suit and tie, a preference inherited from his grandfather who also loved wearing suits while consulting. Despite these 'anomalies', Rodney had the reputation of being a very strong healer. He was called 'Mr. Bones' because of his gift of reading patients' fortunes by throwing and reading the bones[22], and his reputation extended well

---

22   Throwing and reading the bones is an important part of some healing traditions (i.e. Swazi, Venda, Tsonga). The bones consist of a number of pairs of bones (usually goat bones, but in earlier times antelope or lion bones were also part of the set), coins, dice, dominoes and shells, with a huge shell serving as the central piece. Reading the bones is based on reading the position of the items in relation to each other and relating them to the patient's condition. Each set of bones (*tintholo*) is different, but a set of objects signifies social types of persons (adults, children, widows, spouses, etc.) or relationships, actions and emotions (jealousy, violence, gossip, etc.). The configuration of the objects and relations are then read after the bones have been thrown onto the mat. This may be repeated a number of times until a full diagnosis can be made. After the treatment that follows the diagnosis has been completed, the procedure might be repeated again to see if any changes have occurred during the treatment (cf. Thornton 2009: 24f.).

beyond his local area. A woman with relationship problems came from Bushbuck-ridge city, for instance, which is about 40 kilometers away from Share, to consult Rodney. Another patient asked him to go all the way to Middelburg, half way to Johannesburg, to cleanse his house against bad spirits. Another patient came from Acornhoek, about 30 kilometers away, to seek 'treatment' against being fired from his job at the Department of Home Affairs after he had been found guilty of ta-king 'extra fees' for the extension of visas for Pakistani businessmen. The diversity of ailments and treatments that Rodney dealt with was extraordinary – and so-metimes dubious – and was very much enhanced by his compassion and healing capacities. The following description of the consultation with the abovementioned woman who came from Bushbuckridge city to see Rodney illustrates his way of "being *inyanga*" (i.e. being a traditional healer).

The woman and her daughter came from Bushbuckridge city to Thulamahashe to consult Rodney. People never come alone for a consultation; usually a family member or at least a friend accompanies them. Rodney was friendly, inviting the two into his *indumba*, which in early March 2012 was still in Thulamahashe. The consultation started with the woman putting a 100 Rand note under the goatskin that was placed in front of Rodney. He took his bag of bones and shook them rhyth-mically, reciting the names of his ancestors. He snapped his fingers, accompanied by the word *siyavuma* (we can see/we agree). He then threw the bones onto the mat in front of him. The large shell turned upside down (a sign of bad energy). The two dominoes had drifted apart (a sign of quarrelling between spouses). Rodney inter-preted the position of the bones as indicating a dispute between the older woman and her husband. The woman started sobbing and told Rodney, who was obviously was on the right track, the full story: "My husband lives with another woman. My daughter is not married. I have pains in my right shoulder since my husband left me in 2004. The situation has become unbearable for me." The woman put anot-her 100 Rand under the goatskin and Rodney continued, throwing the bones three times in a row, always followed by the rhythmic-repetitive snapping of his fingers and the uttering of the word *siyavuma*. Finally, he came to the conclusion that "she needs the whole treatment."

He then disappeared to prepare a *futha* (steam bath with *muthi*). He lit a fire and boiled water before the arrival of the two women. He had added stones to the fire and had prepared the blanket for the older woman to sit under in the separate little shower building next to his house. Meanwhile, he took the stones out of the fire and placed them in an old rusty bowl in front of the woman. The woman covered herself with the blanket and, since Rodney was not allowed to see her naked, he asked me to assist him to slowly pour the water mixed with *muthi* onto the hot stones. The old woman inhaled the ascending steam filled with *muthi* essences and talked to her ancestors. Finally, a mixture of fat coiled up with different *muthi* was burnt under the blanket and the woman inhaled the strong fumes. She sat there for about 30 minutes, inhaling the *muthi* steam and talking to her ancestors.

In the meantime, Rodney mixed another oily mixture consisting of fat and different *muthi*. Back in the *indumba*, Rodney made tiny razor blade incisions on the woman's right shoulder blade, neck and chest – exactly where she described the pain – and rubbed the oily *muthi* mixture into the cuts. Finally, the two sat together, opposite each other, and Rodney threw the bones again. The large shell turned with the open side to the floor (a sign of good luck and good energy) and the dominoes lay closer to each other (a sign of possible peace between the spouses). Both were happy with the new configuration, and the woman was relieved. Her husband might not come back to her, but the treatment could still help her to make peace with her situation, and might lead to the release of the pain in her shoulder. The treatment came to an end and the woman promised to bring the outstanding 700 Rand by the end of the month.

I observed similar consultations over the course of my half-year with Rodney. People rarely came to him for treatment for an acute illness like flu or diarrhea, but mostly for social and interpersonal problems. Rodney's treatment equipment consisted of the bag of bones that he had inherited from his grandfather, a wooden stick from which he bit off pieces to spit into the bag of bones before starting the consultation, a goatskin, and the different *muthi* that he had stored in bottles and bags in his *indumba*. The variety of *muthi* that he had was not particularly large; it consisted of about 20 bottles with differently colored contents, and I had the impression that he used similar *muthi* most of the time. Indeed, his main healing tool was the bag of bones; being known as Mr. Bones, throwing and reading the bones was his strength. He said that he might bequeath the bones one day to one of his children or grandchildren, if one of them also had the gift of healing.

Rodney often went to his *indumba* to ask his grandfather for advice or to thank him for his support. As such, he upheld a regular connection with his ancestral spirits. His knowledge was inherited from his grandfather (and other, never mentioned ancestors) as well as from his training. Rodney never claimed that his knowledge was his own personal knowledge. Only when he spoke for the Kukula Healers, to explain why they engaged in access and benefit sharing agreements, for instance, did he claim that "This is our [the Kukula Healers'] knowledge." To him, knowledge belongs to the ancestors as well as to the community of healers. He knew that his specialization in the bones differentiated him from other healers and that his knowledge about the bones had come from his ancestors. Knowledge thus has an individual and a collective component. His knowledge belonged to him but was received from a bundle of past and present relations, some of which could be shared, and some (such as the capacity to throw the bones) could not.

Charles Mthethwa

Charles Mthethwa (58, Sotho) was, in addition to Adah and Rodney, the third executive committee member of the Kukula Healers. With his grey beard and aura of calmness, Charles looked like a knowledgeable professor, and in fact he was called 'The Professor' due to his exceptional knowledge of medicinal plants. Whenever I met him in Hluvukani, the town where he lived with his wife and other family members, he was riding his old Chinese-style bike, and was always carrying a bicycle repair set, prepared for the many acacia thorns littering the dusty gravel roads. On the day that Rodney and I visited him for an interview, the family was about to prepare for his son's wedding. A huge festivity tent was being erected. But Charles nonetheless had enough time to spare and invited us into his *indumba*. *Muthi* bottles stood neatly arranged next to one another without a hint of dust. *Itshoba*, bead chains and other healer paraphernalia were tidily hanging on the wall. The atmosphere was calm and light. We sat down and chatted for a bit.

Figure 8 Charles's indumba with his displayed muthi

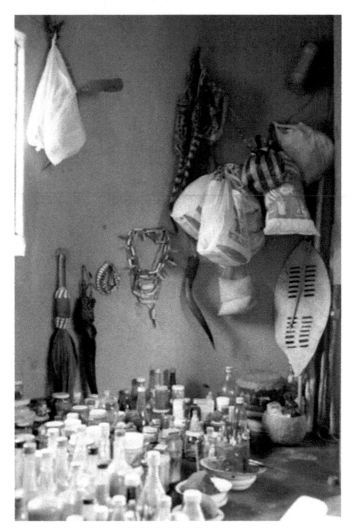

Charles spoke some English; good enough for a chat but not good enough to not give the final word to Rodney, the declared spokesperson, or to his cousin, who joined us after some minutes. Since Charles's cousin and wife both worked as primary school teachers, the family was relatively wealthy and thus not dependant on his healing practice. We sat together for about an hour to discuss traditional healing, knowledge, medicinal plants, politics and religion.

BR: So in terms of heritage (...) can you inherit knowledge?

CM: It depends on the situation. If I am a sangoma, my son might be interested in what I am doing, so he will learn from me.

RS: But another thing, the ancestors, they go to the grandsons. If they become healers, they get it from their grandfathers. But my grandson gets it from me. Maybe he likes the grandson very much, maybe he likes to give him something. You get luck or fortune from where your mother comes from. You can even inherit the bones from your grandfather. (...) [Charles shows me his bag of bones.]

BR: Ah, they are beautiful. But how do you use them?

CM: It goes like this. [He turns the largest shell around so that the open side is facing up, and explains the meaning of the shell falling in this position.] There is a lot of noise, maybe there is a quarrel. This can tell me that there is noise. Maybe if someone wants to kill you, this can tell you. Maybe something bad is coming to you, this one can tell you. And this one [a coin] represents money. It all depends on the position, it speaks a lot. And it is always true. The sticks can tell you whether something is really true or not. That is how we see things. Maybe the child is sick. Then you ask the bones and you learn that the child wants to be called like the grandfather. Then you give the grandfather's name to the newborn and it is ok.

BR: And do you know all the content of the muthi bottles?

CM: Yes I know. I collected everything myself. I pound and grind them. Even from the smell I can tell.

RS: You know it is very important for a healer to do [plant collection] on his own. If you give it to somebody to do it for you, he will make a mistake. It's better you collect them, you pound them and put them in a bottle. If someone else does it, you don't know. And you can even poison people.

BR: And this one [a muthi mixture that Charles and Rodney had discussed earlier] is good for diabetes?

RS: Yes, this decoction, yes. For diabetics. Well cooked. It also helps with coughing.

BR: So, do you share [knowledge and medicine] with each other?

RS: You don't have to be selfish. If somebody can do something better, you can go there. We know ourselves among healers, this one does this, and this one does that. And we refer [patients] to each other. Go to that man, go to that man, help me with this. We share. You can't be the jack of all trades: I throw the bones, I cook the medicine. No. When you find this kind of a healer, he is not honest. He is lying to you.

RS: But this, they use it for cleansing, and you can use it as decoction. And some you use them with a soft porridge. You burn it and use it in soft porridge.

BR: You also burn things? To ashes?

RS: Yes, you burn it and put it in porridge.

BR: It takes a long time, all this knowledge.

RS: That's why I've said that the healers have to train for two years and more. They [who are not well trained] are killing the patients, because once they go out without that knowledge, you are not going to do it properly. And that's one other thing that makes our knowledge run away [i.e. healers losing control over their knowledge].

BR: And who is coming to you? People from the community?

RS: This is a problem. Mostly, people from the community, they don't come anymore. It is mostly people from far away. Also, because people expect you to help them for free. They are family members. They know you. But people from far, from Joburg [Johannesburg], they pay. You know, once they come down from Joburg, you know it is serious and they are willing to pay. And then they take your name and spread it and then other people will also come.

During the interview, issues such as the use of the bones and the importance of maintaining control over the medicine – also to prevent witchcraft accusations and other prejudices against healers – were discussed. If a healer loses control over what he/she does, he/she may, for instance, poison a patient and consequently bring about or exacerbate witchcraft accusations. Charles and Rodney also referred to the fact that the position of traditional healers is threatened within their own communities, an aspect that was repeatedly brought up by many of the healers. This might be one reason why patients in the area may prefer to go to the Hluvukani health clinic than to consult Charles. To avoid stereotyping and prejudices, Charles explicitly claimed that today, openness is very important. Without openness, healers many be even more threatened by witchcraft accusations. Irrespective of this threat, however, the values of knowledge are guarded and protected, and healers use and transform the values to survive and establish a position for themselves in society. Charles mentioned that patients do not come from the community anymore, but from further away places like Johannesburg. Rodney expressed similar thoughts, and his patients indeed came from Bushbuckridge city and even Johannesburg. At the same time, though, Rodney did also have patients coming from adjacent communities.

Healers' narratives about patients were always changing and it was sometimes difficult to determine what was talk and what was reality. Traditional healing is not a fixed concept but is integrated into a web of relations spun around medicinal plants and associated knowledge; it is permeable and adaptable to inner and outer changes. In addition, knowledge is a matter of economic survival. The income generated from the practice as a healer does not have to be shared with others healers, at least not with other members of the *impande*. The only costs that healers have to cover with regard to being a healer are the huge financial burdens associated with the training. This relates back to what was said earlier: knowledge as an inalienable possession is double-voiced. It has a spiritual and emotional value, and at the same time it has an economic value. The spiritual (or sacred) value is highly protected within the boundaries of the *impande*. The economic value is integrated into the everyday life of the healer. Medicinal plants support both. As alienable property, *muthi* helps to maintain the rules of the training and the *impande*, and supports the healer to generate income through the healing practice. As has been shown in the chapter, *muthi*, knowledge, healers, patients, the community, the surrounding environment, as well as the continuation of community life and the healer's economic survival, are all closely interlinked and hardly separabable.

Conclusion and Outlook

The examination of the trajectory outlined at the beginning of this chapter, that started with a plant in nature and led to a plant in a healer's community that is attached with knowledge, offers us an initial conclusion: first and foremost, knowledge is a changing entity. It changes its form and content, and yet has a stable nucleus. The knowledge of traditional healers seems to have its nucleus in the form of ancestral lineages, the *impande*, which assemble many generations and layers of knowledge. This knowledge is always adaptable to and dependent on outer constraints such as changing environmental and political conditions. Draughts, floods and climate change might extinguish certain plants, for instance, the consequence of which might be the loss of certain knowledge. Politics, in particular colonial and Apartheid politics, with the latter being explicitly segregating with regard to the practice and knowledge of traditional healers, has led to a more intrinsic use of the knowledge, for fear of witchcraft accusations and even death.

Such potential negative repercussions have not as yet diminished the belief in and use of healers' knowledge. Knowledge protection schemes that have been passed down through the generations – such as restrictions in the sharing of knowledge outside of the *impande* and the safeguarding of knowledge through customary laws – still prevail. These protection schemes and customary laws protect the aura of the inalienable possession, the knowledge that enables the continuation of the cycle of life from past to present, from life to death. When this cycle is disturbed, the social order of the healers, and consequently of the society that the healers live in, are disturbed. The sharing and transference of knowledge is therefore taught and guarded closely in the *impande*, and may not be transmitted beyond it. Specifically, the art of divination is highly guarded and learned in a close relationship between the trainee healer, the ancestors and the healer trainer. Divination is a learned practice as well as an embodied capability and gift. While some practices of traditional healers may be exposed to the outside world, knowledge about divination remains innate to the healer and inaccessible to outsiders. The connection between the ancestors and the healers in knowledge production cannot be performed or replicated by anyone else, not even herbalists, who have not rained in within an impande.

When outside parties, such as the company Godding & Godding or the IKS Lead Program, are interested in healers' specific knowledge, it is threatened. This is so even if the company is not interested in divinatory knowledge, but solely in the medicinal value of a specific plant. This might be one of the core misunderstandings between healers and companies engaged in bioprospecting when they share knowledge and enter into ABS agreements. The question still remains of how to reimburse the collectively, culturally and spiritually valuable knowledge that is imbued in plants, which a healer may disclose to a third party. Furthermore, we may ask how a company or research institute that is solely interested in the medicinal and economic value of a medicinal plant and its associated knowledge can take the claim about fair reimbursement seriously, given that they are predominantly interested in the medicinal and economic value of a plant, and not its spiritual value. In the next chapter, the trajectory of medicinal plants and associated knowledge continues. The chapter is concerned with knowledge and plants. I do not refer to one specific plant, but to the process of change that plants and knowledge traverse – as they enter the biochemical laboratory of the IKS Lead Program, which basically ignores the above-described cultural values in order to focus on merely extracting plants' medicinal and economic value.

Chapter V
Transformative Science: From Muthi
to Chemical Compound

> I am not interested in the spirit, I am only
> interested in the molecule.
> Dr. Matsabisa, IKS Lead Program

Introduction: "We Go beyond What They Know"

The PhD student and pharmacologist-in-the-making James Mukinda, who, as a visiting researcher, occasionally conducted pre-clinical trials using the IKS Lead Program Laboratory's Liquid Chromatography-Mass Spectrometry (LC-MS) facilities, summarized in brief what this chapter is concerned with:

> Traditional medicine understands from experience, but they [traditional healers] don't know why things work the way they work. That is what we do. We go beyond what they know. Many chemical compounds do not dissolve in water. Many healers, particularly in remote, rural villages, only use water as a dissolvent for plants. But often they need alcohol for splitting up the chemical compound's properties. So, what we do here in the lab is to go beyond their knowledge. Only healers in urban areas have access to other dissolvents. Every compound has a different need as a dissolvent. Until now, we are in the phase of speculation in terms of traditional medicine. This is why I do not believe in traditional medicine. People believe that medicinal plants are safe. They have hope in these plants. So what you now need is deep science to prove the safety. (Excerpt from interview, IKS Laboratory, January 2010)

This chapter continues with the trajectory of medicinal plants and associated (indigenous) knowledge from their place of origin into a biochemical laboratory, and is concerned with the moment in which indigenous knowledge and medicinal plants meet scientific knowledge and practices. In the chapter, I dive into what James Mukinda defines above as "deep science" and "the phase of speculation," with the first attempting to 'overcome' the latter. In this trajectory from *outside* to *inside* the laboratory, medicinal plants and associated knowledge change their meaning, content and value. This chapter therefore sheds light on how laboratory practices and knowledge(s) transform plants and indigenous knowledge by means of scientific, technical, symbolic and political practices (Knorr-Cetina 2001) into objects of bio-value (Waldby 2002) for the pharmacological and economic market. In the tradition of Science and Technology Studies, which in the 1980s engaged in "studying science practice, what scientists actually do" (Pickering 1992: 2) and witnessing "science in action" (Latour 1987) see also Garforth 2012), I investigate the practices, materials and knowledge that scientists use in the scientific process of medicinal plant analysis, which involves networks of non-human actors – i.e. plant material, gravity columns, dissolvents and HPLC (High Performance Liquid Chromatography, or High Pressure Liquid Chromatography) techniques – as well as human actors – i.e. scientists, healers and the government.

Despite Watson-Verran and Turnbull's claim that "[t]here is no term in general usage that adequately captures the amalgam of places, bodies, voices, skills, practices, technical devices, theories, social strategies, and collective work" (1995: 117) that come together in scientific practices, the term 'assemblage' (Deleuze & Guattari 1997) might be suitable to bring all human and non-human actors together under one umbrella term and give space to the IKS Laboratory as "an agent of scientific development" (Knorr-Cetina 2001: 144). But how exactly is this assemblage constituted? The assemblage unleashes perceptions, expectations and hopes that actors maintain about the translation and transformation of indigenous knowledge and medicinal plants into new chemical compounds and therapeutic uses for these compounds. Knowledge, plants and the transformation process are therefore not seen at as neutral and objective, but are loaded with challenges and ambivalent opinions. So which "tribes of scientists" (Latour & Woolgar1986: 17) and other actors are involved in these processes, and what do they really think about the integration of traditional knowledge into science?

Given the fusion of two knowledge systems and divergent materials and the ambivalent opinions and values that come together in the IKS Laboratory, I argue in this chapter that scientific knowledge in this context ought to be seen as a local knowledge system with specific values (cf. Watson-Verran & Turnbull 1995). In this chapter, I will look at the values that are produced and changed in the laboratory and under what conditions. This is particularly interesting because among the highlighted goals on the agenda of the IKS Lead Program are the promotion and support of indigenous knowledge systems, thus it is interesting to question how far indigenous knowledge systems are in fact promoted and supported, and by whom. In addition, in the chapter I will also look at other assignments of the IKS Lead Program, namely the educational aspect and the job creation and poverty alleviation assignments. How do these assignments contribute to knowledge production, as well as to the putative goal of the IKS Lead Program to promote and support indigenous knowledge systems?

The Indigenous Knowledge Health System Lead Program

The Indigenous Knowledge (Health) System (IKS) Lead Program is a sub-unit of the Medical Research Council (MRC), one of the leading South African governmental medical research institutions. It is located in the northern suburbs of Cape Town, next to Tygerberg Hospital, the largest hospital in the Western Cape and the second largest in South Africa. The IKS Lead Program was established in 2000, at which point it was fully incorporated in the MRC. As a governmental institution, the existence of the IKS Lead Program followed the political decisions and directions of the South African government[1]. Especially with the promulgation of the IKS Policy in 2004, this led to a number of new institutions dealing with indigenous knowledge systems, among them the IKS Lead Program Laboratory, erected in 2004/5.

To fulfill the mandate of the South African government, as proposed by the IKS Policy (2004), the IKS Lead Program flagged four priorities: 1) research, discovery and development, with a special focus on developing drugs for malaria, tuberculosis, diabetes, cancer and HIV/AIDS; 2) knowledge development and knowledge management, involving the training of students, communities and traditional health practitioners; 3) the utilization of IKS Lead Program scientific research results, and the development of strategic business plans and cooperation with companies to commercialize the research products; and 4) the application of the social impacts of the IKS Lead Program's findings in public-private community partnership projects to establish sustainable community business enterprises for wealth creation, technical skills development for job creation and poverty alleviation[2].These priorities reflect the activities of the IKS Lead Program, reaching from the biochemical and pharmacological analysis of medicinal plants to the promotion and support of indigenous knowledge systems, from community projects, local development and poverty alleviation programs to giving policy advice to the government. In its scientific mandate, the IKS Lead Program Laboratory follows general drug development guidelines, which comprise: basic research, including collection, extraction, screening for bioactivity and the identification of active compounds; development, which includes identifying bio-validity, analysis and standardization; the

---

1   In 2012, the MRC South Africa discussed whether some research units should be closed down due to the lack of funds (see: www.iol.co.za/news/south-africa/western-cape/mrc-vital-research-units-could-close-1.1393300#.Uayp5JxGBCo). The IKS unit was subject to a larger restructuring process of the MRC in 2014.

2   www.unisa.ac.za/Default.asp?Cmd=ViewContent&ContentID=26715&P_ForPrint=1 (last accessed February 20, 2015).

validation of efficacy and safety, which includes clinical trials; and upgrading and pharmaceutical development, with the latter including manufacturing and the patenting process. The main focus of the laboratory, however, is on basic research and drug lead development. Clinical trials, upgrading and pharmaceutical development are mainly outsourced to other academic institutes or (biotechnology) companies.

The actual biochemical analysis of medicinal plants ensues at the IKS Laboratory. About 20 kilometers from the MRC headquarters, the IKS Laboratory lies in the heart of the Drift sands Nature Reserve. Drift sands is a protected area under the management of Cape Nature, a public institution with the statutory responsibility for biodiversity conservation in the Western Cape[3]. The objective of the Drift sands Nature Reserve is "to transform a nature reserve in the centre of one of the poorest and most densely populated areas of the Western Cape into a safe, multi-purpose urban reserve and a treasured community resource"[4]. The MRC Delft Centre, a huge industrial compound containing MRC facilities, with the IKS Laboratory being just one of them, is part of an urban development scheme that aims to integrate business into poverty stricken areas.

In the following section, I will describe my arrival at the MRC Delft Centre and the IKS Laboratory and recount some of my impressions when I entered the laboratory for the first time, and how these impressions manifested and/or changed over the year.

An Ethnographer at the Laboratory

To reach the IKS Laboratory from the MRC headquarters, I took the R300 freeway that cuts through the Cape Flats and separates the more affluent northern suburbs from the poverty stricken township area. From R300, the turnoff at Hindle Road leads through some squatter shack settlements on the one side and green sandy hills on the other to the entrance gate of the MRC Delft Centre. According to the sign at the entrance gate, a number of other companies and institutions, such as waste management and laboratory animal stables, also reside on the hidden compound. From outside the center, secured with huge barbed wire fences and a security guard at the entrance, I was reminded of the compound's military past, as well as of the generally strict security obligations I often had encountered in South Africa.

Inside the gated compound, a tranquil and almost harmoniously arranged settlement of laboratory and office buildings created a strange atmosphere of busy

---

3   www.capenature.co.za/eco-tourism.htm?sm[p1][category]=718 (last accessed February 20, 2015).

4   www.openafrica.org/participant/Driftsands-Nature-Reserve (last accessed February 20, 2015).

occupation and total isolation. Every time I would enter the compound in the coming year, I would be struck by this ambivalent feeling of nothing happening at all, combined with the knowledge that here was located a highly innovative business and science hub. When I arrived at the laboratory to start the research in February 2009, I left the lively atmosphere of the densely populated Cape Flats behind and managed my way through the entrance gate, equipped with an invitation from Dr. Matsabisa, Director of the IKS Lead Program. Prior to my arrival, the IKS Lead Program had, together with the Institute of Social and Cultural Anthropology at the Freie Universität Berlin, signed a Memorandum of Understanding (MOU), which proposed a focus on conducting research at the IKS Lead Program Laboratory. I entered the isolated industrial area with its laboratories, horse stables, medical waste management factory and a building housing velvet monkeys. Velvet monkeys are invaluable for scientific research and pre-clinical trials, and, as I learned later, they also served as 'scientific currency' in negotiations between the IKS Lead Program and Guangzhou Traditional Medicine Hospital.

I turned right, traversed an alley of blue gum trees, turned right again, passed a small café and stood in front of the medium-sized brick one-storey building with a green tin roof. Opposite the building, behind a wooden fence, was a tiny but neatly arranged garden, with small patches of differently labeled medicinal plants with name tags in isiXhosa, isiZulu, seSotho, English, Afrikaans and Latin, and a crafted wooden table and chairs under a thatched roof. Above it all towered the mast of a high-power floodlight, another reminder of the compound's military past (cf. Green 2008). Later, I would learn that some of the plants in the little garden were endemic to South Africa, while others were botanical migrants from other parts of Africa, as well as Asia and Latin America. The medicinal plant garden served as a rearing ground for plants investigated at the laboratory, as well as an educational site to teach visitors, notably young pupils from the Cape Flats, about medicinal plants.

Dr. Matsabisa awaited me in his office in an office building separate from the laboratory. Straight after my arrival, he took me for a walk through the vast laboratory and introduced me to the other scientific and non-scientific staff members as his "new PhD student." He explained the functions of the different areas of the building and of the technical apparatus, and gave me a taste of a bitter plant powder. "Usually," he explained, "we anonymize the plants we are working with. All plants we use in the laboratory are abbreviated with P21, 22, 23 and so on." But then he revealed the name of the bitter tasting plant as *Dicoma anomala*, a common ground-creeping plant from South Africa. Later, I would learn that the plant was being tested in vitro for its antimalarial properties and that an active compound had been isolated and characterized[5]. Finally, Dr. Matsabisa offered me a desk and a computer in the scientific staff office.

The easy introduction and my fast integration into the research team astounded me (cf. Knorr-Cetina 1999; Garforth 2012). I had expected more questions regarding what exactly I wanted to do and why I had chosen the IKS Laboratory to conduct research. But obviously, the IKS Director considered the research proposal and the MOU sufficient to know my intentions. Dr. Matsabisa was a pharmacologist and politician at heart; social science research was probably not of much relevance to him. Nevertheless, he had invited an ethnographer to conduct research at the laboratory. Perhaps he was interested in gaining a reputation for cooperating with an international university, or perhaps he saw the need to investigate questions about access and benefit sharing that arises from the scientific investigation of medicinal plants. I could, however, never fully figure out what his motivation had been.

Beyond the friendly, assertive introduction, another first impression I had was of the somehow lifeless and empty atmosphere of the laboratory. I could not help thinking that it was more of a showroom than an active laboratory, an impression that would stay with me for the entire year. Julie Laplant described a similar feeling after she had spent a few days at the laboratory as part of her research on *Artemisia afra* (*Umhlonyane*). In her book 'Healing Roots. Anthropology in Life and Medicine' (2015), she said:

> (...) the laboratory did not seem completely real. It was real in a sense of it being there, with all its magnitude, yet it did not seem alive in the sense of a real place to make medicine available to the people who would need it. The Delft facilities seemed to serve the purpose of showing businessmen a good investment that could be made there (Laplante 2015: 89).

This impression was fueled by the vast, state of the art laboratory with its fully equipped laboratory rooms, storerooms, offices and meeting rooms, and the large plantation site behind the building, all well maintained but somehow untouched and overly shiny. Most of the spacious laboratory remained unlived in, even untouched most of the time. A few young researchers worked behind the screen of the HPLC machine, and later, after its installment, behind the screen of the LC-MS machine, but most of the rooms and devices remained unused.

In total, six Bachelor and Master students and three post-doc researchers were working at the laboratory when I arrived. In addition, a general janitor, two cleaning ladies, and the coordinator of traditional healer-related activities, were employed as non-scientific staff members. All IKS staff members were of black origin (Xhosa, Zulu, Pedi, Ndebele, Basotho and Tswana). The only white staff member

---

5   See: http://innovation.mrc.ac.za/malaria.pdf (last accessed October 12, 2015).

was a specialist engineer, who was employed to supervise the LC-MS facilities and to introduce and help visiting researchers, who occasionally came from other research institutions with their own medicinal plant extract samples. The average monthly wage at the laboratory was 5000 Rand – for those who were paid. Most of the young researchers, however, worked as interns without a salary.

The laboratory building itself had different sections and rooms. After entering the laboratory building, the staff members' offices were positioned to the right. To the left, a bit further down the hall, two huge windows looked onto two separate laboratory rooms. One room was filled with centrifuges to extract plant material, scales, columns, an extraction hood to prevent toxic fumes, various liquids in brown and transparent bottles, and samples used in TLC (thin layer chromatography) and HPLC procedures. At the time of my arrival, the HPLC machine located in one laboratory room, was the key technological device used in the laboratory, though this would soon be topped by a newcomer, the LC-MS machine – which the IKS staff members almost gently referred to as "the Ferrari," since the machine was worth 7 million USD and, at that time, was one of only two in South Africa. The LC-MS was placed in the second room, which was still almost empty when I arrived. The two high-tech machines constituted the centers of research attention at the IKS Laboratory. All other scientific practices were preparatory before using one of them. The data extracted by the HPLC and LC-MS machines, in the form of small samples of plant extracts, was itself only pre-phase data, however, used (possibly) in the following pre-clinical and clinical trials, which were mostly outsourced to university laboratories or smaller biotechnological companies. The IKS Laboratory was therefore equipped mostly for basic biochemical research.

Behind the two front laboratory rooms, four extra rooms were equipped with further technical devices. In the first room stood a huge machine for labeling tea bags and another machine producing PHELA labels[6]. The second room was equipped with an extraction hub and a medicinal syrup production area. The third room contained a huge plant grinding machine and a plant-drying oven, and in the last room stood a massive deep freezer to flash freezes medicinal plant material. All of the equipment was impressively shiny and their labels designated them as imported from China and India. Most of the expensive machinery, however, remained untouched over the course of the year. Occasionally, when visiting researchers or other visitors – such as a delegation from the Department of Science and Technology or businessmen from China – came to the laboratory, the shiny machinery would be presented, and sporadically used.

The researchers themselves often addressed the aspect of motionlessness at the laboratory and referred to the fact that "nothing changes." In informal conversations, I gathered that many of the researchers and other staff members were quite

---

6   PHELA was the name of one plant mixture under investigation at the laboratory at the time.

discontent with the work at the laboratory and their feeling of dependency on the sole person in charge, the director, who was, however, rarely present. One of the senior researchers stated ironically with regard to the few changes that occurred: "The more changes are going on, the fewer changes." The changes to which he was referring were the implementation of the LC-MS machine, the extension of the office building to accommodate more staff members (who nevertheless had not actually shown up), and the creation of a medicinal plantation site behind the laboratory building to grow the plants that made up the PHELA mixture.

Although all of the technical devices were presented to me early on, and I quickly got to know about their functions, at the beginning of my fieldwork I was often lost and sometimes felt as if I was not quite in the right place at the laboratory. Observing biochemical analysis is different to actually doing it. I was unfamiliar with the specialized language of biochemistry and I had no experience with laboratory practices beyond the common understandings I had acquired at school. Bruno Latour and Steve Woolgar write in book "Laboratory Life: The Construction of Scientific Facts" a section "An anthropologist visits the laboratory' (1986):

> When an anthropological observer enters the field, one of his most fundamental preconceptions is that he might be able to make sense of the observations and notes he records. This, after all, is one of the basic principles of scientific enquiry. No matter how confused or absurd the circumstances and activities of his or her tribe might appear, the ideal observer retains his faith that some kind of systematic, ordered account is attainable. For a total newcomer to the laboratory, we can imagine that his first encounter with his subjects would severely jeopardize such faith (Latour 1986: 43).

Latour continued that the whole series of questions and answers conducted at the beginning of research in a laboratory would be understood by the anthropologist using his/her common sense, followed by a series of nonsensical impressions, before the researcher could try for a "deeper" understanding (ibid.). In this sense, a social science researcher's arrival at the laboratory is not much different to his/her arrival in a local community. The language spoken in a laboratory is as confusing and as 'unintelligible' as the language spoken in a local community. It takes years of academic training to become an expert in biochemistry and it would be misleading and even arrogant to expect to achieve a full understanding of these complex processes in one year of intermittent participant observation. The following section depicts what I nevertheless learned of the trajectory of medicinal plants and associated knowledge from their place of origin to the biochemical laboratory of the IKS Lead Program.

From Indigenous Knowledge Systems to the IKS Laboratory: A Challenging Translation

A couple of weeks after my arrival at the IKS Laboratory, Dr. Matsabisa introduced me to the extensive research plan that he had formulated for me for the coming research year. The IKS Lead Program's network stretched far beyond mere scientific research, and thus the schedule outlined access that I would have to interview partners such as traditional healers, politicians, lawyers working in the realm of indigenous knowledge systems, and medicinal plant plantation site managers. Although it was a cooperative and helpful gesture, the schedule also made me worried about my independence as a researcher. How much would I be obliged to conform to Dr. Matsabisa's plan and how would I ensure my independence in order to uphold a critical perspective? In the end, it transpired that only a limited amount of the schedule was put into practice. Dr. Matsabisa was away for most of the year on national and international business trips and barely spent time at the laboratory (his ongoing absence was noted among the disgruntlements of the IKS Laboratory's employees, as mentioned above). In contrast to my concern of being overly controlled, I was in fact left to my own devices much of the time, and oftentimes there were periods where nothing happened at all. Occasional invitations to meetings of political and/or scientific significance – such as a telephone conference on the amendment of the MRC intellectual property policy or trips to follow up medicinal plant claims – made up for the lack of supervision.

Medicinal plant claims are actually only one of the many ways in which a medicinal plant and its associated knowledge can enter the laboratory, alongside the re-screening of already existing libraries and databases for new chemical compilations, or the analysis of randomly collected plant material. Yet such claims provide a higher chance of detecting new compounds, methods or therapeutic uses, and are the most promising way in which to discover new drug leads from medicinal plants. Medicinal plant claims are the beginning of the trajectory of medicinal plants and indigenous knowledge into the IKS Laboratory.

Below, I cite an excerpt from an interview that I (BR) conducted in March 2009 with Mirranda Javu (MJ), an IKS Lead Program research assistant and assistant to the IKS Lead Program director and my translator from isiXhosa into English, and Ntate Ndeni (NN), a traditional healer from the Eastern Cape. The excerpt illustrates the ambiguous transition of medicinal plants and indigenous knowledge from the realm of traditional healing to the realm of biochemical research in a laboratory. It is ambiguous due to the meeting of two different systems of knowledge, meaning and value, with vastly differing ontologies and epistomologies, meaning that sometimes the two sides cannot find a way talk to and understand one another:

MJ: The Medical Research Council has a unit called IKS [Lead Program]. It focuses on traditional medicine. Even if you are not a traditional healer, even if you are not a herbalist, if you know about herbs, you are welcome to deliver your information on, let's say, a medicine against cancer. Then you will be involved in a process, so first they give you an agreement; if you agree, you understand; and if you understand, you let us know: 'I am ready to disclose this and that information based on this evidence'. They give you money, and the IKS makes pre-clinical trials and capsules.

BR: And do you think this is a useful approach?

NN: To me it makes sense, although I never claimed a medicine. There are people who don't want to be seen using our [traditional] medicine. Eh, maybe one would love to have capsules or tablets, because other people don't want to be embarrassed. Uh, they think we are bewitching them. You see, so people will feel free to take capsules or tablets. There are people, even those people in the parliament, doctors, lawyers, they come to us, but other people, they don't want to be seen using our medication as it is. Now they will feel good. I remember, we went to parliament for an exhibition, so, no embarrassment from now on. You'll be using your traditional medicine freely, no embarrassment.

BR: But then [traditional] medicine does not have anything to do with the work of the healer anymore.

MJ: OK, if Ntate Ndeni is giving out medicine or his plants to IKS, definitively he will not just give his plants; there is something he has to do.

BR: What is it he has to do?

MJ: Something. He cannot just give his plants to IKS, because he has got ancestors.

NN: I have got ancestors. I cannot just do it freely as I want or wish to. Because that medicine is not mine, it's from my ancestors. So I have to ask permission from them first. Pray to them.

MJ: Otherwise they won't show you the plants. You go there and don't see it. The plant is there. You go there and see it, I go there and don't see it.

NN: Because they [the ancestors] say: 'You do as you like with what we have given you. But not without our permission.' If they don't want, they don't want.

BR: But (...) let's say there is a sangoma, he knows a mixture of certain plants and he realized for himself that it works, because 20 patients already got healed with it and he is not listening to the ancestors (...) and he is ignoring what the ancestors say and will in any case go to IKS. Do you think he will be punished later?

NN: Ju, very bad. Very bad. Not supposed to do the thing. He even can be killed. You have to do certain rituals. It is not easy. You have to be correct with the ancestors.

The transition of knowledge from the realm of traditional healing to the laboratory is, according to Ntate Ndeni, impossible without ancestral guidance and consent. In the previous chapter, I described the strong relationship between medicinal plants, traditional healers, the ancestors, patients, the community and the environment. Hardly any transaction of knowledge in the realm of traditional healing is supposed to be practiced without the (ritual) inclusion of the ancestors. The disclosure of knowledge to a scientific institution also requires ancestral consent. This is a moral and ethical obligation. As Mirranda Javu, a staff member at the IKS Lead Program and a trained healer, told me: "Well, you first have to consult the ancestors. When they agree on the disclosure, then you can do it without problems. When you don't ask them, they can get very upset and they might even harm you" (Informal conversation, Delft, February 2009).

Once knowledge is disclosed to a scientific institution like the IKS Lead Program, or any other research institution[7], the future of this particular knowledge is unpredictable. It might terminate in a dead-end without yielding further results, or it might enter the global market in the form of a new chemical compound and/or pharmaceutical product. The main objective of the IKS Lead Program Laboratory is the biochemical analysis and transformation of traditional medicinal plants into medically viable and economically valuable research results for the treatment of the core diseases of HIV/AIDS, TB, malaria, hypertension, cancer and diabetes. In addition, medicinal plants are used for poverty alleviation, socio-economic development and job creation, for instance through the development of plantation sites for the breeding of medicinal plants. The IKS webpage presented its mission as follows:

> The IKS mission is to promote and advance indigenous knowledge systems through research, research and development by making it a valued health model in the global environment and to redress health traditions, which until now have neglected health priorities and issues[8].

It might seem curious that the IKS Lead Program, in its stated mission, proposed the advancement of indigenous knowledge systems, while the IKS Laboratory itself was mainly interested in the analysis of medicinal plant mixtures, irrespective of

---

7   The IKS is only one of many scientific laboratories in South Africa that at this point in time analyze medicinal plants. The University of the Western Cape's TICIPS (The International Centre of Indigenous Phytotherapy Studies) Program, the South African Herbal Medicine Institute, the University of KwaZulu-Natal South African Research Chair in Indigenous Health Care Systems and the University of Pretoria Phytomedicine Program all also work with medicinal plants. In addition, biotechnology laboratories work in the commercial analysis of medicinal plants. University laboratories and Biotechnology Labboratories often cooperate.

8   http://www.mrc.ac.za/iks/indigenous.htm (this webpage expired after the MRC underwent a huge restructuring process in 2014).

the origin of the knowledge. The fact that the medicine and associated knowledge of traditional healers often contained a viable traditional medicinal product already – i.e. a product that had been used as a medicinal cure over the course of generations by local traditional healers – is beside the point of the mission statement, since the IKS Laboratory was only interested in traditional healers' knowledge if it contributed to the impending biochemical analysis and the development of a pharmaceutical product.

But what does the advancement of indigenous knowledge systems – in the context of the IKS Lead Program's mission statement – mean? What entitles science to claim that it can make indigenous knowledge systems into a "valued health model," given that many already consider these systems valuable? These questions create an ambivalent picture of the relationship between the scientific knowledge system(s) used at the IKS Laboratory and the indigenous knowledge system(s) brought into the laboratory. The program's name ostensibly indicates an integrative approach, as it highlights the support, promotion and protection of indigenous knowledge systems. However, when looking at its mission statement, the IKS Lead Program instead seems to claim a hegemonic power to advance and improve indigenous knowledge in accordance with global standards by means of science and technology. Lesley Green asserts that "indigenous knowledge is tacit knowledge and therefore, not easily codifiable. It is dynamic and based on innovation, adaptation, and experimentation, thus codifying indigenous knowledge may lead to the loss of some of its properties" (Green 2008: 136). While indigenous knowledge may be valuable for tracing new products, the aspect of spiritual and socio-cultural background, or cultural and social capital (Bourdieu 1986) – in the form of integrating the ancestors into the transmission of knowledge to third parties, for instance – is left behind in the allegedly integrative approach of the IKS Lead Program.

Indigenous knowledge entails the entire cosmology of ancestral connection between plants, knowledge and people, which is neither transferred into the laboratory, nor can it be tested for efficacy. It is basically carved out at the doors of the laboratory. Consequently, the trajectory of medicinal plants and associated knowledge from their place of origin into the laboratory is paved with challenges, which is not only, but also, caused by misunderstandings or misinterpretations between the interacting representatives of the respective knowledge systems. The next sections deal with the challenges that emanate from the trajectory from indigenous knowledge systems into the IKS Laboratory and makes the transition from *muthi* to molecule not impossible but more unlikely. The first suspense occurs right at the beginning, when a knowledge holder decides to disclose knowledge of a plant or plant mixture to the IKS Lead Program.

First Challenge: How Muthi Does(n´t) Enter the Laboratory

New resources for scientific investigation can be found in abundance in the public domain. Medicinal plants are available at urban or rural markets, as weeds on the side of the road, or as knowledge on plants published in anthropological articles, all of which offer an array of investigative trails (Hayden 2004: 11). These publicly accessible sources and resources have one advantage; they are freely accessible. This changes, however, the moment that (indigenous) knowledge is involved, and when this knowledge enters the domain of commercialization. Generally, the role of indigenous knowledge in new drug discovery cannot be underestimated. Of all prescription drugs derived from natural products (which constitutes around 25%), about 80% were discovered based on knowledge obtained from the use of traditional medicines and indigenous knowledge holders (Kate & Laird 1998; Laird 2002). Unsurprisingly, bioprospectors increase their chances of finding new leads from 1:10,000 to about 1:2 by consulting indigenous knowledge holders; this, at least, was claimed by Dr. Matsabisa during a presentation that he gave to visiting members of the Department of Science and Technology (DST) at the IKS Laboratory in October 2009. Whether this was a true figure or a 'wishful estimation' remains unclear, though the fact that indigenous knowledge holders do increase the likelihood of detecting valuable new drug leads is certain. Therefore, next to screening already existing libraries and databases for 'old' plants to analyze for 'new' healing properties, new plants or plant mixtures are tested for as yet undiscovered chemical compounds. Medicinal plant claims, i.e. claims that promise new healing properties in a plant or plant mixture, can be proposed to the IKS Lead Program by anyone – whether a citizen of South Africa or another African country as well as non-African citizens – but traditional healers and their extensive knowledge on plant-based medicine are, logically, the most significant target group.

In the exploration of new plant-based products and medicines, the IKS Lead Program aimed to establish a trustful, open and transparent working relationship with indigenous knowledge holders, so that they would consider voluntarily disclosing and submitting their medicine for further scientific investigation. As of 2010, the IKS Lead Program had received over 200 voluntary medicinal plant claims from traditional health practitioners and other indigenous and non-indigenous knowledge holders. The IKS Lead Program director and his team would then decide upon the potential of the submitted claim and whether it was worth following up. When decided positively, the journey would lead all over South Africa, to speak with the claimants and evaluate the scientific value of the claim. This value would thus also depend on the further information disclosed by the claimant.

Of the four medicinal plant claim follow-ups that I had the opportunity to join, only one claim came from traditional healers. Claims, in my experience, were actually proposed more often by people who had regular access to the internet or similar sources of information; traditional healers in rural areas, on the other hand, mostly got their information from the huge countrywide network of different healers' organizations. For the discovery of a new chemical compound, *muthi* has to go through all relevant biochemical analyses, as well as through safety and efficacy tests. Against this background, the imagined hopes and expectations linked to knowledge disclosure and to handing it over to the realm of scientific investigation (cf. Brown 2003) could not always be fulfilled. So how are the claims made at the IKS Lead Program linked to the hopes and expectations of the claimants? Below, I describe two claim follow-ups made in Beaufort West in December 2009, starting with Mrs. Dihara and then moving to the Mdehle Inyanga Healers Association of South Africa, both of whom had very different aspirations for their claims. Describing these claims helps to demonstrate the (un-)likelihood of *muthi* finding its way into the laboratory.

Hope in 'Rohelia': A Plant Claim for HIV/AIDS

The journey brought the IKS Lead Program Director Dr. Matsabisa, Mirranda Javu and me to Beaufort West, a road town and trading center in the middle of the semi-desert Karoo, situated in the inner part of South Africa. December is one of the hottest months in South Africa, but Dr. Matsabisa's air conditioned Volvo left the heat outside. After five hours of driving, we arrived in Beaufort West, also known as the 'Capital of the Karoo'. The Karoo is one of the main biodiversity hotspots of South Africa, rich in potent and medicinally valuable succulents and thorny bushes (Pinhaar 2009). Thundering trucks passed by the town along the N1 on their way from Cape Town to Johannesburg and back. Cheap 'Fong Kong'[9] shops, a KFC, a Chicken Licken and a liquor shop, which was already well frequented in the early afternoon hours, dominated the scenery. The backstreets were filled with Dutch style houses and churches, a relic of the Boere trekkers and the Dutch Reform Church that settled in Beaufort West in 1818. Today, Beaufort West does not offer much work and the unemployment rate among the black and colored population is high. White people own Saxon Marino sheep breeding farms. The contrast between black, colored and white lives was most visible in terms of housing. White people live either in the city center around the churches or on huge farms outside of town, while the colored and black populations live in more dilapidated and bleak settlements and townships at the town's margins.

The first claimant we met was the Afrikaans speaking Mrs. Dihara, a 60-year-old white middle class woman. Mrs. Dihara had gotten to know about the claim making opportunity at the IKS Lead Program after she had searched the internet

---

9   Fong Kong refers to products made in China, but also has the connotation of being cheap, low-quality and counterfeit.

for an institution that might be interested in her plant mixture. On the webpage of the Department of Health she had found a link to the IKS Lead Program's call for claims and had contacted Mirranda for more information and an appointment to exchange information on the claim. When we arrived, Mrs. Dihara was expecting us. Excitedly, she hugged Mirranda and greeted us enthusiastically. Her house was filled with pictures of Jesus, holy crosses, crocheted couch and table covers, and most strikingly, two organs next to each other in the corner of the living room. After she served us sweet, artificial Mango syrup, she started telling her story. She had come to Beaufort West after her husband had died 17 years ago to help "the people in the name of the lord." With this ambition, she had developed a mixture made of aloe vera and other ingredients that she would not disclose, but which are available in the supermarket, she emphasized. "Rohelia," said the label on the bottle, which contained a yellow, viscous liquid, "medicine against HIV/AIDS, TB, Cancer and Anorexia." Due to official laws of the South African Medicinal Control Council (MCC), it is not allowed to claim healing properties without the official certification of the MCC.

Nevertheless, Mrs. Dihara had great hopes in the potential healing properties of *Rohelia*. She believed that through the invention of *Rohelia*, God had given her a wonderful opportunity to help people with HIV/AIDS and at the same time make a bit of money. She had even made a record of the patients she had treated with *Rohelia* and had invited two of her patients to demonstrate the results. The two men reassured us that their wounds and shingles had gotten better and that their general health had improved as a result of the treatment with *Rohelia*. It was part of the requirements for claim making to make a record of patients' treatment histories. Although Mrs. Dihara had followed these instructions, I had the feeling that the longer we stayed in her house, discussing her claim and sipping the sweet mango juice, and the more the IKS director explained the procedures of making a successful medicine claim, the more quiet, almost disappointed she became. *No, she did not know that the IKS Lead Program does not automatically finance the scientific analysis of medicinal plants*. A funding agency or institution would have to be established, unless the claimant would want to pay out of their own pocket. "Where shall I get all the money from?" she asked timidly. "I am not a rich woman. You know, I am in debt, I even sold my car." "Well, if it is a strong and successful claim, we can find funding," replied Dr. Matsabisa, trying to cheer her up. But he knew already that this claim was a lost cause. The mixture contained no new chemical compounds. It probably contained Aloe vera, olive oil and lemon juice, well known and generally available ingredients. Mrs. Dihara's dream "to help people" and concurrently make a bit of money might not come true, at least not with *Rohelia*.

Hope in Helping People: A Plant Claim for Diabetes

Making traditional medicine available to the public to help suffering and sick people was another motivation for considering making a medicinal plant claim. This, at least, seemed to be the motivation of the other claimants whom we visited that same day. On the way back to Cape Town but still in Beaufort West, we turned off the main road and stopped at the Mdehle Inyanga Healers Association of South Africa. All previous claims visits that I had joined had been with 'non-indigenous' people[10]. The three traditional healers of the association were the first claimants whom I encountered with an 'indigenous background'. The conversation between the healers and the IKS Lead Program team was held in isiXosa, with little time for translation into English. The following description is thus considerably shorter and only based on my observations and the short explanations of Dr. Matsabisa.

The three women who welcomed us at the small building of the Mdehle Inyanga Healers Association of South Africa were all dressed in sangoma attire, with the sangoma cloth around their waists and beads around their necks and wrists. The room we entered was slightly damp and dark due to the lack of windows. It was sparsely furnished, with only two chairs, one sofa, a table and a cupboard. The smell of imphepho drifted in from the neighboring room. A huge five-liter bottle containing a green transparent liquid stood on the low table. The spokesperson for the three healers explained that their claim was a plant mixture against diabetes consisting of the extraction of five different medicinal plants collected in the Karoo. But they did not wish to enter into an ABS agreement if the claim transpired to be successful. They did not know who in the association the original holder of the knowledge was. They only wished to make their medicine available to the public for the benefit of sick people. They had learned about the opportunity to scientifically analyze traditional medicines through the huge healers network that the IKS Lead Program had established.

Dr. Matsabisa first briefly introduced the three healers to the biomedical profile of diabetes. They listened attentively and added their knowledge about diabetes and why they thought their mixture was effective against it. As in all claims, the healers would not disclose their knowledge on any of the ingredients and the IKS Lead

---

10   The other two claims follow-ups that I joined, but do not have the space to describe extensively here, had been made by the Tim Jan company and by a private colored man. Tim Jan is a mix of port wine and aloe ferox, which helps against constipation. The company also claimed that Tim Jan has antimalarial properties. They said that it had been tested on tourists in malaria infested countries. The tourists had used Tim Jan as an antimalarial, taking a tablespoon of it every day. Allegedly, none of the tourists had contracted malaria. The second claimant, a colored man in his 40s, offered an ointment consisting of eight essential oils. He had gotten the recipe from an old man and had developed it further, with the help of information he had found on the internet.

Program would never ask for it. The only information that Dr. Matsabisa asked for was regarding the purpose of the claim, the diseases treated with the claim, and the history and success of treatment, usually documented in patient records. The healers, however, could only offer undocumented information on their claim. Later, they also showed us a small bottle that contained a transparent liquid and a white fleshy worm. "*Nyoka* medicine," one of the healers said, "medicine against pollution in the body" (cf. Green 1994, Green et al. 1994). The healers did not consider proposing the *nyoka* medicine for scientific analysis, however. Perhaps they were too aware of the limits of science, which would only be able to detect chemical compounds and not the power of spiritual healing.

All in all, this meeting was very different to the previous meeting, as at no point was there any intention for or expectation of an ABS agreement. Additionally, of the claims that I attended, it was actually the only one that contained potentially unknown medicinal plants, and it was the only claim that Dr. Matsabisa was fully interested in. He took the huge five-liter bottle back to the laboratory. Also because he was diabetic himself, as he told me on the way back to Cape Town, he was curious about the biochemical value of the green liquid. This claim, at least, seemed to offer some hope for a future product.

Hope and Reality in Claim Making

The examples of Mrs. Dihara's claim described above, and of the plant exchange in Thulamahashe described in chapter I, show how in many cases, the likelihood for plants to end up in the biochemical laboratory is quite slim. Even the future of the more promising claim of the Mdehle Inyanga Healers Association was, at the moment of knowledge disclosure, unpredictable. It could release unexpected findings and transform into a viable diabetes (or any other) product one day, or it could be just another of the many claims that lead to a dead-end. And yet, something had motivated Mrs. Dihara and 2000 other people to disclose their knowledge to the IKS Lead Program as of 2010. The fact that plant analysis is a long and cost intensive process was not known and not taken into account by the enthusiastic claimants. The quest of the healers in Beaufort West to make their knowledge and plant material available to the public seemed an honorable motivation. Even Mrs. Dihara's quest, driven by the hope of supporting sick people as well as benefiting economically from *Rohelia*, was understandable. However, both altruistic and idealistic motivations on the one hand, and economically driven hopes on the other, may finally turn into an illusion. It would not be the first time in the field of bioprospecting for an enthusiastic hope to come to a dead-end (cf. Rutert 2010). Nevertheless, despite these challenges, sometimes a new compound will be discovered or a new cosmetic adjuvant developed.

The unpredictability of a claim and the expectation of an emerging biovalue produced through the biotechnological intervention and manipulation of plant material creates hopes and a "dynamic of expectations" (Brown 2003: 3) in knowledge disclosers and scientists alike. To some degree, it is the "intense future orientation that is essential to the rehearsal of the many possible prospective presents embedded in biotechnological research and discourse" (ibid.: 4). The hope when disclosing knowledge is to make an investment in a better future, for oneself and for others. Mrs. Dihara hoped to help people with HIV/AIDS, and to help herself with some additional income. The healers of the Mdehle Inyanga Association hoped to help people overcome diabetes. This future orientation has its basis, amongst others, in a knowledge economy, in which "expectations are loaded with value, they are tradable and therefore form the basis of exchange relationships with 'communities of promises'" (ibid.: 5). In the interaction between the knowledge disclosers and the IKS Lead Program staff members, the exchange of information is an investment into the future, an oscillation between present problems and future solutions. Future solutions, at least for the larger public, can only be provided by science and biotechnology. Carlos Novas described this as the "political economy of hope" (Novas 2006: 290):

> The scientific discoveries and technologies breakthroughs associated with the new genetics have created the potential and hope that cure or treatments for many human ailments will be found in the near future (...) the hope invested in science is not only an aspiration, but can also be thought of as having a political and economic materiality that seeks to bring to fruition the many future possibilities inherent in the science of the present (ibid.: 289).

The investment of the knowledge disclosers is the giving away of individually held (in Mrs. Dihara's case) or collectively held (in the healers' case) knowledge for the health benefit of the public. The Mdehle Inyanga Association healers gave their knowledge away without any expectations of personal benefit. They gave it as a 'pure gift' (Nakozora 2015), giving without taking, as the benefits were unpredictable and not even wished for. This is not a general stance of all healers who disclose knowledge. The plant exchange in Thulamahashe shows that some traditional healers are interested in benefits, as well as in political leverage arising from ABS agreements and intellectual property rights. The 'pure gift', then, transforms into an object of commercial and political value. The green diabetes *muthi* remains, as long as it is not a marketable product, a non-commercial entity; this counts for Mrs. Dihara's claim and for the exchanged plant material of the Kukula Healers as well. But they may become commercial products at some stage in their trajectory. Medicinal plants and knowledge are thus neither pure gifts nor pure commercial objects. They are caught between the two poles of the hope to help people and the hope to benefit economically, and thus wander *in* and *out* of the economic market and gain "value through conversions from non-capitalist transactions" (Tsing 2013, 2015).

In the end, due to the unpredictability of biotechnological research, most of the hopes and expectations placed in medicinal plants and knowledge remain unfulfilled. As the above descriptions of voluntary knowledge disclosure reveal, such actions and encounters are guided by tension and challenge In the next section, I will show how these expectations and hopes are further challenged by the doubts and ambivalent positions of both traditional healers as well as scientists.

Second Challenge: "Why Does Science not Believe in Our Knowledge"?

The disregard for the cultural and social capital (Bourdieu 1986) of indigenous knowledge, once that knowledge enters the biochemical laboratory, was summarized pointedly by one of the leading South African politicians and scientists in the field of traditional healing and medicine, Dr. Isaac Mayeng, director of the Traditional Medicine Group at the Department of Health in Pretoria, South Africa". During a brief conversation in the little office room at the IKS Laboratory, he elaborately addressed the conflicts that come with knowledge disclosure to the IKS Lead Program:

> Look, traditional healing is holistic in nature due to the existence and context that is provided by a cycle of healing. The circle brings about balance in environmental, physiological, mental, social and spiritual well being to attain a state of heath. It is influenced by factors such as history, personal attitudes, belief systems, philosophy and social systems. The core elements of this healing cycle are the stages of life and beyond, like pre-courting and courting, conception and pregnancy, labor, disease, cultural situations, sanitation, dream management, death and post-death. A traditional healer would figure out which stage the patient is in during a counseling session and apply muthi according to need. The Western scientific system, however, is only concentrating on a very small cutout of this circle. Science is actually only interested in the disease part; all other social factors are not interesting for science. Nevertheless, I do believe that there are strong links between Western science and traditional knowledge. And, I think, anthropologists can depict these links[11] (from fieldnotes, August 2009; see also Mayeng 2009).

I met Dr. Mayeng, a scientist who had trained as a Western doctor and pharmacologist at the University of Cape Town and New York State University, during National Science Week at the IKS Laboratory in August 2009. During his youth and

---

11   Dr. Mayeng gave a presentation at the 'Contested Ecologies Seminar Series' at the University of Cape Town in October 2009, where he extended these ideas (Mayeng 2009).

educational years, he had little exposure to African traditional healing. But to his own surprise, he had the calling as a healer in 1978, when he had just turned thirty. Later, he worked for the first South African traditional medicine database (TRA-MED) at the University of Cape Town before finally being appointed director of the Traditional Medicine Group at the Department of Health (see Campbell 1998).

His triple role as a healer, politician and scientist was well recognized, but not always well regarded, by his fellow healers. A healer whom I met independently of the IKS Lead Program at a gathering of healers in Oude Moulen[12], Cape Town, said about Dr. Mayeng: "This Mayeng is working on both sides, he is working for science and then at the same time he jumps to the healers' side. He is not trustworthy." And, he added, when I asked him about his views on cooperation between the IKS Lead Program and healers: "Well, the MRC takes all names and the use of plants for their pharmacopoeia without giving us something back" (Informal conversation, Oude Moulen, Cape Town, August 2009). This healer referred to fundamental problems in the transfer of plant materials and associated knowledge from the realm of traditional medicine to the biochemical laboratory, in particular (lack of) trust, imbalanced reciprocity and the reduction (or transformation) of values.

Dr. Mayeng was very aware of the suspicions aroused against him. As revealed in the quote above, he was also very cognizant of the friction and challenges between 'science' and 'traditional healing', two realms that seem far removed from one another, but are nonetheless closely interlinked in post-Apartheid South African research institutions like the IKS Lead Program. Although both realms fight to maintain their own ground, they nevertheless seem to be attracted and attached to each other. An obvious difference, however, is that "they [biochemists] have a laboratory" (Latour & Wolgar 1986: 257), which reinforces the existing power imbalance between the two systems in terms of technical superiority. Unfortunately, I did not have the chance to ask Dr. Mayeng to elaborate more on the links between traditional medicine and Western science, though the idea never left me, and indeed it has followed me throughout my research, thinking and writing processes.

The following conversation with a traditional healer, John Nxumalo, also took place during the 2009 National Science Week in the small herb garden next to the IKS Laboratory. John was taking a cigarette break from teaching young pupils from nearby townships about traditional healing and medicinal plants. His almost furious statement underpinned the tension between science and traditional healing:

Tell me, why does science not believe in our knowledge? Why do we have to prove something that has been proven over so many years? If I want to get a patent on

---

12   The meeting assembled Xhosa traditional healers who were discussing the possibility of claiming Oude Moulen as land that belongs "to them." Oude Moulen is a large piece of land in the southern suburbs of Cape Town. Such land claims are not uncommon in post-Apartheid South Africa, but due to their complexity they cannot be discussed in detail in this thesis.

a medicine or plant that really works, how can I prove it without science? I was working with a plant that helped children with stomach problems, and it always worked. I worked with patients since 1980 and none of my patients ever complained or came back to me because he or she did not get healed. They all got healed. And now, suddenly, everybody is interested in us. If I give my knowledge away, someone will take the knowledge and use it for [his or her] own purposes. (...) Our knowledge came from our ancestors. If I want to make a patent, how can I, as an individual person, claim a patent on knowledge that belongs to many of us, that belongs to our ancestors? (Informal conversation, August 6, 2009)

John displayed his annoyance quite frankly to me as a stranger, and was not shy in making his almost provocative statements about science. Maybe his annoyance had been brewing inside of him and other fellow healers for a long time and had never really found a voice beyond the circle of healers? Maybe it was not real anger but simply a summary of thoughts that many healers had about the interaction between science and traditional healing? He did, nevertheless, in the rather exposed, semi-open space of the herb garden, definitively summarize some of the main problems in the field of bioprospecting, namely the contradictions, challenges and frictions between indigenous peoples and their rights versus the hegemonic power of scientific, political and legal systems, with the sentence: "Why do we have to prove something that has been proven over so many years?" This supports the argument that traditional medicine becomes one element of what Laguerre (1987) has called "rejected knowledge": "[t]he status of rejected knowledge relies more on questions of power than on standards of truth and effectiveness" (ibid.: 11). The knowledge of traditional healers is not rejected due to its lack of effectiveness, but because of the power imposed by biotechnological intervention and scientific truth claims.

The protests and resistance of the healers against this fact-oriented system shows that scientific facts are mingled with values that are beyond science and state interests, and the mutual co-production of bioscience and politics (Jasanoff 2004). With regard to the inclusion of traditional healers in the bio-scientific analysis of medicinal plants, this poses fundamental questions of ethical justice. What role do citizens, here primarily traditional healers, play in a context where "science does not believe in our knowledge" and where the director of the IKS Lead Program claimed straightforwardly that "I am not interested in the spirit, I am only interested in the molecule" (from personal communication, IKS Lead Program, March 2009)? Such a statement leads to the impression that the IKS Lead Program basically does what Cori Hayden, in the Latourian tradition, formulated as "speaking for" (Hayden 2007: 732; Latour 1993). That is, "authoritative science both represents or 'depicts' nature and represents, or speaks for, the dense webs of interests of those people and things that have been gathered-to, enrolled, or 'interested' in the fact in question" (Latour 1993: 27, cited in Hayden 2007). In this regard, the IKS Lead Program basically aims to *speak for* indigenous knowledge systems and its representatives. And yet cooperation and integration are an officially proclaimed and practically applied part of the IKS Lead Program's agenda.

Marilyn Strathern (2000: 292–294) pointed to the challenge of including people in bio-scientific processes (such as clinical trials or the Human Genome Project; cf. Petryna 2009) in terms of differentiating between "'including people' and 'including them *well*' (that is, ensuring that their participation does not become a form of exploitation or mistreatment)" (cited in Hayden 2007: 733). This implies that scientific knowledge should also represent the 'social interests' of the people and institutions who become wrapped up in its production (Latour 1993), which makes science a political matter (Latour 2004). The partial inclusion of citizens in the bio-scientific process speaks for what Rabinow (1996) has called "biosociality" or what Rose and Novas (2008) have defined as "biological citizens" (see also Petryna 2003), which entails not only the enclosure of citizens within bio-scientific processes, i.e. clinical trials, but also the question of on what basis these people and their claims shall be attached to the inputs and outputs of the research (see Hayden 2007: 736)

Consequently, the question is whether the IKS Lead Program, with its mission to advance indigenous knowledge systems, includes people well enough (Strathern 2000)? The statements of the healers above would suggest that inclusion does occur, but perhaps not well enough, for it basically ignores the social and cultural context of the knowledge and knowledge holders.

The next section looks at the third challenge that disrupts a straight trajectory from indigenous knowledge systems to the IKS Laboratory and a newly discovered chemical compound. This third challenge is about the scientific process and those who execute this process – i.e. the biochemists or pharmacologists – who, at the IKS Laboratory have distinct positions regarding their work and the items that they work with, namely medicinal plants and associated knowledge.

Third Challenge: "We Go beyond Their Knowledge"

Biochemical or pharmacological scientists work with a different set of knowledge than traditional healers. The scientists at the laboratory, mostly educated in South African, and sometimes European or North American universities, apply the scientific knowledge system(s) that they learned at university. Susan Leigh Star and Griesemer (1989) and other scholars such as Latour (1986), Collins (1983), Rouse (1986) and Hacking (2000) have shown that the kind of knowledge system we call 'Western science' depends on a variety of social, technical and literary devices and strategies, assemblages that move and engage local knowledge (Turnbull 2000: 20). Susan Leigh Star has suggested that we look at scientific theory and practices as deeply heterogeneous: different viewpoints are constantly being adduced and reconciled (...) Each actor, site, or node of a scientific community has a viewpoint, a partial truth consisting of local beliefs, local practices, local constants, and re-sources, none of which are fully verifiable across all sites. The aggregation of all viewpoints is the source of the robustness of science (Star 1989: 46).

The theories and practices used in biochemical analysis at a laboratory may seem neutral in terms of the application of specific techniques, materials and a robust academic canon of knowledge. However, the interaction of these 'neutral' aspects with the analyzed plant material and (some) information from the indigenous knowledge system from which it originates (both of which are reduced to a specific extract), as well as the technical devices used and the opinions and knowledge(s) expressed by the scientists, are not always as 'rational' as may be expected in an 'objective laboratory'. Scientific analysis is highly technical, but it is simultaneously deeply intuitive and coincidental work. Michael S. Fischer provocatively proposed that when

we watch carefully (...) we can see Alice in Wonderland and other worlds beyond the residues (the numbers, models, laws, arguments) by which we claim to under-stand what science is. These other worlds are lively: full of quirks and rituals, su-perstitions and fetishization, all-too-human transferences, competitions, and col-laborations, all collaborations, mentoring styles and politichicking games, trans-lations and shifts in scale, and financial incentives and other surprises (Fischer 2012: 386).

When taking into account these all too human aspects in the assemblage of what is represented in the laboratory, it soon becomes clear how and why science can be regarded more as a local knowledge system than a universal benchmark against which all other knowledge systems should be compared (Turnbull 2003). The di-chotomy between scientific and indigenous knowledge is less of a rational con-struct and more of a multilayered discourse of creating scientific facts, decision-making, personal opinions and beliefs, dreams, intuition and educational back-ground. As Knorr-Cetina (2001) has stated:

How does a scientist decide to make a particular technical decision? By translating a choice into other choices. The point about translation is that they often impli-cate non-epistemic arguments and show how scientists continually crisscross the border between considerations that are in their view scientific and nonscientific (Knorr-Cetina 2001: 154).

A conversation between two scientists working with the LC-MS machine at the IKS Laboratory that I observed in October 2009 quite explicitly reveals the crisscrossing of scientific work with traditional medicine. At first, the conversation was about "deep science." One of the two researchers, James Mukinda (JM), said that he did not trust traditional medicine and believed that his job as a scientist was to prove the safety of medicinal plants. His colleague, Jaco van Zyl (JZ), agreed. When I went on to ask what they personally thought about traditional healing methods, they became almost agitated:

> **JM:** Oh, that is when you cut [the surface of the skin] and put medicine into the cuts, to become as strong as the medicine. Then you open your body to the evil forces that can then work in your body. You sacrifice your blood to the demons. I can't believe in it. The movie Harry Potter is true. It is reality. It is the evil spirit that can lift you up. In witchcraft, the body can control the spirit. The ancestors are the evil spirits. It is pagan praying. A pagan is an evildoer. Their soul will go in trouble [JZ nodded approvingly]. A tattoo is a mark of Satan.
>
> **JZ:** First, everybody should listen to the word of Christ. If you don't believe in Christ, then there is no belief.

The conversation continued onto illuminati conspiracy theories and the idea that Satan controls the United Nations. War making is necessary to sacrifice blood to Satan, hence there will always be war in the world, because Satan wants to rule the world.

The turn in the conversation was obscure. I had expected a rejection of traditional healing practices. Most of the scientists whom I interviewed said that they personally never visited traditional healers. But this fierce, almost enraged expression of denial of the practices of healers, by bringing witchcraft together with conspiracy theory, seemed farfetched. The supposedly 'rational' act of extracting compounds was mingled with religious beliefs. The two researchers were practicing Christians and regular churchgoers. In a side conversation, James would later elucidate that his life was basically divided between the laboratory, his bed at home and church. He said that he often dreamed about new directions to take, or about the next solvents or plant combinations he should try. The approach he took to science was thus an interesting mixture of intuition (dreams), ritual (the daily, repetitive structure of his day, combining religion – going to church – and science – performing scientific processes), personal beliefs and scientific work. A couple of months later, in February 2010, I had the chance to interview James Mukinda individually at the IKS Laboratory, and to return to his opinions and perspectives. He elaborated on his thoughts on traditional healing:

> **BR:** Do you think witchcraft does exist?
>
> **JM:** When you are Christian, a true believer, the sangoma can't have power over you, can't reach your spirit. It does not have the power to control you. But when you are not a Christian, these guys can play around with your spirit, can play around with your life. He can cast on you what you can call black demon, spirit, to disturb

your life. (...) Because when people are not Christians, they don't have a strong faith, they believe in anything that comes. Some of the guys are just lying, they want to cheat [people out of] money, they scare you. (...)

BR: And what do you think about a healer who is a sangoma and Christian?

JM: It can't be. Because when you are a Christian, you cannot be a sangoma. You are pretending. Because as a Christian we have Commandments, and Jesus or God cannot allow doing that. You do contrary to what the Bible says. (...) You see, the knowledge of old people, I believe in that, I accept it, because this was passed on from generation to generation. So it was a fruit of trial and error. They have done well, but that was done in human beings. So now, today, we are trying to take it at that level and to scientifically prove it, to have proof of that knowledge, because that knowledge is still a theory, without any scientific proof. We take that knowledge as just speculation, and then we try to prove it. If it is provable, then we accept it. (...). One of the plants has been used for many years. But that plant is toxic, it is affecting the kidneys, it is affecting the liver, it is destroying them, but the people, because [of] what we call chronic toxicity, it's not acute, it is something that comes back if you take the plant regularly, then after 3 to 6 months, then the symptoms are back[13]. People say I am used to the plant. But they don't know that bit by bit it is destroying their bodies, but by now [that they are sick from the medicine] they are looking for a scapegoat.

James maintained his 'anti-*sangoma*' and 'pro-Christianity' position. Being a Christian and a traditional healer simultaneously was, according to him, impossible. In addition, it was clear for James that scientific work is necessary to prove the efficacy of medicinal plants, that an upgrading of scientific methods to ensure the safety of the medicine is necessary, even though he admitted that the knowledge of "the old people" does have some value. "The old people," according to James, does not necessarily refer to "the ancestors" but to the older generation, a strong reference point in African traditions. Cases of intoxication induced by medicinal plants are not rare (i.e. Steenkamp 2002, Steward 1996). The fact that intoxication and incorrect dosage also occur in biomedical treatment did not seem to play a role in James' personal argument. He represented the idea of a hierarchical imbalance between the knowledge of traditional healers and science, with the latter being the one that could 'upgrade' the first. His argumentation moved in and out of personal, subjective interpretations and rational, medically based reasoning about the efficacy and

---

13   James was referring, among others, to the then recent example of the plant mixture Ubhejane, which it was claimed could cure HIV/AIDS. A truck driver named Zeblon Gwala was the original 'inventor' of Ubhejane; he alleged that he had dreamed about the mixture. The case led to heated debate, since the 'remedy', rather than curing HIV, in fact caused liver failure among those who took it (Levine 2012: 56 ff.).

value of medicinal plants. His argument can neither be called purely scientific nor purely non-scientific.

It must be pointed out that James cannot be taken as representative of all of the researchers at the IKS Laboratory. First of all, he was not directly employed at the IKS Laboratory but was a visiting researcher tasked with conducting research using the LC-MS machine. Second, he was the only non-South Africa (he was from Kongo), whom I interviewed. Third, his religious views were almost radical, particularly when compared with many of the other researchers, who had much more balanced views regarding their work and interactions with traditional healers, their knowledge and medicinal plants. Brian Sehume (BS), for instance, a Master student whom I interviewed at the IKS Laboratory in January 2010, expressed an almost diametrically opposed opinion to James:

> **BR:** Do you believe in the medicinal power of medicinal plants?
> **BS:** Yes, I believe they work.
> **BR:** And do you believe that they have the solution for, let's say tuberculosis?
> **BS:** Yes, I do believe that. It's just the reason why I can't find something on the market. I am following Western procedures of isolating [chemical compounds]. Those procedures are not really the right procedures, because we need new protocols on medicinal plants than those protocols that are dictated to us by Western society.
> **BR:** And what could be the alternative?
> **BS:** The alternative? We must do research in our own way. In South Africa, if I want to do research on traditional medicine my own way, there is no way that any university teaches it. We are trying to mix, but then we lose it somehow.
> **BR:** But what is an alternative way? How does it look like?
> **BS:** Well, look, plants have always been used by our forefathers or whatever, and the problem now with medicines, even the antibiotics that are on the market, is the dosage, and that is why in most cases you develop a resistance. My personal belief towards this is: the old people used to know the dosages, the medicines and how to prepare them. And we don't know that [anymore]. You know, even the machines in the back, I actually felt bad when those people [plantation site workers from De Doorns] were here and the machines, I just wanted them to be quiet. One of them even said: "But you are changing something in the plant." And it is true, we are changing something in the plant. But this is the scientific way of doing it. But we shouldn't even be doing stuff in test tubes to test these medicines. I think these things [medicinal plants] are meant for human beings and should be tested in human beings. The thing is you then start testing toxicity. You prepare the medicine and give it to people and see if there is any toxic effect, and if there is nothing and then you go on and check the efficacy of this (...) Then the same way it was prepared, that's how you should have [traditional] medicine on the market.

Brian claimed that African traditional medicine calls for new protocols that should support research conducted "in our own way," namely an African/traditional way. The scientific methods used at the laboratory were based on standardized (Western) academic practices and knowledge. These practices and knowledge manipulate the medicinal plant to detect a viable compound. An 'African way' would rely more on the methods and knowledge of the "old people," on the knowledge and trial and error experiments that exist already. "The same way it was prepared, that's how you should have the medicine on the market," claimed Brian. Despite these idealistic notions, he nevertheless followed the common methods of biochemical research for his Master studies, knowing that he had no other choice; he saw the manipulation of medicinal plants for the purpose of research and product discovery as inevitable. He might also have known that research and development is driven by failures of the industry to seek alternative methods and approaches such as combinational chemistry or the better study of already existing natural products (see Koehn & Cater 2005; Handelsman 2005; Wynberg & Laird 2009). Despite this, he did what his research project expected him to do. An adjusted African model of research would probably take years to establish in African laboratories, if at all.

Nchinya Benedict Bapela (Benni), a post-doctoral researcher at the IKS Laboratory, had yet another different stance with regard to traditional healers and traditional healing when I interviewed him at the IKS Laboratory in January 2010. I asked him whether he himself ever consulted *sangomas*. He replied:

> No, I don't. But I will be honest with you. I don't really want to know what my future will look like, my destiny is in my hands, I don't think it is in their hands, or whatever. And a second thing: I think their trend is more about trying to make you feel small or making you afraid in a way. If I have to go and say I am sick, so I have cancer, and they say ok let's take a look and they throw their bones and say, we can see your disease is cancer. And they will then prepare a medicine against cancer, and then it is good. But in most cases it is not like that. Why do you go there and you have to tell them you have cancer or they throw bones and they will tell you that you have cancer or they will tell you lots of stories and say people are bewitching you. But also I think they believe that they are in contact somehow with the people that are dead and they are getting messages from those people, and me as a scientist I cannot prove [this] and as a black person I cannot disapprove. Because there are people that are like that. You as a white wouldn't really understand, because they [dead people] don't even exist. (...) When I am sick, I am not going to a sangoma. If I am sick I rather go to a herbalist. I tell him, 'I have this problem, can you give me medicine?' The herbalist knows that for this disease you give this medicine and they tell you how to prepare it. I don't go there to be told about my ancestors. Well, I also don't believe in those people who read palms. Because first they tell you how good you are and how smart and they go on and then take your

money. And you can't argue against their ancestors, saying no. So, there is still fear and then they start controlling you, play with your mind. So that is why I don't really like this kind of healers. One time we were traveling in the Eastern Cape with the IKS [Lead Program] and this man wanted to scare us. He is a big doctor who wants us to come into the room, we are sitting there waiting with Gilbert and he comes back with a long snakeskin. So he asked us, 'Do you know what this is?' and we said 'Ya, this is a snakeskin.' He said, 'Ya, I killed it myself.' So, I got so angry I just stood up and went outside and let Gilbert talk to him. And another one, my interest was always in TB, so I asked: 'Do you know what is TB?' and he said 'Ya, I know, it's germs that are in you.' So I asked, if he has a patient that has TB, what is he doing? [He replied] 'That person, you just give something to vomit and he will vomit these germs out.' But they do also good to other people. I mean, personally, first of all, I must say there are sangomas that are really gifted. They do not exploit people. But I think they [people visiting sangomas] are scared, and especially in urban areas you find a lot of crooks.

Benni's concern about traditional healers was about the potential manipulation that may occur during a consultation. He also referred almost angrily to the lack of knowledge that some healers had with regard to the most pertinent diseases in South Africa, namely tuberculosis and HIV/AIDS. Benni still believed that there are gifted traditional healers with great healing capacities, but at the same time he warned against the many crooks, particularly in urban areas, where the lack of social control enables the uncontrolled 'training' and practice of traditional healers. He therewith highlighted and confirmed one of the pertinent challenges in the realm of traditional healing, namely the lack of control over teaching methods, particularly with regard to the preparation of medicine and quality of *muthi*, a problem that the government has endeavored to address with the THP Act (2004).

Manipulation in the interaction between healers and scientists, in both directions, seemed to be a major concern of many of the scientists at the IKS Laboratory, though people expressed their concerns differently. Another post-doc researcher, Duduzile Mofele (DM), a female chemist in her 30s, seemed to have a more diplomatic view about traditional healers and their practices when I spoke to her at the IKS Laboratory in January 2010. She was passionate about her research area of medicinal plants, which probably made her particularly careful about not being too judgmental. She took a standpoint in defense of traditional healers, and even more so medicinal plants. She even claimed there to be commonalities between traditional healing and the natural sciences.

BR: Do you personally believe in the power of muthi or in traditional medicine?
DM: I believe in the plant, as a chemist. As a chemist, all the structures we eventually synthesize were all discovered from plants.

BR: But [you do] not [believe] in the other part of the medicine, methods like cuttings?

DM: Well, you know, hmm, not really. But people are diverse, people differ (...). But with the medicinal plants, it is something I can work with and I know what is happening in it. With this other one, cuttings, they perform their own rituals; I won't understand what is it exactly, but I respect them in that way and we work with them. You know, for me to be able to work with them, at least one should try and listen and understand and not to judge. We once went to the African Traditional Medicine Colloquium, it was researchers and traditional healers, so they performed their ritual prayer, burned their incense, sang their songs and did all these things. So for me, although I don't believe in them, I have to respect.

BR: Ya, and you can learn from them and the other way round.

DM: Ya, but they don't like researchers much. Because they feel manipulated by them. Because I remember when we were there, they kept on saying, 'The researchers steal our knowledge'.

BR: And do you think working with them is useful?

DM: Ya, partly, because we need parts of their knowledge, hmm, information. Healers, they have a long [history of] traditional knowledge, created over generations, that is almost similar to what scientists know. I went to sangomas and they explained that they burn poisonous plants to reduce the poison and then they mix it with fat and so on. They have got trial and error methods over centuries. Got them to points where scientists ended up over years of research. I think there is a lot of interaction between these two worlds [science and tradition]. There is lot of common things. We can end up integrating the two. That's why I am focusing on the common things that we have.

Duduzile took a totally different position here than some of her colleagues. "I have to respect" their way of being different, she insisted. She even saw some commonalities between traditional healing and science, such as burning plants to remove their toxicity. Therefore she preferred to focus on finding new valuable medicines with the help of indigenous knowledge, since she knew that the knowledge and information of traditional healers is indispensable for the discovery of new products. She even acknowledged that healers have come to equivalent points in their knowledge development through trial and error as reached by scientists through their own research. And she admitted, conversely to what Benni said, that traditional healers also feel manipulated by scientists (and not only the other way around, that healers are the ones doing the manipulating). In general, she preferred to look at these communalities instead of building up extra boundaries. Adam Ashforth, in his book 'Witchcraft, Violence and Democracy in South Africa' (2005), cited a similar comment from a young high school student whom he interviewed:

To my personal point of view, I think physical science, or physics, goes hand in hand with African physical sciences. Why am I saying this that physical science, well it is approved, and it is done by different nations, like Greeks, Americans. But it is in a modern way. There are labs, there are laboratories. With us, we don't have laboratories. It is done in an old way. But it goes hand in hand (Ashforth 2005: 146).

I have chosen to highlight these interview excerpts with IKS staff members (Brian, Benni and Duduzile and a visiting researcher (James)) to show how ambivalent the position of the scientists was towards indigenous knowledge system(s) and their representatives (see also Verran 2001). With the exception of James, the researchers did not have a clear-cut anti-traditional healing position. It seemed clear for them that indigenous knowledge systems are a vital and valuable contribution to the discovery of new medicines, enclosed in the plant material. Knowledge, in this sense, is a path towards the better use of the plant material. It seemed more that the aspect of the abuse of power and manipulation attributed to traditional healers was regarded as most threatening by the scientists; something that they might have experienced in their private lives, and not only or necessarily in their professional encounters with healers. This might be one reason why the researchers claimed that they did not seek advice from traditional healers for private purposes. But even their professional encounters were loaded with emotions (and not only positive ones), as Benni's almost angry account of "crooks" and their lack of knowledge on diseases revealed.

Obviously, the interaction between science and traditional healing is pushed forward by the efforts to find common ground. But at the same time, this interaction is loaded with misunderstandings and stereotypical judgments. In sum, the excerpts present the mainly subjective antagonism between acceptance and respect on the one hand and distance and neglect on the other. The researchers did, however, worry less about the value of their scientific knowledge and more about the validity of traditional healing knowledge. This complies somehow with the comment of the healer above, who seemed concerned about the implications of the cooperation between scientists and traditional healers and the lack of belief in indigenous knowledge. Although interaction between the two realms is sought for, it remains an ambivalently connoted cooperation.

Partial Connection and Mutual Dependency: One System Needs the Other

As was shown, scientific knowledge and practices, like all other knowledge systems, have particular local manifestations (Watson-Verran & Turnbull 1995). The knowledge and practices produced at the IKS Lead Program are the products of a certain moment in time and particular political, socio-cultural and economic (power) configurations. Other outside influences discursively co-produce and shape this sci-entific knowledge, like the traditional healers and their knowledge systems, politi-cians and politics, as well as pharmaceutical companies and the economic market. The IKS Lead Program, with its mission, staff members and equipment, represents a very particular form of scientific knowledge production and scientific facts; not as a solitary nucleus cut off from but rather formed in relation to other – specifi-cally indigenous – knowledge systems. In both sides' attempts to collaborate, they ideally ought to *speak to each other*, instead of one system *speaking for* the other.

So far, the impression might have come up that traditional healers are basically "databases for potential identification of sources that may yield lead compounds with bioactive properties" (Ntutela et al. 2009: 34). This reduction of healers to mere "databases" obviously creates tension, but maybe also provides opportunities. The engagement of a healer with the IKS Lead Program represents new efforts in post-Apartheid South Africa to at least establish a form of communication between the two systems. At the IKS Lead Program, traditional healers have the chance to con-fidentially share indigenous knowledge on plant material, which, in case valuable chemical compounds are detected in the laboratory and transformed into a phar-maceutical product on the market, might be followed by an ABS agreement. This is a laborious process that, on the scientific side, is time and cost intensive with a low chance of discovering the needle – i.e. a new compound – in the haystack due to the endless combinations of possible compounds in a medicinal plant or medicinal plant mixture. The opportunity for healers is less about the product and more about the integrative dialog that may arise from this disclosure of information, a dialog that was previously completely impossible due to the repressive Apartheid politics in South Africa. The healer whom I spoke to in the IKS Laboratory's herb garden questioned this endeavor with the assertion that indigenous medicinal knowledge already heals effectively. Although the healer pronounced his discontent clearly, he was nevertheless still voluntarily cooperating with the IKS Lead Program as a tea-cher, as well as in terms of receiving the offered training opportunities (such as in tuberculosis prevention). He, like many others in the field of bioprospecting, re-presented the dialectic interplay between protecting and evaluating (indigenous) knowledge and medicinal plants, and the wish to get a piece of the cake (including educational and financial benefits). He questioned this situation, but also seemed, due to his attendance at the IKS Lead Program, to be intentionally interested in being part of it; a stance he shared with other healers who worked with or for the IKS Lead Program, or other similarly oriented research institutions.

Obviously, the two systems are based on differently enacted practices, concepts, methods, materials and actors. At the same time, the involved actors have the uti-lization of the material properties of medicinal plants and their effects on human health in common. There are "partial connections" (Strathern 2004) between the two systems, in which the one system cannot be enacted without the other. The

IKS Lead Program would not exist without the indigenous knowledge systems of traditional healers. Medicinal plant screening and analysis is much more efficient when it includes the pre-existing knowledge of traditional healers. Traditional healing knowledge and its material, in turn, can only be made available to the market when it is disclosed to and 'advanced' by scientific practices and knowledge systems. The two knowledge systems co-exist in an interrelated mutual dependency, but are nonetheless caught in a power discourse, with the scientific realm posing hegemonic claims over indigenous knowledge systems. Some healers accept this claim. Others, like the healer in the IKS Laboratory's garden, feel inadequately heard and represented. His claim called for a more thorough understanding of the cultural and social value of knowledge, instead of only looking at the economic and scientific value. But at the same time, he was also aware of the fact that economic value can only be made through scientific intervention.

Accordingly, the trajectory of medicinal plants and associated knowledge from *outside* to *inside* the laboratory is paved with ambivalence and juxtapositions. But what exactly, after all, really happens in the laboratory? What practices and knowledge are used to transform *muthi* into a new chemical compound? What eventually is the "deep science" that James spoke about?

"Deep Science": The Biochemical Transformation of Muthi

The previous sections showed that the path to the laboratory is a stony one full of ambivalent challenge Once a claimed medicine has nevertheless managed its way into the laboratory, a long and tedious process of research and development begins, which involves an assemblage of human and non-human actors. So what instruments, materials, knowledge, actors and practices are used to make traditional medicinal plants and associated knowledge viable and legitimized biochemical information?

Again, Duduzile Mofele (DM) explained in brief words the assemblage of scientific practices that a medicinal plant or plant mixture must traverse, the methods, practices and theories used, and the thing being searched for: the smallest unit of a medicinal plant, the chemical compound.

> **BR:** What is your assignment at the laboratory?
> **DM:** I am working as a chemist. We extract and analyze them [medicinal plant compounds], we are trying to analyze the chemical constituency, or the compounds that are found in that particular plant. By knowing them we know they are doing some bioactivity, and then we check if there is a compound that induces biological activity.
> **BR:** What does biological activity mean?

DM: Microbiological activity, that is when they are doing these tests, or maybe during clinical trials when they are doing safety, toxicity and check other biological activity. For example, when you do the extracts and then they will test the extracts without purifying it first. And then, after purifying it again, I mean they test the extract of it that shows any activity. And then they will purify it further. And then test different fractions that have been collected and if there is one or two that shows interest you go further and do in-depth now to find out exactly what compounds are in that extract. So basically it is structural investigation.

BR: That is what Jaco [Jaco van Zyl, employed at the IKS Laboratory as an LC-MS technical engineer] is doing?

DM: Ya, that is what Jaco is testing. Because for structural elucidation you need to know the molecular weight of that particular compound. So basically, his instrument [the LC-MS machine] is determining that. So it is an essential part of the structural elucidation. We also need this information in order to say 'This is a pure compound' and 'This has this particular molecular mass'. So once you come up with a structure, you need to come up with the molecular weight and then you have to match it with the data, which comes from Jaco to say, 'Yes this is the one, no this is not the one'. (...)

Duduzile outlined a number of the actors, practices and parameters that were involved in the assemblage of human and non-human actors at the IKS Laboratory, namely the LC-MS machine, the process of structural investigation, the plant material and Jaco, the technical engineer. They were involved in processes called *particularization*, the identification and separation of useful knowledge (Agrawal 2002: 290) and *abstraction*, the identification and separation of useful material, to be tested and validated using criteria deemed appropriate by science (ibid.: 291). Abstraction discards spirituality, rituals, language, practices, sensations or interactions between healers and patients of indigenous medicine and replaces them with scientific rituals, language, practices, technologies, materials, sensations and intuition. The use of scientific criteria to test and examine in clinical and pre-clinical trials and the documentation of these tests can be called a *validation* process (ibid.) to ensure and secure "scientific facts" and "objective truths about efficacy", as Vincanne Adams claimed (Adams 292: 659). Waldram (2000) has reasoned that the clinical trial (and I would also add the pre-clinical trial here) is the "gold standard" in terms of determining validity and efficacy, asserting that

> statistics, rather than human experience, become the only acceptable means through which efficacy can be established. Studies of traditional medicine that do not employ the gold standard or that assess efficacy in culturally meaningful terms tend to be quickly dismissed as unscientific romanticism (Waldram 2000: 616; see also Edgerton 1992; Eisenberg & Kleinman 1981; Hahn 1995).

The above procedures are also politically manifested. According to the WHO (2000), every herbal medicine available on the international market has to be standardized according to basic criteria for the evaluation of the quality of herbal medicines[14]. The laboratory therefore aims to substitute a 'disadvantaged' medicinal plant or plant mixture with standardized and more 'advanced' plant extracts and compounds. This approach also supposedly provides 'safe' medicines that protect patients from drug toxicity[15]. The scientific validation process transforms the original plant, method and knowledge and substitutes it with a standardized product with biovalue (Waldby 2002), applicable to the global market (WHO 2000).

> Biovalue refers to yield of vitality produced by the biotechnical reformulation of living processes. Biotechnology tries to gain traction in living processes, to induce them to increase or change their productivity along specified lines, intensify their self-reproducing and self-maintaining capacity (it takes place not in vivo but in vitro, a vitality engineered in the laboratory, where, as Rabinow puts it, the biological fragment is constituted as a 'potentially discrete, knowable, and exploitable reservoir of a molecular and biochemical products and events' (Rabinow 1996: 149) (Waldby 2002: 2000).

The following sections will show that the pure scientific work, which is supposed to be independent of any subjective influences, is, beyond all objectivity, influenced by politics and, as was described earlier, subjective knowledge production. This situation contributes to the scientific assemblage that produces biovalue, which implies the transformation of a 'living process', a medicinal plant and its living knowledge, into a scientifically valuable product. Particularization, abstraction and validation are the main steps in the production of a viable new compound, or the validation of already detected compounds. The following two sections dive into the politics and practices, materials and investigations of chemical compound extraction and the validation of existing compilations such as PHELA.

The Quest for Validity and Safety: PHELA, a "Crude" Plant Mixture

In the process of structural investigation, the plant material is analyzed for its constituents, in particular the molecular mass that characterizes the weight of a specific chemical compound. Traditional medicines are complex mixtures, often made

---

14   For the WHO guidelines (2000), see http://apps.who.int/medicinedocs/pdf /whozip42e/whozip42e.pdf.

15   Studies have shown that the detection of toxins in products of a botanical origin can be problematic (see Steenkamp et al. 2005). This does not mean that medicinal plants are not toxic, but that the identification of such toxic events in patients is not easy to do (Stewart 1999). There is, however, no evidence that traditional medicine is per se toxic.

of more than two constituents. To structure these complex processes, the IKS Laboratory works with three approaches to new drug discovery. The first approach is the standard extraction and isolation techniques used to find single new chemical entities. This approach is generally known as the *reductionist approach* and is best used for the study of single medicinal plants. The second approach is to develop products that can be used as an adjuvant[16] to current prescription drugs. The third approach evaluates the whole product for its safety and efficacy (informal conversation with Dr. Matsabisa, March 2009).

Most of the Bachelor and Master students at the IKS Laboratory were using the reductionist approach for their research. Brian Sehume, on the other hand, was using the third approach for his Master thesis, entitled 'Pharmaceutical Evaluation of PHELA Capsules Used as Traditional Medicine' (Sehume 2010). In his research, he aimed to evaluate the efficacy and safety of the plant mixture PHELA, a "crude" botanical product consisting of four different plants collected in four different regions of South Africa, but originating from countries outside of South Africa (Mexico, tropical Africa and Asia, tropical East Africa and Brazil)[17]. In an unpublished paper and his thesis, Sehume describes how the original plant combination provided in liquid form revealed "disadvantages," and thus required "further investigation" and ultimately "upgrading" through the provision of PHELA in capsule form.

> A claim will experience scientific upgrading ending in a measured product in capsule, tablet or syrup form (…). In general, the traditional dosage forms some disadvantages: Firstly, they are not easy to keep free from microbial contamination. Secondly, the large volume of preparation required may not be comfortable for patients. Thirdly, the traditional doses measures of a plant medicine are not exact (e.g. half a cup full, two spoonfuls etc.) (Sehume 2009: Document without page numbers).

"Such inaccuracy," Sehume claimed, "will affect the uniformity of the dosing in the individual users" (ibid.). His aim was to overcome these disadvantages and make use of the knowledge of original knowledge holder of PHELA and its potential to "increase energy and the treatment of the disease "muyaka," a disease that causes chest problems, pimpled tongue, high temperature, headaches vomiting and

---

16   An adjuvant is a pharmacological or immunological agent that modifies the effect of other agents.

17   In both an unpublished draft paper (Sehume 2009) as well as his Master thesis (Sehume 2010), Brian anonymized the plants using the letters RM, PT, CG and S, according to intellectual property rights requirements. The four plants were bred in the IKS Laboratory's herb garden and later on at the larger plantation site behind the laboratory building. I also do not mention the plant names for intellectual property rights reasons.

finally a slow and painful death. [To do this] A new dosage acceptable according to pharmaceutical standards needs to be developed" (Sehume 2010: 6ff.).

'Disadvantaged' medicine is a critical term that determines medicinal plants as only valuable once 'upgraded' by science, even though plants often contain value irrespective of the scientific process (which nevertheless helps to detect this value). In a study, (more details on study) it was found that around 81% of 300 evaluated medicinal plants contained biological activity (Fourie et al. 1992). In another study on antimalarial properties detected in South African plants, it was shown that extracts of 49% of all species exhibited promising antiplasmodial activity (Crouch et al. 2008: 356). Obviously, the biochemical pursuit of new compounds is promising, even though it is not the only way to find new compounds. Screening already existing medicinal plants for new compounds is also an often taken pathway to new discoveries. In addition, the documentation of treatment methods of traditional healers or other knowledge holders, as proposed in the 'Traditional Knowledge Documentation Toolkit' (WIPO 2012), for instance, could also lead to successful new discoveries in herbal medicines. But the core problem with herbal medicine remains safety, and safety can only be guaranteed when tested scientifically and according to WHO standards, i.e. for "microbial contamination, pesticide and fumigation agents, toxic metals or other likely contaminants and adulterants" (Sehume 2010). To stick to safety requirements, basic criteria like time of harvesting of the plant material, stage of growth, and drying and storage conditions should also be documented (see WHO 2004). If these safety requirements are complied with, the new discovery will be further analyzed for different aspects, such as toxicity or "the mechanism of action by which PHELA boosted the immune system" (Lekhooa 2010), as was stated in the paper of another researcher who later also worked on PHELA. Others might investigate "the pharmaceutical quality and its sustainability for use in clinical trials" (Sehume 2010). These processes can, however, only be applied when, prior to safety and efficacy tests, the basis for all tests has been found: the chemical compound.

The Quest for the Peak: Detecting Chemical Compounds

Detecting a new chemical compound requires thorough analysis, a process that can take many months and even years of repetitive, tedious work. Researchers have to go through the same procedures again and again to eventually detect a valuable chemical composition. But what actually happens in the process of identifying a molecule?

The density of molecules and chemical compounds in one plant or a plant mixture is extremely high. The separation methods for molecules must therefore also be very powerful and refined in order to detect new compounds. For the analytical process, separation methods are required on a preparative and analytical scale

(Manz et al. 2004). Before plants enter the biochemical process of microanalysis using HPLC and LC-MS techniques, they have to go through some preparatory steps. First, the plant material is cut into pieces, then ground or pulverized; practices that traditional healers also conduct, yet using less refined and high-tech machinery. The crushed plant material then progresses through further micro processing procedures, performed with further technical devices such as the HPLC and LC-MS.

A note from the blackboard in the staff office of the IKS Laboratory gives an indication of the steps that take place in this process and the sort of language, methods and materials used. The steps below do not explain all work done in the biochemical process. They only introduce first steps, which will then be further proceeded, i.e. in a gravity column, the HPLC/ LC-MS.

DCM 24 (I)

1. Weigh 5 grams of DCM 24
2. Dissolve this completely in MeCn
3. Decant the filtrate (supernatant 200 ml)
4. Re-dissolve the white residue
5. Mix all supernatant of 4 for 5 min
6. Spin the supernatant in 5 for 5 min @ 2 RPM [revolutions per minute]
7. Mix all the supernatants
8. Re-dissolve the residue and repeat step 6

DCM 24 (II)

1. Measure volume of supernatant
2. every 30 ml of supernatant add 70 ml water (distilled)
3. maximum of 300 ml of step 2 into round-bottomed flask
4. Evaporate the MeCn – white milky solution will be final product
5. Slowly freeze only this solution (do not put into -80 freezer)
6. Freeze dry the material
7. Pool all freeze dried materials together

Practices such as measuring, dissolving, evaporating and freezing are common instructions in bio-analytical chemistry. But what do the terms DCM 24, supernatant, filtrate, MeCn and RPM mean? DCM, to begin with, stands for *dichloromethane*, a solvent commonly used in biochemistry for its capacity to dissolve organic material. DCM 24 stands for a medicinal plant (Plant 24) dissolved in DCM.

MeCn (*Acetonetile*) is a chemical compound commonly used as a mobile phase[18] in TLC, HPLC and LC-MS. Another commonly used solvent is, for instance, ethanol (C_2H_6O or EtOH), generally known as (drinking) alcohol. In an interview, the PhD researcher James explained during an informal conversation at the IKS Laboratory in January 2010 that "Traditional healers also mostly use alcohol as a dissolvent. These solvents are miscible [mixable] with water and help to separate other chemical compounds of a chemical composition." With reference to the instructions on the staff blackboard, MeCn was diluted in distilled water and was then used to dissolve DCM 24. To separate out the chemical compounds of this complex, crude mixture, the mixture should then go into a centrifuge to be spun for five minutes at a rate of two RPM. The above instructions stopped at this point but the analytical process still continues. It commonly continues with the evaporated liquid being then filled into a gravity column for gravity chromatography.

Gravity chromatography is a separation method where the analyte (the substance or chemical constituent being analyzed) is contained within a liquid or gaseous mobile phase, which is pumped through a stationary phase. The compounds of the analyte interact differently with the two phases. Depending on their polarity, they spend more or less time interacting with the stationary phase, and thus the compounds can be separated from one another according to the speed at which they pass through the gravity column (Manz, Pamme & Iossifidies 2004: 29). In the gravity column, chemicals are separated according to weight; those with less weight come out of the silicon column first. For a chemical compound like $C_{12}H_3O_{16}H_1$, for instance, the numbers represent the molecular weight of the chemicals.

One of the researchers explained to me "Generally, it is not easy to find new chemical compounds. Often they have the same molecular mass, which define chemical compounds. But they nonetheless look completely different." He quickly drew a diagram of two similar compounds that have a totally different molecular mass to explain the difficulty to distinguish them. For the minor differences it takes such long time to detect a new chemical compound. The two diagrams show two compounds of similar molecular mass, which yet are totally different.

---

18   A 'phase' in chemistry is a physically distinctive form of matter, such as a solid, liquid, gas or plasma. "Chromatography is used to separate mixtures of substances into their components. All forms of chromatography work on the same principle. They all have a stationary phase (a solid, or a liquid supported on a solid) and a mobile phase (a liquid or a gas). The mobile phase flows through the stationary phase and carries the components of the mixture with it" cf. www.chemguide.co.uk/analysis/chromatography/thinlayer.html (last accessed February 10, 2016).

Figure 9 Two different chemical compounds

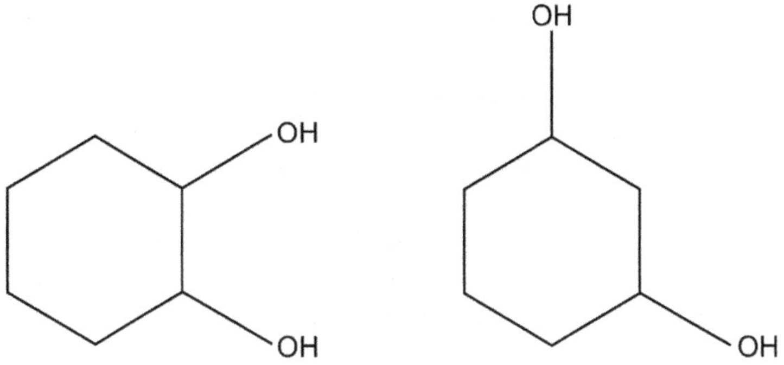

1,2-Dihydroxycyclohexane   1,3-Cyclohexanediol

The solution extracted through the process of gravity chromatography is again only a preparation for further processes. One of these further processes is TLC (thin layer chromatography), a chromatography technique used to separate non-volatile mixtures (Lewis & Moody 1989). It is carried out on a sheet coated with a thin layer of adsorbent material, usually silica gel or cellulose. After the medicinal plant dissolvent that has been extracted in the gravity column has been applied to the plate, a solvent or solvent mixture known as the mobile phase is drawn up the plate via capillary action. Because different compounds ascend the TLC plate at different rates, separation is achieved. TLC can be used to identify compounds present in a mixture, and determine the purity of a substance, including medicinal plants and their constituents (Reich & Schibli 2007).

After all of these more mechanically applied practices, the eventually separated extract will be further processed in the HPLC machine, which was used by most students, and the LC-MS machine, which was used more by the doctoral and post-doctoral students.

HPLC and LC-MS: Identification of Unknowns

Molecules, among others, consist of proteins. These proteins react to specific sub-strates (i.e. ethanol). This happens in the HPLC process and, in an even more accurate form, in the LC-MS machine. Together, these two high-tech chromato-graphic machines are the core instruments used at the IKS Laboratory. Most of the activities that I observed happened in front of these two high-tech pieces of equipment, especially in front of the chromatogram, the result sheet shown on the attached computer screens. Small samples of previously extracted plant material dissolved in different solvents (ethanol or methanol) were analyzed to extract potentially new chemical compounds. Jaco van Zyl, the scientist engineer specifically employed to work with and introduce visiting scientists to the LC-MS equipment, often spent days with visiting or IKS Lead Program researchers working to detect a compound. I observed him and a visiting scientist from the University of the Western Cape's TICIPS (International Center for Indigenous Phytotherapy Studies) program[19] spend hours together in front of the two computer screens attached to the LC-MS machine. A brief excerpt of a conversation that I followed between the two researchers while they were at work provides an insight into the quest for "peaks": accumulated compounds that indicate a "high biochemical value." The LC-MS machine was, at this point, still new to the laboratory and the language used in front of the screen was as unfamiliar to me as was the blackboard instructions cited above.

> **JZ:** (To JM) Look, you can see between 4.5 and 3.5 the peak is high.
> **JM:** So, do you think it is pure?
> **JZ:** 2.85 is a nice peak, but 2.25 is too little. But it can work.

What do the two scientists purport here? And what actually happens in an HPLC and LC-MS machine? In short, what happens is based on the lock-and-key principle. A mixture that contains proteins runs through a substrate, which either recognizes the structure of the protein (like a key fitting into a lock) and causes a reaction, or it does not and thus there is no reaction. To elucidate the structure of a molecule, highly sensitive and very sophisticated methods are needed (Manz et al. 2004: 23), which are offered by the HPLC and LC-MS.

To increase the resolution that has been previously achieved using TLC and to allow for more accurate quantitative analysis, additional enhancements must be done. High performance TLC/mass spectrometry, HPLC/MS or HPLC for short, is a chromatographic technique similar to the gravity column used to separate a mixture of chemical compounds, i.e. an extract of a medicinal plant, with the purpose of identifying, quantifying or purifying the individual components of the mixture. It relies on pumps to pass a pressurized liquid solvent containing the sample mixture through a column filled with adsorbent material. Each component in the sample interacts slightly differently with the adsorbent material. This causes different flow rates for the different components and thus leads to the separation of the components as they flow out of the column (Manz et al. 2004).

In the analysis of the chemical components of traditional medicine, the HPLC technique is usually used for the separation and identification of a variety of similar structural compounds. It separates according to the molecular mass of the chemical, with the larger compounds taking longer than the smaller compounds to run

---

19   The TICIPS program is a joint venture of the University of Missouri-Columbia, the University of Western Cape and the Missouri Botanical Garden, St. Louis.

through the column. This scheme of molecules will appear on the computer screen attached to the HPLC machine as "a peak of compounds," which are represented as a chromatogram on the computer screen known as a "fingerprint" (Sehume 2010). A valuable compound (or as Jaco said above, a pure compound) will show as a high peak on the computer screen. A fingerprint design below shows the density of potential compounds, presented as peaks. A spectra exhibits peaks of the same plant material dessilved with different dissolventsdetected in an HPLC chromatogram of PHELA material[20]. The work at the HPLC is not only to find new compounds, but also to detetct how compounds react on changes. The illustration below, for instance, indicates on the change in chemical compounds after storage time of 24 weeks. This helps to understand loss of efficacy of medicinal plant products.

To reach an even higher level of accuracy in terms of molecule separation and identification, the analysis of plant material is continued in the LC-MS machine, which offers analytical specificity superior to that of conventional HPLC techniques for lower weight analytes (Grebe & Singh 2001). LC-MS is an analytical chemistry technique that combines the physical separation capabilities of liquid chromatography (LC) with the mass analysis capabilities of mass spectrometry (MS). LC-MS has a very high sensitivity and selects, separates, detects and identifies chemicals of particular masses in the presence of other chemicals.

Jaco van Zyl, the LC-MS technical engineer, was mostly occupied with introducing researchers from national universities (such as the University of KwaZulu-Natal and University of the Western Cape) as well as international universities (including Guangzhou University, China) to the complex processes of the LC-MS machine. They often spent many days in front of the computer screen detecting peaks of compounds.

---

20   For detailed information on the peak samples, see Sehume (2010). It is beyond the scope of
      this thesis to go into further details of plant biochemesty and analysis here.

Figure 10 The HPLC machine

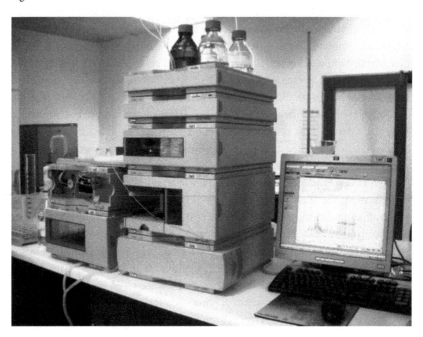

It is actually the pure compound that the researchers are searching for in their daily, often interminable quest behind the screens of the HPLC and LC-MS machines. Finding such a pure compound is, however, very rare. And if such a compound is detected, it still has to go through further analytical steps in order to determine its value and use in terms of its specific healing applicability. A new compound may be viable for the treatment of obesity or malaria. The plant *Dicoma anomala*, for instance, is a well known and well described medicinal plant in South Africa (see van Wyk et al. 2009: 118). After long-term investigation at the IKS Laboratory, a compound was finally detected that was deemed valuable for its antimalarial properties. But the detected compound then had to be tested in pre-clinical and clinical trials for safety and efficacy (see also the example of PHELA above)[21]. These further processes are outsourced to universities, the pharmaceutical industry or private biotechnology companies.

---

21   Pre-clinical and clinical trials are not the main focus of this research. For more detailed literature on clinical trials, see i.e. Lurie & Wolfe 1989; Petryna 2005, 2007, 2009; Pogge 2006.

Transformation of Indigenous Knowledge into Scientific Knowledge

What was eventually detected is the pure compound; the micro-component of the multi-complex constituents of a medicinal plant or medicinal plant mixture. The process of dissecting the compound not only separates "useless" and "useful" biochemical material, but also replaces one knowledge system with another knowledge system. The strong rejection of the old people made by James or the idea of replacing Western scientific knowledge with African systems as proposed by Brian are both part of the knowledge production at the IKS Lead Program. This knowledge production can, as such, hardly be defined as objective and rational, but more an assemblage of specific moments of production, produced by people with distinct backgrounds – i.e. traditional healers of different traditions, scientists with different ethnic and religious backgrounds, machinery from different countries and a continuously changing policy landscape (influenced by national policies as well as international WHO guidelines) – all of which shape the IKS Lead Program. In the transformation process of medicinal plants and indigenous knowledge into a new chemical compound, the knowledge passes through many different steps of abstraction, particularization and validation and is the knowledge passes through many different steps of abstraction, particularization and validation and is dependent on the multiple influences that create the space of the IKS Laboratory dependent on the multiple influences that create the space of the IKS Laboratory.

Figure 11 below elucidates the trajectory of the knowledge of medicinal plant material that comes from indigenous knowledge holders into the laboratory. The cultural values attached to the knowledge basically remain outside of the laboratory's walls. Although largely replaced by scientific knowledge systems and practices, a marginal part of the original knowledge does, however, remain in the discovery process of the compound and may eventually lead to further developed products. It is not the knowledge in its original form but a reduced part of this knowledge. This knowledge hardly matters for the scientific process. And yet, in ABS agreements, which will be discussed in the following chapter, such knowledge plays a major role, since ABS agreements deal largely with the cultural value of knowledge, and not only with the biovalue that derives from scientific investigation that is detected *in vitro* or the economic value of a potential product. ABS agreements deal with the remains of the cultural value inherent in all products that have their origin in indigenous knowledge (even though the scientific process essentially removes this cultural value).

Figure 11 The transformation of indigenous knowledge at the IKS Laboratory

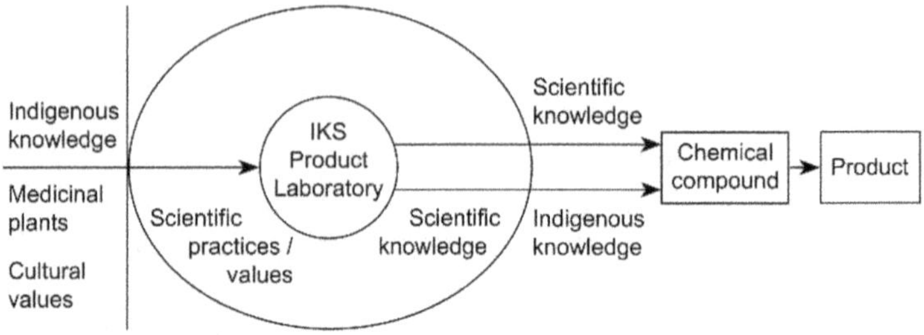

© B. Rutert.

In the goals and mandate of the IKS Lead Program, indigenous knowledge played an ambivalent role, especially under the auspices of the program's mission to support and promote indigenous knowledge systems. So how far is indigenous knowledge integrated into the educational and job creation mandates of the IKS Lead program?

Additional Mandates:
Educate, Use and Develop

The IKS Lead Program has flagged the support and promotion of indigenous knowledge systems among its primary goals. Promotion includes education. The educational mandate implies teaching traditional healers about prevalent diseases such as HIV/AIDS and tuberculosis, as well as teaching pupils, students and other citizens about traditional knowledge, medicinal plants and biochemistry. Among others, the IKS Lead Program participates in National Science Week, which forms part of the IKS Lead Program schools outreach program, which

> (…) is committed to educating our communities and bring science back to the villages. We at IKS believe strongly in developing our foundation of science and traditional knowledge at the foundation phases. The Lead Program's outreach program aims at educating pupils about their traditional knowledge and to value such knowledge[22].

These objectives pose questions. Why would the IKS Lead Program deem it necessary to teach pupils about knowledge that many will have grown up with? It does make sense for a scientific institution to bring "science to the villages" and also to choose young people as a target group for developing "our foundation of

---

22   www.mrc.ac.za/iks/iksclinical.htm (last accessed August 8, 2004).

science and traditional knowledge," but why should a scientific institution teach about traditional healing? With these questions in mind, the next section shows how the IKS Lead Program put its educational mandate into practice.

Educating the Neighborhood: National Science Week at the Laboratory

The Cape Flats are mostly populated by black and colored people. The unemployment rate is very high[23] and future job perspectives for young people are limited, especially when it comes to academic education and a later academic career. Usually, access to the compound of the IKS Lead Program is restricted and it is fairly isolated, with researchers or other appointed visitors only occasionally coming to the laboratory. But for one week in August 2009, the compound changed into a vivid fusion of the world of scientific biochemistry and the world outside of the compound, represented by young pupils of the surrounding communities and other invited guests, among them traditional healers. This gathering took place during the South African National Science Week, where about 1500 young pupils were invited to visit the IKS Laboratory to gain insight into biochemical and pharmaceutical research. For this event, the IKS Lead Program's staff members had thoroughly prepared the laboratory facilities. The technical equipment had been arranged, the laboratory rooms cleaned, the herb garden in front of the laboratory weeded and watered, and a huge festivity tent was built next to the laboratory buildings. National Science Week is a nationwide annual event in which various scientific or science-relevant institutions bring science closer to South African citizens. In 2009, the IKS Laboratory in Delft invited pupils from secondary schools in the neighborhoods of the Cape Flats to visit the facilities, also as an opportunity to explore science as a potential career.

For the whole week, staff members showed student classes around the laboratory. They explained the functionality of the technical equipment, introduced some of the chemical solvents and described the biochemical processes that a medicinal plant must traverse from being a raw plant, or part of a plant, to being a detected chemical compound of pharmaceutical interest. The usually quiet and secluded atmosphere of the laboratory turned into one of activity and engagement between scientists and pupils. For most of the students, it was their first time seeing a biochemical laboratory from inside. I followed some of the classes through the laboratory and felt reminded of my own school excursions to art exhibitions or old churches, where boredom, heavy limbs and tired eyes would suddenly turn into silly giggling with classmates while others absently stared into space. A few pupils,

---

23   In 2011, the unemployment rate was estimated to be at 38%. See: www.capetown.gov.za/en/stats/2011%20Census%20%20Planning%20District%20Profiles/Cape%20Flats%20Planning%20District.pdf

however, did listen attentively and asked interested questions. Possibly, the lack of attention of the others was due to the overwhelming novelty of the subject and basic language problems. The pupils' main language was isiXhosa, while English, their second language, was spoken by many only with difficulty. Since none of the presenting IKS scientific staff members were native Xhosa speakers, the presentations were held in English.

After being shown around the laboratory and being introduced to the main facilities and techniques, the students moved to the adjacent office building, where two traditional healers awaited them in seminar rooms to give lectures on traditional healing and traditional medicinal plants. I had the impression that the pupils were more attentive in these lectures and discussions with the healers than they had been with the scientists, perhaps because of the closer proximity in terms of language and subject matter (one might assume that most of the pupils had heard of traditional healing practices before and could thus more easily connect with the topic). Later, Dr. Mayeng of the Department of Health also gave a short talk about the importance of traditional healing for South African society and the national health system.

National Science Week was one of many activities carried out by the IKS Lead Program. My observation of the events in 2009 revealed the entanglement of science (represented by the scientists and the laboratory), politics (represented by Dr. Mayeng), the public domain (represented by the pupils), indigenous people and knowledge (represented by the traditional healers), technical equipment (represented by the laboratory itself) and medicinal plants (represented by the plants in the adjacent herb garden as well as the plant material in the laboratory). To enable this implicit synthesis between science and traditional healing, the IKS Lead Program collaborated with traditional healers from all over the country. The assistant to the IKS Lead Program director, Mirranda Javu, a Xhosa and English speaking 42-year-old traditional healer, represented this integration like no other staff member. As a healer and member of the Western Cape Healers Association, she had access to a huge national network of healers. Resulting from this network, the IKS Lead Program and traditional healers were engaged on various levels. Firstly, healers worked as educational trainers during events such as National Science Week, as well as being facilitators during trainings outside of the laboratory, where they transferred the knowledge they received at the laboratory to the communities.

This led to the second engagement. The IKS Lead Program trained healers in courses such as the Traditional Health Practitioners Awareness Training Program on Tuberculosis, HIV and AIDS (see Matsabisa et al. 2009). The huge tent erected next to the laboratory building for National Science Week was to celebrate the healers having attended a program on tuberculosis. In the late afternoon hours, the tent was filled with about 200 healers who had come from the surrounding townships to receive the certificate that indicated their participation in the training course. Dr. Matsabisa handed over the certificate to each healer individually, always followed by the enthusiastic applause of the other healers. Finally, the IKS Lead Program continually worked on the integration of indigenous knowledge systems into national policymaking. For instance, Dr. Matsabisa and Dr. Mayeng were engaged in advising the government on the further integration of indigenous knowledge systems into legislation.

Another way of reading these integrative efforts could be to look at the superiority that science demonstrated with regard to indigenous knowledge systems, as they integrated indigenous knowledge and traditional healers into the scientific realm; a task that was promoted with the promulgation of the IKS Policy in 2004. At the IKS Lead Program, science fused with indigenous knowledge systems. The healers were allowed to represent their own knowledge system – as teachers about traditional healing, for instance – but they remained dependent on the framework and requirements of the IKS Lead Program. Science did therefore include indigenous knowledge systems, but the inclusion was ambiguous and, when listening to the voices of the healers, was not done "well enough." Teaching the same content in a township, independent of the program, would possibly not find so many listeners. Indigenous knowledge thus experienced an 'upgrade' by being taught in a governmental scientific institution. The statement of the healer above shows that this authority was not necessarily perceived as integration, but was questioned as evidence of paternalism. Furthermore, the focus group discussion that I conducted with healers at the IKS Lead Program revealed a certain disdain for the interaction between the scientific and the indigenous realm. The interviews with scientists about their perceptions of healing also revealed a similar sense of disdain, ranging from the total denial of traditional healing to ambivalent acceptance. On the other hand, the healers made use of this integration by being taught about prevalent illnesses, such as HIV/AIDS and tuberculosis. The IKS Lead Program, in turn, profited from the input of the healers in new drug development and by integrating them into their mission of "educating communities." While this could be read as a win-win-situation, for both sides it seemed to be more of an ambivalently perceived encounter.

The next section deals with the additional mandate of the IKS Lead Program: the use and production of medicinal plants for local economic development and job creation. To do so, the focus will shift away from the laboratory to a *Sutherlandia* plantation site in De Doorns, Western Cape.

"Sowing the Seeds of Hope": Sutherlandia Plantation Site Project

The sowing of the first seeds of *Sutherlandia frutescens* was celebrated at the opening ceremony of the 'La Serena' project, a *Sutherlandia frutescens* plantation site in

De Doorns, in June 2009[24]. La Serena was located in the Hex River Valley, surrounded by the Hex River Mountains, the second highest mountain range in the Western Cape. These particular surroundings create a Mediterranean climate, which serves for the cultivation of wine as well as medicinal plants. La Serena was a vineyard before the two-hectare plot of land was transformed into a plantation site for *Sutherlandia*. It took me a substantial amount of time to receive permission to conduct interviews with the plantation site workers from the IKS director. I could not at the time understand why he was so reluctant to let me visit the plantation site, though I realized later that it was for political reasons (of which I only came to understand small bits and pieces, as they were never disclosed to me). But in August 2009, eight months after my arrival, I was finally allowed to join Gustavo, La Serena's project manager, on one of his weekly supervisory visits to the plantation site.

The La Serena plot lay within sight of De Doorns, a small settlement in the Breede Valley Municipality, roughly 140 km north of Cape Town. In 2009, De Doorns was known in the South African news for xenophobic violence against immigrants from Zimbabwe. The Zimbabweans were evacuated to a refugee camp next to the N1 national road to Johannesburg after being chased out of De Doorns following violence based on job competition. The (mostly) colored population of De Doorns was habitually employed in the wine industry, with seasonal employment during the grape picking season in autumn. For the seasonally dependent wine industry, additional workers are always in demand during the summer and autumn months. The general wage of the workers at the time was about 60 Rand (6 Euros) a day. Immigrants from other African countries, however, would work for less, given that this amount was still more than any wage they would get in their home countries. "Residents called the Zimbabweans dirty, accused them of practicing witchcraft and said they offered themselves as cheap labor, leaving locals unemployed," reported one news article[25]. This particular situation partly stemmed from the fact that De Doorns had the highest unemployment rate of the entire Breede Valley Municipality, with 60% of residents being unemployed or having only seasonal employment. The level of economic insecurity and poverty was high and poverty alleviation one of the targets of the municipality in its long-term growth and economic development strategy[26]. One project that manifested in this strategy was based on public-private partnerships between groups of organized entrepreneurs, private sector

---

24   www.mrc.ac.za/iks/seeds.htm (last accessed May 1, 2012; the link was deleted with the liquidation of the IKS Lead Program in 2014).

25   See Lewis (2010)

26   See: www.mrc.ac.za/iks/seeds.htm (last accessed May 1, 2012; the link was deleted with the liquidation of the IKS Lead Program in 2014).

companies and research institutions. The project particularly focused on medicinal plants as an income generating strategy.

La Serena was one of three pilot projects in the Breede Valley, all of which fell under the title of 'New Entrants into the Pharmaceutical Industry Initiative'. It was based on a partnership between the Breede Valley Municipality, the Western Cape Department of Social Development, the Medical Research Council and the private company Zizamele Herbs[27]. The project was organized under the lead of the IKS Lead Program. La Serena was implemented as an "Empowerment and Poverty Alleviation Program to facilitate economic growth and to develop interventions that will create sustainable employment and ownership"[28]. Ten people were employed on the plantation to sow, grow and harvest *Sutherlandia frutescens*. But the project had experienced ups and downs since its initiation, and on the day that I finally received permission to visit La Serena in August 2009, I only found George, the project coordinator, Thomas, the co-coordinator, and George's two daughters (all of whom were colored people) as the sole employees. All of the other employees (black people) had left the project, aggrieved. When I asked George where the other workers were, he claimed:

> They didn't want to work with us. They only work with themselves. You see, they worked on that side [of the plantation] and we worked on that side. That's how they worked. They are Xhosas. The family lives in the Eastern Cape, Queenstown. And then they just stayed away. But they all still get their salaries. They get the salaries and we do all the work (Excerpt from fieldnotes, December 2009).

According to George, the black people had left "because they don't like to work." The Department of Social Development paid a monthly salary of 800 Rand. Initially, George and his co-workers were promised 1900 Rand per month, but "the Social Department came and they said that we only get 800 Rand," explained George in a later interview.

George lived right next to the plantation with his wife and two daughters. He and his family lived a simple life without much comfort. But although the income he received from the plantation was relatively low, it was at least stable compared to the seasonal salaries paid on the surrounding vineyards. George was proud, enthusiastic and passionate about more or less being his own boss on the plantation site. For him, "*Sutherlandia* is the global solution. Plants are very important, because most of the people, they are born with the cancer and that's why *Sutherlandia* is there to help them. *Sutherlandia* is a solution, not only for Africa, but for the whole world" (informal conversation, December 2009). When emphasizing the fact

---

27   www.zizamele.com (last accessed September 12, 2014).
28   See: www.mrc.ac.za/iks/seeds.htm (last accessed May 1, 2012; the link was deleted with the liquidation of the IKS Lead Program in 2014).

that he was helping "the whole world," his eyes sparkled. He disclosed later that he wanted to be the project manager of a huge medicinal plantation site, which would provide the "whole world" with plants from De Doorns. He was unaware of the fact that *Sutherlandia* had so far not gone through all of the necessary safety and efficacy tests and clinical trials in order to be exported internationally.

Figure 12 The plantation site with George, Site Manager

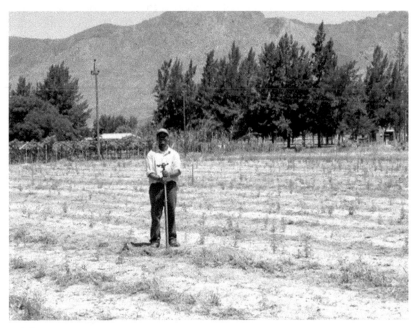

© B. Rutert.

George had been trained as a social entrepreneur at Zizamele Herbs in Barrydale in the Klein Karoo region, about 200 km away from De Doorns, and he planned to continue with further training. He even had future plans beyond his employment at La Serena: "I now go for another training course. I do this and then I have experience, and then I start my own project." He knew that one needs to be prepared: "If you start a business, you need to know your market. You must have a market. If your market is ready, then you get your business." George understood himself as a businessman, who had nothing to do with traditional healing. "We are crazy with medicinal plants, not with these astrologies and *sangomas*. That is not my interest, because I know nothing about this. My training was about medicinal plants" (from focus group discussion with the plantation site workers, February 2010). In case he and his family became ill, he said that they consulted a medical doctor. George simply wanted to be a successful entrepreneur, for which medicinal plants were a means to an end. Access and benefit sharing and intellectual property rights played no role for him, since he did not work with the knowledge of indigenous people. He learned about plant breeding at workshops at the small Zizamele Herbs company. Plantation site workers were simply suppliers of plant material. For George and his family, medicinal plants had an economic value. The emotionality that arose in him with regard to medicinal plants as "the global solution" may be related to the fact that medicinal plants provided a means of survival.

With the La Serena project, it could be said that the developmental mandate of the IKS Lead Program was, to some extent, accomplished, but with only limited success. It basically fed one family. And yet the IKS Lead Program director believed in the value of medicinal plants as providers of economic development. Medicinal plants like Buchu (*Agathosma*) or aloe vera feed a large industry in South Africa. The Breede Valley Municipality had other plantation sites with rosemary and thyme for the cosmetic and food industries; an easier terrain, as these plants do not require further scientific approval. However, *Sutherlandia* may still become an economically highly valuable plant, similar to aloe vera or Buchu, and be sold internationally, once all relevant tests have been done.

La Serena was affected deeply by many challenges, including ambivalent positions towards medicinal plants and indigenous knowledge, personal misunderstandings between Dr. Matsabisa and the overall project manager Gustavo Alfaro, as well as the inter-ethnic problems between the colored and black workers. Nevertheless, at the end of the season in February 2010, Zizamele Herbs did buy the harvested plants and George was proud about "his" project, which enabled him to feed his family independently of the wine industry.

The point of La Serena for all involved participants, and its limited success, was economically-oriented: to generate income in an economically deprived area. In this context, the knowledge of *Sutherlandia* did not come from indigenous knowledge holders, nor was such knowledge sought; rather it derived from the Zizamele Herbs company. As the following chapter will show, however, even knowledge about a common plant like *Sutherlandia* could also become contested.

Conclusion and Outlook

At this point, the transformation of *muthi*, or any other relevant plant mixture, comes to a first pause. At the IKS Lead Program Laboratory, the interest in indigenous knowledge was essentially based on the quest for chemical compounds, and the identification of their efficacy, safety and patentability. The formal national and international market prefers standardized capsules and tablets to raw and crude medicinal plant mixtures that may contain toxic elements (from pesticides, for instance). Thus "[i]n the very moment that indigenous knowledge is proved useful to research and development through the application of science, it is, ironically, stripped of the specific characteristic that could even potentially mark it as indigenous" (Agrawal 202: 292).

This particularization, abstraction and validation process is, basically, a process that promotes the biovalue of medicinal plants for the economic market. (Indigenous) knowledge and plant material may thereby be turned into a globally accepted and commercially viable product. Lesley Green, associate Professor at the University of Cape Town, who together with students also visited the IKS Laboratory in 2008 asked the previous manager of the IKS facilities "Are there plans, once the efficacies of plant medicines are proven, to promote low-cost health care by teaching people to garden with medicinal plants and dose themselves appropriately?" "No!" he responded, "this is a capitalist company" (Green 2008: 48).

The standardization process is, however, influenced by the subjective interpretations, intuitions, views and attitudes of the involved scientists. This does not imply that all scientists working at the laboratory are against indigenous knowledge systems or their representatives per se. Indeed, their opinions about traditional healers and traditional healing were ambivalently positioned along a continuum ranging from respect and acceptance to rejection and even anger. Indigenous knowledge was similarly accepted by some, but nevertheless also treated like "rejected knowledge" (Laguerre 1987: 11). This implies that even a practice such as scientific investigation, which is often defined as 'objective', is liable to subjective interpretations as well as influences from other knowledge systems, an observation that defines science as yet another local knowledge system (Watson-Verran & Turnbull 1995).

The additional mandates of the IKS Lead Program were also ambivalently torn between the (ab)use of indigenous knowledge holders and medicinal plants, and the attempt to make use of medicinal plants and associated knowledge for the benefit of the knowledge holders or other less powerful citizens (like George and the other plantation site workers). This is not to say that all activities at the IKS Lead Program were conflictive. But it does show that all activities were driven by the good intention to "promote and support indigenous knowledge systems," but turned out to be ambivalently town between making use of medicinal plants and indigenous knowledge on the one hand, and the more idealistic attempts to support them on the other, and between adjusting to market-driven needs and the attempt to promote African values and cultural heritage. This balancing act continues (to an even greater extent) in ABS agreements, which are essentially an attempt to bridge the two systems with adequate politics. The next chapter will deal specifically with this balancing act. It continues to follow the trajectory of medicinal plants and associated knowledge, this time out of the laboratory and into the politics of access and benefit sharing and intellectual property rights, and examines how these challenges the divergent actors involved.

Chapter VI
ABS – A Stony Path Towards Sharing: The Chances and Challenges of Access and Benefit Sharing

Gift or Commodity?
Mark Osteen (2002)

ABC in South Africa: The "Best Case" Hoodia Gordonii

Hoodia gordonii is a thick, fleshy succulent plant that grows in the Kalahari Desert, a region that stretches from South Africa via Namibia to Botswana. For generations, the San people have chewed the edible plant on their hunting trips through the Kalahari to stem off thirst and hunger. In 1963, the Council for Scientific and In-dustrial research (CSIR) – which, aside from the Medical Research Council (MRC), is one of the largest research institutions in South Africa – used knowledge gathe-red on *Hoodia* during colonial times in a research project into the plant. After a long research period, the CSIR finally extracted a new chemical compound called P57, which was patented in 1996. Further development was delegated and licen-sed to the British pharmaceutical company Phytopharm. After Phytopharm closed down their Natureceuticals group, the further development was licensed to the US pharmaceutical giant Pfizer, and later to the consumer giant Unilever. Unilever developed a SlimFast product containing P57. In the meantime, *Hoodia* traders in South Africa and Namibia were engaged in the cultivation of about 300 hectares of *Hoodia* plants. Some even changed their cultivation program from other plants to focus exclusively on *Hoodia*. Unfortunately, Unilever suddenly dropped completely out of the production of the *Hoodia* SlimFast product after clinical trials found it to cause vomiting, high blood pressure and other side effects, but no weight loss[1]. A study initiated by the CSIR, by contrast, showed that the succulent's extracts were "generally safe and well tolerated" (Starling 2011). However, since Unilever's with-drawal no other company has been interested or become involved in continuing

---

1   "Would-be fat-fighter Hoodia nothing but side effects", October 29, 2011 (www.reu-ters.com/article/2011/10/28/us-hoodia-idUSTRE79R6AI20111028).

research on *Hoodia* and associated products, and thus the *Hoodia* market came to a standstill, or one could even say breakdown. Those plant traders who had put their hopes in the hype created around the succulent experienced serious financial losses. The challenge is that without the necessary continuation of research, the plant does not have much of a chance on the international market. While this might seem like a normal story of research and development, patenting and licensing, the interesting and unique part is that the CSIR decided to participate in an ABS agreement with the San community in the year 2003. The negotiated royalties were set at 3% of all benefits that the CSIR would receive from *Hoodia* products. Before Unilever dropped out, the San community had received around 500,000 Rand. After their dropout, no further benefits were passed to the San community. Those who had placed their hopes in the commercialization of the plant now had to realize that there was no market future, at least not in the formal pharmaceutical and dietary market. The market basically came to a standstill. However, the ABS agreement between the CSIR and the San Council was referred to as "historically significant in symbolizing the restoration of the dignity of indigenous societies" (Ngubane 2003).

In 2009, *Hoodia gordonii* was the only ABS agreement in South Africa, which – to a limited extend – released monetary benefits. And it is probably the most discussed plant in the academic and political debate around bioprospecting for traditional medicinal plants (Wynberg et al. 2009; Wynberg 2004; Vermeylen 2007; Flint 2012). In 2009, Rachel Wynberg, a leading environmental scientist at the University of Cape Town, Roger Chennels, the lawyer who supported the San in their ABS agreement, and Doris Schroeder, a professor of Moral Philosophy at the University of Central Lancashire, took *Hoodia* as an entry point to discuss ABS in their book 'Indigenous Peoples, Consent and Benefit Sharing. Lessons from the San-Hoodia Case' (2009), a subject that until then academically had been little discussed in South Africa. The book is a milestone in the South African discourse on traditional knowledge, medicinal plants, and ABS. It was launched in January 2010 at Kirstenbosch Botanical Garden as part of the ABS training course that I attended. The book showed that *Hoodia gordonii* is a plant, which is the product of many discussions, controversies, meetings and political exchanges that directed the field of bioprospecting into a socio-political arena concerning human rights, access to natural resources, law, equity, human rights and environmental sustainability (Wynberg 2003). Hoodia *gordonii* thus stands exemplary for the chances and challenges access and benefit sharing agreement politics offers, for failings in ABS, but also for new opportunities and ways forward; chances and challenges not only for local communities like the San, but or traders, scientists as well as for the nation state.

Introduction

I chose to start the chapter with the *Hoodia gordonii* case, because it was a recurring example during the first research year and it stands exemplary for the failings, but also for the chances ABS offers. The previous two chapters illustrated how medicinal plants and associated knowledge are transformed from properties bound to social relations into scientifically and commercially usable property in science. In traditional healers communities, a property given away by someone (or a group of people) is imbued with the identity of its owner(s), which causes the property to have an authority, that compels the recipient to reciprocate. This exchange inevitably leads to social bonding and deepens social relations as well as obligations. Once knowledge and plants become involved in an exchange beyond the cultural rules of knowledge exchange within traditional healers' communities, they transform from having a gift status to a commodity status, bound to political and legal regulations.

The current access and benefit sharing (ABS) legislation attempts to bring these two types of property and exchange systems together. In ABS negotiations, like the one above on *Hoodia gordonii*, these exchange systems meet, and sometimes collide. People who work in the field of bioprospecting, such as scientists and medicinal plant traders, generally expressed their struggles with implementing and applying the legal and political ABS regulations. These struggles have their origin in the political attempt to overcome past inequalities and injustices and to integrate indigenous knowledge holders equitably in ABS; for instance, by seeking solutions for how to substitute spiritual and healing value in an economy-oriented value system. In a market predominantly interested in economic values, this endeavor poses a number of challenges to the stakeholders involved in bioprospecting. This chapter looks at these challenges that come with the well meant but difficult to apply ABS regulations.

The chapter continues with looking at moment, when the two systems meet in ABS agreements. It is a meeting of two different ways of experiencing law, and leads, in case of success, to a fusion of these two systems. The chapter then moves on to an ABS training course in Cape Town, where ABS implementation was taught and discussed among stakeholders from mostly African countries. The course displayed the political and legal relevance of and expectations contained within ABS. Moreover, the views of representatives of the Medical Research Council's (MRC) Intellectual Property Unit and of the IKS Lead Program, traders working with medicinal plants, as well as a description of a *Hoodia* Task Force Group meeting dealing with the *future* of the *Hoodia* market, will all bring to light the challenges that ABS regulations bestows on its actors, but also the ambivalently discussed opportunities for business as well as local community empowerment that come about with its implementation on the ground. These different cases and its actors might first seem to lack coherence. But in fact, all three – the ABS training course, representatives from the MRC and IKS Lead Program, and the *Hoodia* Task Force Group meeting – must deal with similar challenges and questions, which will be discussed in this chapter: How do or can stakeholders implement the politically enforced ABS regimes, if at all? How do or can they make use of ABS and what challenges do they come across? How and in how far are benefits shared, if at all? What needs to be improved to make better use of ABS?

When looking at these accounts of the different stakeholders, ABS at first comes across as inapplicable. And indeed, there remain a number of obstacles and challenges that have to be overcome. But as has already been hinted at a couple of times before, the mélange of different values, open questions and vague directions in ABS also produces facts and hopes, which may fail and turn out to be an illusion, or they may find a way into application and new forms of local empowerment and agency, and national (economic) development. The chapter continues with illustrating how stony the path towards ABS agreements is, and why these agreements seldom materialize. This opens the space for chapter VII, which will then illuminate the opportunities that ABS and also the protection of indigenous knowledge under the current intellectual property law offers.

ABS: A Stony Path Towards Sharing

Politically defined tools to protect knowledge have, in the last two decades, become obligatory for all bioprospecting activities. At the international level, this came with the CBD in 1993 and the Nagoya Protocol on Access and Benefit Sharing, which South Africa ratified in January 2013, and at the national level in South Africa took shape in the Biodiversity Act in 2004 and the regulations on Bioprospecting, Access and Benefit Sharing (BABS) in 2008. With these new regulations, bioprospectors have to conform to the following regulations: 1) Prior informed consent (PIC) has to be sought before any bioprospecting activity can start. This guarantees the consensual agreement of the knowledge holders to share their knowledge. PIC is thus the first step to guarantee that the knowledge holder is informed about the procedures of product research and development. 2) A non-disclosure agreement (NDA) stipulates the confidential treatment of transferred information, and ensures that it is only used for the agreed upon purposes[2]. The knowledge discloser agrees that the respective information will not be disclosed to any other institution. Ownership of the knowledge is at all times vested in the discloser(s). 3) When a product emerges from the disclosed information and material, an ABS agreement has to be negotiated, which acknowledges the value of the shared information and ensures the

---

2   See, for instance, the NDA agreement between the Kukula Healers and the Company Godding & Godding, chapter VII.

redistribution of this value. 4) Finally, a co-patenting agreement is made, with the original knowledge holder having rights to the patent.

From Gift to Commodity Exchange

The objectives of these ABS tools are to prevent biopiracy and allow for the protection of the disclosed knowledge, the knowledge disclosures, the knowledge receivers and the fair sharing of benefits. They also replace traditional forms of knowledge protection, as they were laid out in chapter IV, with new, politically enforced knowledge protection schemes. But the (indigenous) knowledge that is protected under these new protection schemes still contains the values of the ancestral past and the spiritual and healing values of the present. The knowledge, once disclosed and thus opened up for the public, thus comprises both the traditional and the enforced political protection schemes. Both schemes are thus cohesive when ABS is negotiated. This process can be compared to what Anna Tsing claims when she says that a commodity is never a commodity without its pre-commercial status, and that it will always slip in and out of a commercial state:

> Capitalist commodities gain value through conversions from non-capitalist transactions (...) despite the power of capitalism, all capitalist commodities wander in and out of capitalist commodity status. (...). Capitalism always requires non-capitalist social relations to accomplish its goals (...) despite all the apparatus of private property, markets, commodity fetishism, and more, taking the gift out of the commodity is never easy (Tsing 2013: 22ff.).

Hence, in ABS, a commodity-to-be is would never have gotten to the point of commoditization without the pre-commercial status, the actual value of the disclosed knowledge and the exchange system attached to it. As described in chapter IV, the knowledge exchange system in a traditional healers community, predominantly organized along gift exchange principles, happens within the boundaries of the *impande*, with the ancestors serving as moral guides controlling the exchange process. This protective and regulatory space is no longer relevant once the plant material and knowledge are given over to a commodity-oriented and economic value-based system, at least not for the companies or research institutions working with it. This space is basically carved out at the moment of knowledge disclosure to the third party. With the turnover of plants and knowledge to this commercial value system, the plants and knowledge shift to having the status of commodities, and thus further exchange will be organized according to the rules of the economic market.

The transition from gift to commodity exchange therefore entails the cutting out of former social relations and replacing them with political regulations, which stipulate new forms of interaction and engagement between knowledge discloser and knowledge receiver. Social relations do, however, still play a significant role in these new modes of knowledge protection. The plant exchange in Thulamahashe, for instance, illustrates how much the creation of mutual trust between the healers and the K2C committee and Natural Justice was an integral part of the exchange. ABS can thus be regarded as a commodity exchange system that comprises parts of a gift exchange system, with PIC, NDA, ABS and co-patenting acting as political and legal synonyms for securing the values of gift exchange against economic abuse within the commodity exchange system.

The Comaroffs framed this substitution of local legal structures by political and legal instruments using the term *lawfare*, the use of law to achieve political and economic ends (Comaroff 2001; Comaroff and Comaroff 2006: 30f.). Lawfare pushes local communities to "render cultural identity into the language of copyright, sovereignty, and patent" (ibid.). This description makes it sound like everything that is based on the commoditization of property leads to a digestion of cultural traits into the capitalist system. As proposed above, I would rather suggest looking at these processes as synergetic, where local communities adapt to enforced political requirements, but nevertheless aim to keep their own structures alive. Engaging with PIC, NDA, ABS and co-patenting does not automatically lead to the giving up of local legal and political structures.

However, it is the expected economic value of the potential benefits that arouses expectations, hopes, desires and protective measures among the actors involved in bioprospecting (even when, as has been described in the previous chapter, the chance of discovering a new chemical compound, method or cosmetic product is relatively low). In the new political system of post-Apartheid South Africa, the idea flourished that everyone would be able "to speculate and accumulate, to consume, and to indulge repressed desires" (Comaroff and Comaroff 1998: 284). This was stoked by the anticipation that everyone would be able to participate in the wealth and new entrepreneurial enterprises (Comaroff & Comaroff 1999, 2009) promoted by neoliberalism, even though for the vast majority, these hopes would pass them by without offering any visible enrichment (Comaroff & Comaroff 2001). "New situation[s]," Evens-Pritchard wrote in Witchcraft, Oracles and Magic (1937), "demand new magic," and so the new global bioprospecting era aimed to "yield wealth without production, value without efforts" (Comaroff and Comaroff 2000: 313f.), simply by opening up secrets that for millennia had been protected by tradition and customary rituals. Hope and desire to participate is nurtured by the image of the "magical moment" of a "millennial capitalism" that "presents itself as a gospel of salvation: a capitalism that, if rightly harnessed, is invested with the capacity wholly to transform the universe of the marginalized and disempowered" (ibid.: 292)[3].

In the case of bioprospecting, these hopes and desires are wishfully projected onto a field where maybe only one in hundreds of screened medicinal plants may offer a chance for such dreams to come true. An even then, the path remains brittle, as the *Hoodia gordonii* case showed. The salvation promised by financial participation in the big cake of the knowledge economy will for most remain unfulfilled, with such hopes created through potential – but most probably never materialized – ABS agreements. In chapter V, I described the unlikelihood of a plant or plant mixture that is submitted as a claim to the IKS Lead Program ending up in the laboratory. The plant exchange in Thulamahashe, which represents many other similar cases, also shows that the likelihood of getting involved in ABS is very limited. The expectations and hopes rest not only in indigenous communities, but also in the nation state and all other relevant stakeholders working in the field of bioprospecting. But where there is hope, one also finds frustration, disappointment and dead-ends. The following sections illustrate why these hopes so rarely materialize.

What and Where Is 'the Community'?

In an interview conducted at the IKS Lead Program Laboratory, the post-doctoral student Nchinya Bapela (Benni, NB) briefly summarized some of the central challenges and opportunities that ABS agreements bestow on a scientific institution like the IKS Lead Program (as well as other institutions). He was the first to clearly define the difference between a medicinal plant as alienable property and knowledge as inalienable property, and both of their roles in ABS agreements. The focus on knowledge as an inalienable possession inevitably links ABS to IP protection. It is therefore difficult to separate the two:

> **BR:** What is property for you? In terms of plants, do plants belong to anyone?
> **NB:** You see, this is what people are confusing in terms of intellectual property. Property is the knowledge of using that plant. Everyone can see the plant, which is growing there. It is God who put it there. But the knowledge of using that plant for a certain thing, it is if I know something that others don't know, then it is my property. So put, I can't stop you from harvesting [it], but the knowledge for using [it] is my property.
> **BR:** Healers say the knowledge comes from the ancestors. So to whom does knowledge in the end belong?

---

3   This hope can be compared to the hopes projected in millenarianistic movements or cargo cults, where hope was bound to religious leaders or 'white ancestors' bringing goods and messages that would redeem suffering on earth (Cohn 1970; Jebens 2004; Kaplan 1995; Rutert 2010).

NB: Well, if my ancestors give me that knowledge, say of using that medicine for this [problem], don't you think that they are giving that knowledge to me, [it] is my property? The other thing is, if my forefathers give it to me, it means it is my family's property. And that's how property has been passed on from one generation to the other.

BR: But when the same plant grows in the next community as well, then there is a problem because a plant does not grow at one specific place.

NB: Yes, but my community, where I come from, there is somebody or people in the community that had that knowledge of using that plant or this herb and other communities they don't know this. The 'community access' way is not perfect, but [it is] the way they are going to do it in South Africa. Look, if then by 'communities' [it] means putting schools in poor communities and not only giving money, putting infrastructure for them, then it will work.

Benni differentiated between the actual plant material, which basically belongs to the public or to a private landowner, and knowledge, which belongs to the respective knowledge holder(s). ABS mostly involves the intangible property – knowledge – and not so much the tangible property – medicinal plants. With the focus on knowledge in ABS agreements, some initial obstacles appear, including how to identify a community of knowledge holders. According to Benni, the approach initiated by the National Biodiversity Act of 'community-based access', though not perfect due to the difficulties in defining community, is currently the best way to apply ABS in South Africa. What exactly a community is, however, is still only vaguely defined in the act[4]. When a community is finally detected or defines itself as being a knowledge holder – as, for instance, the Masakhane community in the *Pelargonium sidoides* case – another question arises, namely with whom in the community the benefits should be shared? Furthermore, what sort of benefits should be shared, and under what circumstances? Politically, such issues are only vaguely defined. Should communities always claim financial benefits? The Biodiversity

---

4   In the National Biodiversity Act, 'indigenous community' is defined as "any community of people living or having rights or interests in a distinct geographical area within the Republic of South Africa with leadership structures (...)" (NEMBA 2004: 9): www.environment.gov.za/sites/default/files/legislations/nemba_regulations_g30739rg8831gon138.pdf.

Act proposes monetary, non-monetary and 'in kind' benefits[5]. Benni deemed non-monetary benefits (in the form of building schools or hospitals) most appropriate.

In actual ABS negotiations such as the *Hoodia* case, this remains a contested realm. Some communities prefer monetary benefits while others also realize that money is difficult to deal with (among others, some local communities lack the infrastructure to deal with large amounts of money). Communities are, furthermore, oftentimes insufficiently prepared to engage in ABS negotiations, particularly since they are habitually held using highly technical legal language. Also, impoverished communities with low levels of education are commonly unprepared to communally manage a large injection of cash. The unexpected prosperity may end in conflicts and corruption, as Roger Chennels, the lawyer who worked with the San Council on the ABS agreement between them and the Council for Scientific and Industrial Research (CSIR), commented in an article on 'Sharing Benefits Fairly: Decision-Making and Governance' (Wynberg et al. 2009: 231ff.):

> I got buy-in from the San Council (...) but I think it would be fair to say that they were completely in the dark about what was right and what was wrong with regards to intellectual property, so at that stage I had a stronger role than I had [with] modern (sic.) clients, whose leaders are fully aware of everything (...) I am intensely conscious of the fact that a lawyer can easily say that my client has decided when you actually forced them to make that decision (Roger Chennels, Upington 2006, in Wynberg et al. 2009: 240).

Representatives of the San Council commented in a similar tone: "We were sitting there and [had to] rely mostly on our lawyer as we had no knowledge" (ibid.). Indeed, a core issue is that in ABS negotiations, local communities can hardly lead or engage in them without the support of a lawyer or legal institution knowledgeable in this matter. This naturally creates a form of dependency. These lawyers or legal institutions are, in turn, dependent on the demands of the negotiating party. Again Chennels:

> If I could have built up better NGO links and better funding arrangements and all of that it would have been made easier (...) we did not consult enough, we didn't have enough time to talk (...) because it was all was done in a rush. I was forced into a Western system that required very quick answers for the stakeholders –

---

5   According to the National Biodiversity Act (2004), Annex 8, non-monetary, monetary and 'in kind' benefits may include: sharing research results; conservation support; species inventories; student training and support; scientific capacity and development; technology transfers; joint research; information, equipment and infrastructure; access to international collections by South Africans; community development projects; and environmental education (to name but a few) (NEMBA 2004: 59–66): www.environment.gov.za/sites/default/files/legislations/nemba_regulations_g30739rg8831gon138.pdf.

Pfizer [a large pharmaceutical multinational interested in developing and marketing Hoodia] not prepared to go ahead until there was clarity. So, if this thing
was going to be a success for us, we had to reach an agreement quite soon. Yet (...)
there was this whole world of people who had not had the opportunity to understand this collective thing. So more time and more support would have been good
(ibid.: 242).

Whether benefits are monetary or non-monetary was, for Mr. Sechaba, whom I
interviewed in Pretoria in February 2009, less relevant. He was more concerned
with the also prompting question of how benefits may be shared with a community,
especially when a community spreads across national borders. He added a concern
that he had about the government's approach to ABS.

> **BR:** Hmm, and how is the government working with these issues?
> **MS:** I think the way that the government is going about [it] is the Biodiversity Act
> (...). But if things grow [and] cross borders [i.e. when the knowledge holders are
> not bound to a single nation state], whose consent is needed? So, those are the
> issues that I think need to be addressed and you need benefit sharing arrange-
> ments with the communities. But what is a community? You cannot identify the
> communities, so the solution that the government then provides is to set up a na-
> tional trust. You need a permit basically under the Biodiversity Act to do research
> [that leads to] commercialization' research commercialization. So in that way you
> will be able to control it in terms of biopiracy. But you will not be able to stem
> it entirely, because people cross borders, they visit traditional healers, the tradi-
> tional healers can give them a cure, whatever it is.
> **BS:** Is the benefit sharing agreement always negotiated with communities?
> **MS:** Ya, it is stemmed with communities, because traditional knowledge, unlike
> intellectual property, in the traditional sense is not the property of one person.

With the CBD, sovereignty over biodiversity was handed over to nation states, and
it offers no politically manifested rules on how to deal with cross-borders issues. In the *Hoodia* case, the problem was that the San could not be framed as *one*
community, but rather as an ethnic group consisting of different communities
spreading across South Africa, Angola, Namibia and Botswana (Vermeylen 2009).
To make the issue of communities more complicated, a community – or what is
defined as a community – will often have a complex, hierarchical structure, with
chiefs, sub-chiefs and community councils, as well as other authorities such as
church members and other citizens with strong, authoritative voices. Internal conflicts, such as those between the chief and traditional healers, may, for instance,
cause differences about the distribution of funds, in the event that such funds ever
reach the community.

Obviously, ABS, though a well-meant initiative to appropriately share benefits, is not easy to apply in practice. The problems begin with the application process for bioprospecting, which, with the commencement of the Biodiversity Act, became administratively strenuous and politically thorny. The challenges that come with ABS reach into all corners of bioprospecting, as the remainder of the chapter will show. In most cases, the exchange of knowledge hardly ever reaches the point of an ABS agreement. PIC and an NDA may be negotiated, but the negotiations will hardly ever go further. Given such a low success rate and lack of certainty, is ABS even really worth consideration as a tool for local and national development? Examples of stakeholders and institutions grappling with ABS will show, that the answers are as ambivalent as the field of ABS, where hope interchanges with disillusion. I will start with describing the challenges coming with ABS in the scientific realm.

Science in Distress:
Navigating Spurious Inventions

In 2009, bioprospecting legislation in South Africa posed severe difficulties for scientific institutions during the discovery phase, particularly with regard to ABS[6]. The problem was not the sharing of benefits alone, but the protection of scientific knowledge and research results that comprise indigenous knowledge. Although research and development activities are taxing with regard to time and money, and thus require appropriate protection via intellectual property law (in the form of patents), when indigenous knowledge is involved in scientific inventions it too cannot be ignored, and intellectual property law and patents are insufficient in this regard. This poses a fundamental question about how to identify the knowledge that should be protected with regard to scientific inventions, and how. Again Nchinya Bapela (Benni, NB) at the IKS Laboratory illustrated for me the implications of these challenges:

> **NB:** (...) you're doing research on this and you patent the stuff. So if you patent it, you patent the stuff you want to do further research on and you don't want other people to know what you are doing. Once you publish, it is for public consumption. And anybody who comes across will say, I can do this for this and this and this and they will beat you [to it]. This is one of the reasons why the IKS is not publishing. This work is not meant for publication. Pharmaceutical companies also don't

---

6   In a follow-up conversation in March 2012, Dr. Matsabisa told me that the law had changed and that basic research institutions no longer not had to get involved in ABS. According to the new law, only those institutions and companies that deal with the commoditization of the product have to engage in ABS agreements.

publish their work. You don't go to journals and find their publications, unless it's been done by an accreditation institution. (...)

BR: So, do you think the protection of [indigenous] knowledge is necessary?

NB: I think intellectual property should be protected. If you go to, say, to a German company and they make weapons and they (...) want to be the sole suppliers [of those weapons] and protect the knowledge, or [a] KFC recipe, because that knowledge gives them money to survive. Now, if our knowledge makes other people rich and we keep staying poor, that's useless. That's why we need to protect [knowledge holders]. (...) Personally, I think it is more important to protect the knowledge holders. So for me, doing that type of work [scientific analysis of medicinal plants], I am not really the knowledge holder. I mean, I get paid. Those people who provide the knowledge, they don't get paid. I can live a better life than the person who gave me that knowledge.

Benni asserted that intellectual property should be protected. He did stress that scientific inventions also require protection, but according to him, it should be less the scientific knowledge and more the knowledge holders that should be protected. This is also because the knowledge holder(s), in case he/she or they are of indigenous origin, are generally (financially) disadvantaged.

Sharing and Protecting 'Property' at the Medical Research Council

The Innovation Center (IC) is a special unit at the MRC established to process MRC patent applications. The IC has the assignment to "drive innovation opportunities emanating from MRC research discovery so as to commercialize and implement sustainable health technologies for the benefits of the MRC, the inventors and society in general". It is responsible for the identification of research with commercial potential and/or social value, for providing assistance and advice to MRC researchers on various intellectual property related issues, for the marketing and licensing of intellectual property, and for developing and implementing policies, procedures and systems for effective intellectual property management and technology transfer. In an interview with Michelle Mulder, manager of intellectual property and business development at the IC in August 2009, she briefly summarized the core challenges of IPR provision and in particular addressed issues regarding the interface between traditional knowledge and intellectual property:

Look, combining the two worlds of traditional knowledge, including cosmologies, spirituality, on the one hand, and science, and its very own construction of reality, on the other hand, is a very difficult task. The challenge is to meet the different needs of all stakeholders in legal policies and regulations. At least one of the involved parties might always feel neglected. (...) Also, the process of intellectual property rights and benefit sharing in bioprospecting is still very young. Things still have to be balanced out. The whole process basically only started in mid-2000. One has to consider that plant analysis and extraction of active pharmaceutical substances is a highly cost-intense and time-consuming process. It can take years to really find a valuable component and the investments often remain without any output and success. The question [of] how to share benefits arising from this long-lasting process ends in the unresolved questions: what, in a 'fair' benefit sharing [agreement], is fair, and what isn't?

Dr. Matsabisa underpinned Mulder's argument during a conversation we had at the IKS Lead Program in August 2009. He explained, "There is no comprehensive intellectual property regulation with regard to indigenous knowledge. Also, so far, we have no fully developed access and benefit sharing case in South Africa, apart from the *Hoodia* case." Research at the IKS Laboratory was at that time still in its infancy and was at not at the point of filing a patent[7]. However, at the time of our conversation, he was nevertheless curious about the question of how to appropriately share the benefits of upcoming research results.

He presented an interesting case to me. A *muthi* mixture that was under investigation at the IKS Laboratory consisted of a combination of four plants derived from different parts of South Africa. The knowledge holder who shared the mixture with the IKS Lead Program originally came from Kenya, but had been living in South Africa for 10 years, until his death in 2006. He did not have any known heirs nor could a community be located where the knowledge of the plant mixture had initially come from. Against this background, Dr. Matsabisa asked, how and with whom should the benefits that may accrue from this plant mixture be shared? Dr. Matsabisa asked me to think about the problem and offer a solution in the form of a PowerPoint presentation in a few days' time. His request astounded me. I could hardly follow the complexity of the stakeholders and interests that he was presenting in the illustration, and I am not a lawyer concerned with intellectual property law and ABS agreements. From what I understood I was not at all qualified to present 'solutions' for how to determine a fair and appropriate benefit sharing agreement for a complicated problem that an entire unit at the MRC was engaged with. What his request did demonstrate to me though was that ABS poses a significant problem for scientific institutions that only do basic research.

---

7   A patent on *Dicoma anomala* was filled in 12 countries 2005 on the "Treatment of parasitic Infections in humans and animals" by Dr. Matsabisa, William Ernst Campell, Peter Ian Folb and Peter John Smith (all Cape Town), see: http://patents.justia.com/inventor/motlalepula-gilbert-matsabisa. The research on *Dicoma anomala* was continued and released a patent claim for *Dicoma anomala* as a novel therapeutic against malaria: http://innovation.mrc.ac.za/malaria.pdf (last accessed February 12, 2016).

I assumed that the case Dr. Matsabisa presented to me was for PHELA, the plant mixture on which Brian Sehume was conducting research. Perhaps further research would lead to the finding that PHELA contained viable antimalarial properties. But this remained an assumption on my part; Dr. Matsabisa maintained the rules of anonymization and did not reveal the names of the plants about which the illustration spoke. According to the illustration the plants came from different parts of South Africa (North Western and Limpopo Province), and beyond (Swaziland and Lesotho). The illustration roughly illustrated the estimated distributed percentages of the benefits deriving from the production of a 4mg capsule of the plant mixture. Fifty percent of the profits should go to the communities and 50% to the MRC. The 50% meant for the community would be allocated and redistributed by a national trust fund. Commonly, 5–10% of this money ought to go to the knowledge provider, usually the community of a knowledge provider. Of the 50% set for the MRC, one-third should go to the investor who paid for the research and development, one-third to the MRC and one-third to the IKS Lead Program. As was explained before, when a mixture consists of four plants from different regions of South Africa, or from other African or non-African countries, the question of how to share the benefits becomes complicated, in particular when the focus of the South African government so far is on sharing with a community. Benefit sharing with a community is only possible when ownership is clearly defined, which was not the case in the illustration.

The illustration exemplifies why ABS so rarely turns out to be an applicable solution. Firstly, the distribution of benefits is, politically speaking, still not clearly defined. The illustration offered a vague summary of possible distributive measures, not a thought through solution. Secondly, the many stakeholders involved make distribution very convoluted. When distribution is so complex, the likelihood of some stakeholders being unsatisfied is very high. A simplified approach like a national trust fund may offer a better way of distributing funds. Thirdly, at no point did the illustration take into consideration the value of inalienable possessions; that is, the cultural and social value of the intellectual property. It was purely interested in the distribution of financial revenue. This, however, posed a key problem. The original knowledge holder had died and a community was not detectable. The plants, furthermore, had no clearly definable place of origin. Hence all of the measures proposed by the National Biodiversity Act to ensure an appropriate ABS agreement were inapplicable. Dr. Matsabisa never came back to me to ask for the PowerPoint presentation offering my proposed solutions. And indeed, I actually could not see any solution for the complex case for which, even on a political level, there seemed to be no sufficient answers.

Databases: A Possible Solution?

One possible solution to protect knowledge, and that has been applied in many countries, is to set up medicinal plant databases (Gupta 2005; Reddy 2006). Databases might be a useful tool since when ABS agreements are negotiated, the origin of the discussed knowledge must be provable. As the above illustration showed, proof is not always easy, especially when knowledge is largely undocumented and only orally transferred, as it is in many African countries. If the knowledge was documented in a database, this would constitute a useful resource for those attempting to set up an ABS agreement[8]. National patent offices could scan these databases for already existing or new knowledge.

According to Reddy (2006), databases in this context involve the process of "writing, codifying, translating, or digitizing a tradition (and the making of cultural objects)" (Reddy 2006: 163; see also 2008; Bowker & Star 2000, Foucault 2002 [1966]). In China and India, databases such as the Indian Traditional Knowledge Digital Library (TKDL) have a long tradition, also because of the fact that plant-related knowledge has been documented over centuries (Reddy 2006: 162ff.). Ownership can, in this instance, be more easily defined. Much hope and work is put into such documentation projects, which are also aimed at ensuring security of the knowledge. It is, however, not always an uncontroversial undertaking. Questions such as "What kind of data is fed into databases and what is cut out?" or "How far do indigenous people have rights over the knowledge once it is fed into a database?" are pertinent. Mr. Sechaba also critically reflected on the idea of knowledge protection in databases:

> **BR:** But, ya, there must be a means of protection in the globalized world.
> **MS:** Ya, but you see, that would be partly protected by the Biodiversity Act because it is plant material that leaves the country, so therefore they need an export license or permit. But then in terms of the mixtures, that's where the Indians talk about databases. They put together databases. South Africa is talking about databases as well.
> **BR:** Ya, they started a database project already.
> **MS:** But databases do not provide protection. They say they provide protection against biopiracy, because then those databases are made available to the patent offices round the world and when they do novel research they can be able to follow up on these things and they say 'No, you cannot get a patent for this because it is already in databases'.

---

8   The lack of documented or written knowledge in turn poses a challenge, however, for those attempting to set up such a database.

In South Africa, the idea to attempt to protect knowledge via databases was realized with the Traditional Medicine Database (TRAMED), started in 1994. The University of Cape Town's Traditional Medicines Research Program in the Department of Pharmacology and the University of the Western Cape implemented the database. To this day, TRAMED aims to assemble and archive traditional medicinal plants and indigenous knowledge to ensure their long-term accessibility to the public – for scientific research, the pharmaceutical industry and traditional healers – without being confronted with claims of biopiracy. It is also intended to serve as a measure against decreasing biological resources and the loss of indigenous knowledge.

TRAMED was also designed with the plan to include the knowledge of traditional healers, making them equal partners in contributing to the database. At the beginning, traditional healers were invited to share and publish their knowledge in support of TRAMED, enticing them with promises of shared benefits in the event that bioprospecting would lead to successful developments. The cooperation resulted in the publication of the 'Traditional Healers' Primary Care Book' (Felhaber 1997; see Flint 2012: 260). For most contributing healers, however, the knowledge they offered that was fed into TRAMED remained unrewarded, as one of the participating healers, Philip Kubukeli, resentfully told me during an interview in Cape Town in February 2010. The ownership of the knowledge also basically rests in the database itself and those who organize it, not in the healers, even though the knowledge belongs to the healers. This has led to frictions between contributing healers and scientists, and ended in the refusal of some healers to further contribute to the database (Flint 2012).

In this context, TRAMED has been criticized by the US-based group 'People's Health Alliance Rejecting Medical Authoritarianism, Prejudice And Conspiratorial Tyranny' (PHARMAPACT) for illegitimately disclosing local knowledge. The group disseminated the concern about a traditional medicine sell-out (Reihling 2008: 5) by publishing a long letter in 1999 to Dr. Isaac Mayeng, who was the Senior Medicines Control Officer at the Medicines Control Council of the Department of Health at the time. The letter began: "Say NO! To the Tyranny of Monopolistic PHARMACEUTICAL EXPLOITATION of Natural Health Substances"[9]. It was an outcry against biopiracy and the illegitimate use of databases without the appropriate integration of knowledge holders. The Nyanga Traditional Healers Organization for Africa also openly expressed their discomfort over TRAMED. On their webpage they claim "scientific institutions, such as the University of Cape Town's TRAMED project seek access to traditional medicine knowledge for the primary purpose of developing

---

9   www.gaiaresearch.co.za/pharmapact/Mayeng%20Dec%2099.pdf (last accessed October 20, 2014).

profitable products"[10]. They announced their position in an article on their website entitled 'Biodiversity and Intellectual Property Rights – Implications for Indigenous People of South Africa':

> (...) once indigenous peoples share traditional health information or plant material they effectively lose control over those resources, regardless of whether or not they are compensated. If formulas using traditional medicine knowledge are eventually patented, access to these cost effective and freely available materials can be legally restricted by monopoly patents and registrations by means of registering health claim benefits. The current South African Medicines, and Medical Devices Act (SAMMDRA) and it's (sic.) regulations will empower the bio-pirates (sic.) and not the people, as the healers have not got the technical or financial resources to enter the playing field of traditional medicine production which should be their right. No matter what the circumstances, indigenous communities must have the right to say "no" to bio-pirates and legitimate bio-prospectors (...) Many healers are now joining in a new struggle to preserve their cultural integrity and are actively canvassing for support in holting (sic.) the expropriation of natural health substances by the pharmaceutical industry, the Medicine Control Authority, TRAMED, and the WHO[11].

With 29,000 members, the Nyanga Traditional Healers Organization for Africa is one of the largest in the country, and they are probably the most influential healers' association in South Africa. Dr. Maseko, former CEO of the organization, and his daughter Phepsile Maseko, now the National Coordinator, are strong public voices fighting for the rights of traditional healers in South Africa. The organization targeted Dr. Mayeng in particular, accusing him of being actively involved in traditional medicine research at TRAMED without adequately informing and supporting traditional healers. Dr. Mayeng, who in 2009 had become director of the Traditional Medicine Unit at the Department of Health, is trained as both a traditional healer and a pharmacologist. He previously worked at the Department of Pharmacology at the University of Cape Town and was, among others, co-responsible for the initiation of TRAMED. On their website, the Nyanga Traditional Healers Organization for Africa write:

> Dr. Mayeng is known by our organization as a "biopirate", because he has been actively involved in traditional medicine research at the University of Cape Town's Traditional Medicines Research Project (TRAMED). This specialized research de-

10   www.traditionalhealth.org.za/t/documents/biodiversity_and_intellectual_property_rights_
      02.html(last accessed January 25, 2016).
11   www.traditionalhealth.org.za/t/documents/biodiversity_and_intellectual_property_rights_
      02.html (last accessed July 14, 2014).

partment have (sic.) been actively screening our regions (sic.) traditional plants for potential drug development, under the auspices of anti-malarial research[12].

This was the second time that I encountered serious accusations made against Dr. Mayeng by traditional healers. When I interviewed him in his office at the Department of Health in Pretoria in 2009, however, he seemed very considerate and concerned about his profession, traditional healing, and about the protection of medicinal plants and indigenous knowledge. During the interview, which was short and felt that it remained somewhat superficial, Dr. Mayeng assured me: "Look, I am a healer myself and I believe in the power of traditional healing. I do everything within my power as the director of the National Department of Health to support traditional healers and their needs" (from interview, Pretoria, October 2009). Despite this, it would appear that his peers view him more as a politician and scientist who "is working on both sides".

Databases like TRAMED, or the knowledge documentation project initiated by the World Intellectual Property Organization (WIPO 2012)[13], comprise certain aspects of traditional knowledge, but leave out most of the ontological, spiritual and socio-cultural background to the knowledge. WIPO tries to overcome this by adding visual material such as video, photo and audio documentation like narratives, stories and descriptions to the documentation process.[14] The objective and benefit of the NRS is, according to the CSIR, to create opportunities "for benefits to flow back to the communities," in the form of community recognition, sustainable livelihoods, economic value and improved quality of life.

The crux of indigenous knowledge protection remains that knowledge that is collectively held, is embedded in a socio-cultural and spiritual context, and is continuously changing. Databases can only fix a very particular part of this knowledge and has to leave out most others. Therefore, I suggest, and in agreement with Mr. Sechaba, that indigenous knowledge protection requires not one but multiple means of protection. Instead of abolishing the idea of databases, other measures of protection should be added, in particular those that deal with the socio-cultural value of indigenous knowledge. Databases are a defensive protection tool that enables scientists to scan already existing data, partly in order to check whether the knowledge has already been patented or not. These defensive measures of protection then have to be complimented by proactive measures of knowledge protection,

---

12   See: www.traditionalhealth.org.za/t/documents/biodiversity_and_intellectual_property_ rights_02.html (last accessed July 14, 2014).

13   See: World Intellectual Property Organization (2012): The World Intellectual Property Organization Traditional Knowledge Documentation Toolkit (www.wipo.int/export/sites/ www/tk/en/resources/pdf/tk_toolkit_draft.pdf).

14   With the 'National Recordal System' (NRS) launched in 2013, South Africa is trying to put this documentation scheme into practice.

one being ABS agreements, where the specific knowledge of knowledge holders is legally protected. The example of TRAMED and the 'Traditional Healers' Primary Care Book' showed, however, that while this is an interesting approach on paper, it is rather controversial in reality. According to Phepsile Maseko and the Nyanga Traditional Healers Organization for Africa, PHARMAPACT and others, the promised benefits never materialized.

This was at least the case at the beginning of the 2000s. In the year 2009, however, it seemed that the situation had progressed. The ABS workshop that I attended in Cape Town, which I will describe in the next section, and other similar workshops and conferences – such as a workshop on the Traditional Knowledge Commons in Cape Town in March 2012 (see chapter VII) and the Third Global Congress on Intellectual Property and the Public Interest and Open A.I.R. Conference on Innovation and IP in Africa in Cape Town in December 2013, to name but a few – demonstrate the global and national relevance of the subject and the hope for development, that comes with ABS. The next section will look at the ABS workshop in particular, also to show that ABS does have relevance with regard to the proposal of ABS being an issue of national and local development.

ABS – Three Letters for Development?

Coming back to the question whether ABS does have an impact factor for development, the answer must provisionally be yes, at least when looking at the efforts put into the development of ABS. Knowledge protection and benefit sharing has become a significant 'market of hope' (Rutert 2010) promoted by several large global networks. One such network is the ABS Capacity Development Initiative, begun in 2006 and managed by the Deutsche Gesellschaft für Technische Zusammenarbeit (GTZ, now Deutsche Gesellschaft für International Zusammenarbeit, GIZ), which has as its core focus on the question of "how to harness and make use of the moment of knowledge disclosure and ABS for local development and poverty alleviation"[15]. In this context, innovation in Africa is regarded as a central part of pushing development forward. How to protect these innovations and how to share the benefits that may arise from these innovations is crucial in this context.

An online report from 2010, under the headline "Southern Africa: Region Failing to Innovate, Says Study,"[16] cited a study conducted by the United Nations Educational, Scientific and Cultural Organization (UNESCO) that concluded that "Countries in southern Africa are producing so few scientific publications and patents that

---

15   See: www.abs-initiative.info.
16   "Southern Africa failing to innovate, says study", August 13, 2010 (www.scidev.net/global/policy/news/southern-africa-failing-to-innovate-says-study-1.html).

[the] region's social and economic progress is threatened" (Campell 2010, citing UNESCO 2010, cited in de Beer et al. 2014: 6). Scientific publications and patents are generally taken as a sign of innovation and development. The more patents a country owns, the more innovative and developed it is seen to be. But is it really as simple as this? The huge, economically strong companies of the Global North hold most of the patents worldwide because they can afford the expensive production and patenting procedures (cf. Robinson 2010; Shiva 1997, 2007). In addition, innovation is not measurable by patents alone, as if a patent was an innovation currency, but rather by the mere fact that something new has been developed – a process that often happens not in laboratories but 'on the ground'. And this innovation on the ground was realized as having huge potential as a means of local development, when properly harnessed.

An ABS Training Course in Cape Town

The challenges and potentials of ABS, and its importance as a developmental tool for the African continent, were intensively discussed during an ABS training course entitled 'Training Course in Access and Benefit Sharing from Genetic Resources and Associated Traditional Knowledge' that I attended on January 24–29, 2010 at the stylish Breakwater Lodge Waterfront in Cape Town. The foreword of the Course Manual and Resource Book made the following proposition: "ABS – THREE LETTERS FOR DEVELOPMENT." This was both directive and assertive; setting a clear imperative for the idea that ABS will benefit national and local development. The GTZ ABS Capacity Development Initiative and the Environmental Evaluation Unit of the University of Cape Town hosted the workshop. The participants were primarily from the African continent, with the exception of myself and a researcher from the Northern Research Institute in Norway, who came together to discuss the current legal and political situation of ABS and (indigenous) knowledge protection. In total, 37 delegates from southern and eastern African governments, NGOs and the private sector – including the South African Department of Environmental Affairs and Tourism (DEAT), the Namibian Ministry of Environment & Tourism, the Tanzanian Commission of Science and Technology, and the Southern Alliance for Indigenous Resources in Zimbabwe – were present to learn about ABS and take the message back home to their countries[17]. The overall aim was not only to discuss local challenges but also to put larger developmental goals into perspective and thus contribute to a greater balance of justice between North and South. The ABS Capacity Development Initiative's website describes the potential of the CBD and ABS as having been 'carved in stone' with the adoption of the Nagoya Protocol:

---

17   The ABS training course was also offered in Ghana for western African countries and Cairo for northern African countries.

This international agreement is without doubt a major milestone in the efforts to ensure justice in the protection and sustainable use of biological and genetic resources worldwide. It is also well integrated into the global context of sustainable development: reaching the Millennium Development Goals (MDGs), ensuring food security, supporting the emergence of a Green Economy and establishing North-South Justice[18] (cf. Maister et al. 2012).

The overall consensus of the training workshop was that Africa, against common images of it being underdeveloped, poverty stricken and war torn, has a lot of creativity and innovation to offer, which only has to be properly valuated and harnessed. The workshop was thus constructed as an awareness-raising event to introduce the stakeholders to the concepts and principles, challenges and opportunities, of ABS. The four days were packed with presentations on international and national ABS regimes and policy frameworks in specific African countries, the legal specificities of ABS, the role of indigenous knowledge for ABS and its legal and customary protection schemes, and finally the ABS negotiation process. Experts working in the field gave various presentations, including Kabir Bavikatte from the NGO Natural Justice, who presented biocultural community protocols (BCPs); Roger Chennels, a lawyer who presented the ABS negotiations pertaining to the *Hoodia* case; and the IKS Lead Program Director Dr. Matsabisa, who introduced the IKS Lead Program. Scholars working in the field of bioprospecting also gave presentations. Finally, representatives of communities who had been involved in ABS negotiations were invited to present their experiences; in this case, a representative of the Masakhane community in Alice in the Eastern Cape spoke on their successful challenge to the patenting of *Pelargonium sidoides*.

The atmosphere among the participants was intellectually stimulating and fact oriented. The workshop was concerned with teaching the participants about ABS, content that they had not known previously or only to a limited degree. ABS legislation was, in most African countries, still in its infancy (in South Africa, it had only existed since 2004) and had not yet been fully incorporated into national application schemes. Controversial opinions were, generally speaking, not discussed as conflictive but as explanatory. Only Phepsile Maseko, the strong-minded and straightforward National Coordinator of the Nyanga Traditional Healers Organization for Africa, announced her discomfort with regard to the cooperation between science and traditional healers, as well as the restrictions that the National Biodiversity Act places on traditional healers with regard to accessing their natural plant collection grounds[19]. Maseko also raised the controversial issue that traditional healers were,

---

18   www.abs-initiative.info/abs-simply-explained/ (last accessed February 15, 2019).
19   An example of this arose during my fieldwork when I visited a *thwasa* (trainee healer) in Mboyti in 2009. He said that healers were no longer allowed to collect plants in the near-

due to the National Biodiversity Act, being restricted from performing traditional healing in the "traditional way", i.e. because they are prevented from collecting medicinal plants in nature reserves or other fenced-up areas. She vehemently proposed the right of healers to participate in nature conservation as well as in science. Later, after Dr. Matsabisa's presentation, Maseko assertively held that "Traditional healers' associations are not integrated in research and development of medicinal plant products and the inclusion of knowledge into databases." Dr. Matsabisa in return announced: "It is true that the MRC has been negligent towards traditional healers in the past. That may have been for the fact that the structures of healers' organizations are not transparent enough. This lack of transparency makes it virtually impossible to approach the relevant healers". Over lunch, Maseko told me "Science does not care about us healers. They only want the knowledge to extend their research and find new products." This short argument between Phepsile Maseko and Dr. Matsabisa illustrates the link between the (lack of) inclusion of knowledge holders and the production of knowledge in bioprospecting, and the fact that inclusion is not automatically applied in the way it is politically claimed. What is missing is a regular monitoring system to control the application of ABS.

These issues were brought up again the following day, when the whole delegation visited the IKS Laboratory in Delft, where traditional healers and scientists presented themselves and their cooperation at the laboratory. The reflections of the workshop participants on this meeting expressed how they had perceived the position of traditional healers at the IKS Lead Program. One participant said, "I could not really see why traditional healers were at the laboratory, besides looking nice and representative." Another participant claimed, "The group of scientists looked as if they don't acknowledge the role of traditional knowledge. From what they said, I could see a bit of dishonesty. It made me feel there is a lot of mistrust among the people." A third voice was annoyed: "You see, when the government puts these policies into place but does not monitor them, they are useless. And also, the MRC is not explicit on how much to share with the traditional healers and how much the company receives, so there is a continuous exploitation of knowledge." ABS was generally perceived as being only superficially monitored, and this was synthesized as one of the main problems facing its successful implementation.

The training course ended with a book presentation of 'Indigenous Peoples, Consent and Benefit Sharing' (Wynberg et al. 2009) at the Kirstenbosch Botanical Garden, and the presentation of the Masakhane community representative who discussed the history of the *Pelargonium sidoides* case. Moreover, Uli Feiter, the director of the medicinal plants and pharmaceutical company Parceval, presented his

---

by forest because nature conservation efforts had restricted access (from interview, Mboyti, October 2009).

perspective on ABS, which was a bit more provocative. He asserted, "ABS is a highly emotional subject, which at times gets out of hand." He also complained:

> It is often repeated that huge pharmaceutical drug giants [are] exploiting rural African communities, which in fact is not the reality, but rather an emotionally charged narrative. It takes lots of effort to take the emotions out of the debate. In the end, the field of medicinal plants is a business.

He then continued:

> The problem remains the definition of community. I chose to closely cooperate with a community in the Eastern Cape, which approached me to start a business on Pelargonium. We signed an ABS agreement with the community and they installed a trust to share benefits. The process is still pending, especially because the ministry (of Water and Environmental Affairs) is slow in approving the papers.

Both, the reactions to the visit at the IKS Laboratory and Uli Feiter's approach to dealing with the 'emotionally charged' field of ABS reveal how contentious and uncertain the field still is. Training courses introduce people to the complexities of the ABS landscape and to its contradictory and emotionally charged application. This contextualization helps stakeholders to implement policies in their own countries, especially those where ABS has not yet been (adequately) implemented. Courses such as the one I attended would not be offered without the belief that ABS holds opportunities for local and national development. The course was surely also meant to close the gap between the ABS rhetoric and the realities on the ground. But still, in 2009 obstacles and challenges pave the way towards fair and equitable benefit sharing, with most of the challenges deriving from restrictive ABS legislation and its application, as the next section – which gives voice to traders working with medicinal plants, and a *Hoodia* Task Force Group meeting, in particular regarding their problems in applying ABS – will show.

People and Plants in Action

South African commercial plant traders are bioprospectors, and as such they are affected by bioprospecting legislation. They cultivate medicinal plants in order to manufacture them in their own factories and/or to supply bigger companies overseas. The medicinal plants and pharmaceutical company Parceval, for instance, situated in Wellington in the Western Cape, cultivates *Pelargonium sidoides* in the Eastern Cape, which it then either manufactures in Wellington or delivers to the German company Schwabe in Germany. This commercial business differs from that of petty traders and so-called '*muthi* hunters' in terms of the size of the business, and very often skin color. All of the commercial plant traders whom I spoke to were white businessmen, while *muthi* hunters are mostly black and engage in the illegal collection of the barks, roots and leaves of medicinal plants to supply the big *muthi* markets in Johannesburg and Durban. The National Biodiversity Act mandates that bioprospecting activities must be permitted by the Department of Environmental Affairs (DEA)[20] and that the bioprospecting rules and regulations have to be maintained at all times[21]. Not upholding these rules is punished by five years' imprisonment (ten years for second offences) and/or a fine not exceeding 5 Million Rand (10 Million Rand for second offences) (Section 98(2) of NEMBA 2004). The benefits may be shared either monetarily or non-monetarily, e.g. providing support to build schools, hospitals or other infrastructure, as well as promoting employment and business opportunities, depending on the parties' agreement. Politically, this sounds like a reasonable approach to bioprospecting. Practically, it unleashes a number of new challenges.

"It's an Awful Lot of Work": Trading Under the ABS Legislation

One of the traders I spoke to was Uli Feiter, the CEO of Parceval. Uli, a trained gardener from Germany, came to South Africa in the 1980s and established the small-scale company as a manufacturer of herbal, homeopathic and natural medicines in 1992. Over many years, Uli taught himself about South African medicinal plants. His company grew larger and eventually became one of the most successful medicinal plant manufacturing companies in South Africa. In an interview that I conducted with him in August 2009 in his office in Wellington, he expressed his concerns about the current South African ABS legislation, as well as his own thoughts on how to survive in this competitive market, which had become more problematic since the promulgation of the CBD and the National Biodiversity Act:

BR: What roles do international organizations and regulations, such as the CBD und the Biodiversity Act, play for you? What position does the commercial sector

---

20   See NEMBA Chapter 6, Section 81(1): "A person may not without a permit engage in commercialization phase of bioprospecting involving IBRs [indigenous biological resources] or export IBRs for bioprospecting or any other kind of research"; and Section 81A: "No person may without first notifying the Minister engage in discovery phase bioprospecting involving any IBR; and a person involved in the discovery phase of bioprospecting must sign a commitment to comply with the requirements of the commercialisation phase of bioprospecting", see: Malherbe C. (2011): Bioprospecting, Access & Benefit Sharing in South Africa, Marrakech (www.abs-initiative.info/uploads/media/Marrakech_ 01-2011_Malherbe.pdf).

21   www.abs-initiative.info/fileadmin/media/Knowledge_Center/Pulications/ABS_Dialogue_042 014/National_study_on_ABS_implementation_in_South_Africa_20140716.pdf (last accessed January 10, 2016).

represent here?

UF: Since the CBD was introduced, working with indigenous medicinal plants became much more difficult. One permanently has to take care of regulations and political requirements. Filling out paperwork and signing lots of documents. It is an awful lot of work. I did try to oppose these regulations, in meetings and workshops, but nobody listened.

BR: And how should a functioning access and benefit sharing agreement look?

UF: The problem is that [indigenous] people think that they have a true treasure chest into which they only have to grab and immediately there is big business. Of course they want to be part of the business made with medicinal plants. However, they do not consider the high costs it takes to produce a commercially valuable product: time, knowledge and knowhow, materials, money. A safety study could easily cost 50,000 Euros. And even then, no benefits are made. It can take several million Euros for a product to really be on the market. Who can pay that, besides Merck or Pfizer? And finally, who can deal with the administration of these products, particularly the complicated administration demanded by the government? Only the big companies will be able to financially maintain the administrative process. My solution would be to think smaller, to find a niche. Why must we always strive to achieve the best and the most? Everyone believes in finding a cure for HIV/AIDS or cancer, particularly for products that are interesting for the European market. I think it is much more useful to find products for the African market, e.g. something that helps to sooth edema, a classic side condition of HIV/AIDS. Why not find an affordable cream for the market here? I think small traders like us can help to loosen up the monopolization of the big companies (Wellington, August 2009).

The requirements of NEMBA and BABS include not only tedious negotiation processes with the respective communities, but also lots of administrative paperwork with the Department of Agriculture and Environmental Affairs. Often, applications remain for a long time on the desk of the administrator or minister who has to approve and sign all bioprospecting applications. This procedure is laborious and keeps small companies away from bioprospecting activities due to a lack of time and/or human and financial resources, a fact that is mostly unknown by the providers of knowledge. For them, their own ideas about benefit sharing, evoked by ABS politics, stand in the foreground. Uli, understandably angry, claimed that the new ABS legislation evokes ideas in indigenous people of simply being able to grab into their "treasure chest" of medicinal plants to release "gold" or "green diamonds" (Wynberg & Chennels 2009). As a plant trader with commercial interests, Uli knows about the challenges that the medicinal plant trade ultimately faces: costs, time and huge competition on the market, especially from the larger 'Big Pharma' companies such as Pfizer. His solution for a small company like Parceval rests in finding a niche, like the production of an affordable cream for the treatment of side effects of HIV/AIDS. Such a medication is probably not as profitable as the 'green diamonds' to treat the world's major diseases, but it would still help people in need.

> We have a sort of benefit sharing agreement with the community in the Eastern Cape, where we currently run a Pelargonium plantation site. But I am neither a development worker nor a social worker. I am a gardener and a businessman. So again, the CBD made everything much more complicated for us (Wellington, August 2009).

Pelargonium sidoides (Geraniceae) is a medicinal plant native to South Africa. It has heart-shaped velvety leaves and a deep purple flower. The medicinally valuable parts of the plant are the thick tubers, which, when extracted, expel the tincture known as *Umckaloabo*® (the name *Umckaloabo* stems from the isiXosa word *ukuhlaba*, meaning "to stab" or "stabbing pain," but is also translated as "heavy cough") (Brendler & van Wyk 2008). The indigenous population of the Eastern Cape and Lesotho have used the plant extract for many centuries against respiratory infections, gastrointestinal problems and ear infections. The plant found its way to Europe via Charles Stevens, who travelled to Lesotho in 1897 to find a cure for his tuberculosis. A Zulu medicine man residing in Lesotho gave him a boiled root preparation containing *Pelargonium* to drink twice a day (Bladt & Wagner 2007). Stevens took the plant back home to England, where he unsuccessfully tried to merchandize it as Stevens' Cure. Years later, in the 1920s, the French-Swiss physician Adrien Sechehaye started using Stevens' Cure to successfully treat TB patients. Then in the 1960s, the plant was eventually analyzed at the University of Munich, and in the 1990s *Umckaloabo*® was finally trademarked by the German company Schwabe, which produces and markets the product (Brendler & van Wyk 2008).

Due to its medicinal value, *Pelargonium sidoides* was extensively harvested in the Eastern Cape and Lesotho, mostly to supply Schwabe. The plant collecting practices in the Eastern Cape – mostly undertaken by vastly underpaid plant collectors (who earned 2–4 Rand, 1–2 Euros, per Kilo) – led to over-harvesting and the near extinction of the plant in the Eastern Cape region, until the Eastern Cape government placed a temporary ban on the harvesting and export of *Pelargonium sidoides* in the wild. For many (female) plant gatherers, collecting plants is their main source of income (Lewu et al. 2006), and small suppliers are highly dependent on much larger buyers (van Niekerk & Wynberg 2013). Illegal harvesting has been prohibited since the introduction of the National Biodiversity Act, but it is still an everyday practice.

The Schwabe company, which is still retailing the respiratory infection medicine Umckaloabo® successfully today, appointed two patents at the European Patent Office in June 2007, one on 'Method for Producing Extracts of Pelargonium sidoides and/or Pelargonium reniforme' (EP 1429795) and the other for exclusive use of 'Pelargonium sidoides and Pelargonium reiforme for treating AIDS and AIDS re-lated diseases' (W 2006002837). In 2008, these patents were challenged by three NGOs – the African Centre for Biosafety in South Africa, Der Evangelischer Ent-wicklungsdienst (EED) based in Germany and the Swiss-based Berne Declaration – in cooperation with the Masakhane community in Alice in the Eastern Cape. The basis for the challenge was, they claimed, that Schwabe had not conformed to the international regulations of the CBD and the South African National Biodiversity Act. Schwabe had not sought prior informed consent to use Pelargonium sidoides and had not agreed upon a material transfer agreement with the community. Schwabe eventually withdrew the patents to avoid the stigma of biopiracy. The Pelargonium sidoides case is one of the few bioprospecting cases in South Africa where a local community, supported by national and international NGOs, was able to dispute a patent.

Beyond these more challenging aspects of bioprospecting, there is, in addition to empowering communities, another positive side effect of bioprospecting. In De-cember 2013, Uli Feiter, who was invited to speak at the 3ʳᵈ Global Congress on IP and the Public Interest and Open A.I.R. Conference on Innovation and IP in Africa in Cape Town, said:

> One result of the tight ABS regulations was that they forced me into benefit shar-ing agreements with the communities I worked with in the Eastern Cape. I had to open up and negotiate ABS with these communities. Ultimately, the long and intense negotiation phase brought me closer to the culture of the Xhosa people. Eventually, I even started having a close friendship with the village chief (sum-marized from presentation at the Open A.I.R. Conference, December 2013, Cape Town).

In the course of understanding the Xhosa people's cultural background, Uli was thus more ready to integrate ABS into his work. This marks a considerable change of tone from my interview with him in August 2009, when he was very critical of ABS legislation. Aside from the complications that ABS legislation has bestowed on Uli, he could, after a long process of interaction and negotiation, also see its be-nefits. One of these benefits is interaction between groups, here a white business-person from Germany and a black community in the Eastern Cape, which would not have cooperated on this level before. ABS, to some degree, may thus be seen to serve as a measure of black economic empowerment, as well as a way for people on different sides of the bioprospecting agenda to approach one other face-to-face as equal partners. In addition, another side effect is a deeper cultural understan-ding by white businessmen of black community structures. This positive approach, however, is not inscribed in the perceptions of all traders, as the following examples will show.

"It's Just an Excuse": ABS and the Expansion of Biopiracy

In a similar way to Uli Feiter, Robby Gass, the owner of Zizamele Herbs[22], a bulk and retail supplier of herbal medicinal plants, expressed his unease about ABS. Robby had a contract with the IKS Lead Program to buy the *Sutherlandia frutescens* plants cultivated at the La Serena plantation in De Doorns and retail them to other traders, shops or private persons. I met him on one of his many visits to La Serena. He was not very keen to be interviewed, but after some persuasion he finally agreed on a short interview.

> **BR:** How do you see the future of access and benefit sharing?
>
> **RG:** Access and benefit sharing agreements, I believe, will never work. It is – and now I am saying a dangerous thing – just an excuse for the abuse [of indigenous people] of the last centuries. But since there is no benefit, there is no sharing. And in the end, the question is: who is they?[i.e. who are the original knowledge holders with whom the benefits should be shared?]. I had so many different San coming to my office in Barrydale [Western Cape], wearing feathers and beads and skins, they came and told me their story, many of them with different stories (...) but in the end, who are they?
>
> **BR:** Yes, it is very difficult to define who 'they' are.
>
> **RG:** The only way [to appropriately share benefits] would be a national trust fund. But with the actual regulations, there will be no fund. It is actually easier to buy plants in China and sell them in South Africa, than breeding and planting them in this country. The regulations don't consider or include the international market, it is almost impossible to put things on the EU market (...) products that have been put before 1993 [year of ratification of the CBD] are still on the market. Beyond that stage, no new product can be found. Until now, only Schwabe did all the necessary work that needs to be done to put a product on the market. The regulations will let the market die. Lucky enough now we have strong cooperation with Brazil. Once the US [has] registered that no one in Brazil or [no] South African citizen dies from our medicine, the US will become interested, and then Europe probably comes and starts to do the necessary research. What are 5 million Dollars [for research and development] for pharmaceutical companies and for the government? But you know, in the end they only want to go for synthetic drugs, not for the natural remedies (De Doorns, January 2010).

Robby was and is very active in the field of bioprospecting. He was not only a plant retailer but was also politically very active, and presented at many workshops and conferences. In the above excerpt of our short interview, he seemed unconvinced

---

22   Zizamele Herbs merged with Afrinatural holdings, see: www.afrinatural.com.

that the 'phyto trade' [trading with medicinal plants] has a real future, particularly under current national ABS legislation. Prior informed consent, material transfer agreements, co-ownership of patents, the strenuous application procedure at the ministry and very strict export regulations discourage traders from engaging in the field. In the end, he claimed that the endeavor to implement the CBD by means of the National Biodiversity Act is nothing but a political excuse for and the expansion of centuries of biopiracy. The idea collapses, in his opinion, due to the fact that after all there will simply be no benefits to be shared.

When looking at past ABS agreements in South Africa, this is not an entirely incorrect assessment of the situation. Additionally, Robby's question of "who are they?" resonates with the concerns of others about how to identify knowledge holding communities with whom benefits should be shared. This continues to be a difficult question in the South African context, with its complex history and multi-ethnic background. Empowered and strengthened San communities, for instance, are more often claiming to have rights to plant-based knowledge in light of their 'first-come' position (see chapter III). But for a trader, identifying "who is San" is virtually impossible. According to Robby, a distributive measure like a national trust fund would help to solve the problem of with whom to share possible benefits.

He also pointed out the dependency of the global South market on developments and movements of the market in the global North. This is mainly based on still prevalent mistrust in countries in the Global North, namely Europe and the US, who maintain that medicinal plants from Africa may not be safe for consumption. Robby thus hopes for a strong development of the phyto-medicinal market in other parts of the world, which might slowly lead to greater trust in medicine from countries in the Global South and to more (global) interest in the South African market.

"There Is no Future for Phyto-Medicine": The Future of Medicinal Plant Trading

Nigle, a botanist and (co-)publisher of several books on medicinal plants in South Africa (i.e. van Wyk & Oudtshoorn & Gericke 200), had himself also conducted extensive research on *Sutherlandia frutescens*. In an interview in August 2009, he told me that *Sutherlandia* is a potent immunity booster supportive in the treatment of HIV/AIDS patients (Gericke 2001). He is also the co-founder of a small-scale phyto-pharmaceutical company that merchandizes *Sutherlandia* tablets. My interview with Nigel took place in the Kirstenbosch Botanical Garden Café. I felt a little uncomfortable with our somewhat secretive meeting. The misty winter clouds covering Table Mountain in the background resonated with my discomfort. First, Nigel was reluctant to meet with me, stating that he hardly ever gives interviews. "Bioprospecting is not an easy field. When you are cited incorrectly, people might attack you," he explained. But Anne Hutchings, a colleague of Nigle whom I had met at the yearly Indigenous Plants Use Forum (IPUF) conference in Stellenbosch, finally convinced him of my trustworthiness[23]. The following summary of the interview is based on my recollections supported by the notes I took during and after the interview. To my question of how he perceives the future of traditional medicinal plant trading in South Africa, he answered:

> **NG:** There is no future for phyto-medicine in South Africa, at least not at present. The regulatory framework of the government hinders research on and commercialization of products. I did try to work with Sutherlandia. The plant grows all over the Western Cape and beyond, most healers know about it. But the current regulations make it almost impossible to work with Sutherlandia. I worked a lot with Sutherlandia on HIV/AIDS patients. I have more than 800 files on the effect of Sutherlandia on these patients. It is very detailed and comprehensive information. But the government does not want to know. You see, I understand that people are waiting for a solution for the major problem of HIV/AIDS. Sutherlandia could really help. But the government does not react. They still seem to wait for the endless money flow coming from phyto-medicine [based on the expectation that it will deliver the solution against cancer or HIV/AIDS, for instance] but stand in their own way.
>
> **BR:** What does that mean?
>
> **NG:** Well, it means that the government needs further changes to really open the market. The government is wishing for the integration of local communities into bioprospecting, but with this integration they make the market very complicated and inaccessible. And then there are two paths that the government could follow, the commercial and the public health path. But they only follow the commercial path. They only want to make cash. Otherwise they would consider Sutherlandia

---

23   Anne Hutchings cooperated closely with Nigel in the research project on the effects of *Sutherlandia* on HIV/AIDS patients. Anne is a retired university research fellow at the University of Zululand and the author of several books and papers on medicinal plants in South Africa (see Hutchings et al. 1996; Hutchings 2007). Next to her herb garden at the university that she cares for passionately, she works as a social worker in the communities surrounding the university town of Empangeni. She uses a homemade cream containing five different medicinal plants, *Sutherlandia* from the Western Cape being one of them, to treat the shingles and open wounds of HIV/AIDS patients whom she visits in her capacity as a social worker. I joined Anne for some days on her routine visits to patients and their families. She recorded the healing processes of the patients she treated with the cream by taking note of their CD4 count, weight and health changes. Anne, similarly to Michael, proposed *Sutherlandia* as an effective medicine for the treatment of HIV/AIDS patients with a low CD4 count, since, according to her observations, CD4 count increases rapidly when patients take *Sutherlandia* capsules and use the cream.

as a potent and important plant for the treatment of HIV/AIDS patients. (Cape Town, August 2009)

Nigel, like Robert Gass above, was also frustrated with the current ABS regulations. As a botanist who believes in and lives off the (medicinal) value of medicinal plants, he advocates for a public health approach for the government. But the government only strives for "green diamonds," economic revenue. Therefore, the government would rather proceed with the "commercial path," which is financially more promising, rather than follow the "public health path" that would support local knowledge systems and communities by utilizing existing local resources for the South African public health system. Michael also realized that he should have patented his research results on *Sutherlandia* earlier in his career. He did not, for reasons of social and ethical justice. A patent comprises the exclusion of the knowledge owners; they are neither part of the patent nor are they allowed to use the 'invention' themselves. The Masakhane community, for instance, was not allowed to use the extraction method of *Pelargonium* after Schwabe had patented it, even though they and other communities had used it for centuries. Today, Nigel regrets his decision. Other, less socially-oriented institutions will claim patents arising from *Sutherlandia*, without the interest of caring for the knowledge holders.

In sum, constantly reappearing obstacles in bioprospecting lies in the fact that ABS regulations are not transparent enough and are difficult to apply. The legislation is subject to constant friction between the government, traders, indigenous peoples and NGOs. Robby's consideration of buying plant material from China rather than cultivate plants in South Africa seemed like a fatalistic attempt to deal with the situation. As a consequence of these obstacles, many bioprospectors would rather not engage in bioprospecting at all, or will do it illegally, rather than engage with the complicated application procedures. While the CBD/Nagoya Protocol and NEMBA/BABS are supposed to balance out past inequalities, the policies and regulations make the work of medicinal plant traders unattractive and strenuous. This may lead to the total breakdown of the market. This, at least, was Robby's and Nigel's take on the situation.

The case of *Hoodia* presented at the beginning of this chapter is an example of the vigorous process that bioprospecting evokes, not only for plant traders but also for indigenous communities, governments and NGOs. And it shows how easily the market can break down, less due to legislative challenges and more because of the actions of those who play a major role in developing and marketing medicinal plant-based products, namely the huge (pharmaceutical and other) companies, mostly from the Global North. The *Hoodia* case shows that solutions for a fair and equitable sharing of benefits are complex, particularly when the knowledge owner is not clearly identifiable and/or spread across borders. The number of stakeholders and countries involved make the case multifaceted (similar to the earlier example of the mixture containing four plants that Dr. Matsabisa described to me at the IKS Laboratory).

Hoodia Gordonii and the Future of Medicinal Plant-Based Trading

The breakdown of the *Hoodia* market was also the subject of a *Hoodia* Task Force Group meeting that was appointed to be held in Cape Town in September 2009 to develop a plan for the future commercial and scientific development of *Hoodia*, which I was invited to attend by Dr. Matsabisa, the Director of the IKS Lead Program (who did not attend). The following observations and quotes stem from my field notes and later e-mail correspondence. The meeting was organized by the NGO Natural Justice and the Department Environmental Affairs (DEA), and was characterized by an atmosphere of urgency to find a solution for how to revive the *Hoodia* market after Unilever's dropout. The commercial (and political) focus of the meeting became clear as the participants mainly consisted of members of national and international plant traders and the commercial industry, the government (Department of Environmental Affairs, Department of Science and Technology, the Provincial Government of the Western Cape, Department of Trade and Industry, Department of Economic Development and the environmental organization Cape Nature), members of the Southern African Hoodia Growers Association (SAHGA), with Robby Gass as a leading representative, and Johanna von Braun of Natural Justice. Significantly, no representatives of the San community were present, but they had apologized for being absent.

First, update presentations were given to the delegates by the DEA on current ABS legislation and the permit application process, by the CSIR on the history of research into *Hoodia gordonii*, and by SAHGA on the climate for commercial growers. The debate brought up the most crucial obstacles for successful bioprospecting in South Africa. Mostly debated was the missing and inconsistent research at the national level, with secrecy being highlighted as discouraging overseas research and development companies from looking for solutions in South Africa. Robby Grass claimed:

> Mistrust exists against the quality of products coming from (South) Africa. Instead, China and India are perceived as better sources of medicinal solutions as they have 5000 years of written heritage. Regardless of the plant wealth, South Africa is still perceived as a third world country with terrible hygiene conditions and low quality products.

China in particular has a much higher reputation for delivering quality products. Although much research was undertaken to make P57 applicable to the formal market, countries in the Global North still do not accept *Hoodia* products. Clinical and pre-clinical trials have to be continued in order to back up the claims that *Hoodia* might serve as an appetite suppressant. Such trials would be subject to less strict rules than pharmaceutical-based clinical trials, since *Hoodia* so far counts as a 'food supplement' and not as a 'pharmaceutical'.

Vinesh Maharaj of the DST/CSIR questioned, "Why is more research needed on *Hoodia*? All necessary research had been done long before 2004 and *Hoodia* should not at all fall under the regulations, and restrictions, of NEMBA or BABS. Why access a bus that already left?" Johanna von Braun from Natural Justice answered: "Unilever dropped out and questioned the safety of P57, new patenting opportunities would need to be discovered. The Western world does not yet pay for all additional costs in the product line". The representative of the DEA, Philemona Mosana, proposed that "Academic and political idealism is in tension with the commercial reality and needs." Furthermore, as Robby Gass pointed out:

> National legislation hinders effective commerce and export of Hoodia from South Africa to, for instance, the European Union or the United States. So far, South Africa exports 1% of all plant-based products, including Rooibos as the strongest commercial plant, to the European Union.

A consensus in the meeting was, however, achieved in the observation that through Unilever's involvement in *Hoodia*'s development and commercialization, the image of the plant, and thus of products coming from the region in general, had increased immensely; though it also dropped again after Unilever pulled out. It was nonetheless advocated as a very positive step to have products from (South) Africa "out there."

Another important aspect was continuously repeated. Medicinal plants are not only vital for trading and commerce, but are also an important means for local poverty alleviation and development. The Farmer to Pharma (F2P) Grand Challenge Initiative of the Department of Science and Technology, for instance, was initiated "to combine biotechnology with indigenous knowledge systems and South Africa's rich biodiversity in an effort to position the country to competitively participate in the emerging bio-economy"[24]. It aims to create jobs for communities by helping to establish small, medium and micro enterprises (SMMEs) to facilitate local communities to initiate projects based on medicinal plants as a means of income generation. The outcry for the revival of the *Hoodia* market was thus not only based on the attempt to revive the economic market, but also went hand in hand with the idea of ensuring a sustainable livelihood and poverty alleviation for local rural communities. The Department of Science and Technology thus promotes community-

---

24   www.gov.za/aboutgovt/programmes/sustainable-livelihoods/index.html (last accessed July 20, 2014).

owned commercial plantation sites to provide economic wealth and job opportunities for impoverished communities. Similar projects are being implemented on the basis of other medicinal plants (e.g. *Pelargonium sidoides* and *Devils Claw*).

This initial *Hoodia* Task Force Group meeting was part of a solution-finding undertaking, but was also dominated by many open questions and was more concerned about coming to basic understandings rather than determining the next steps[25]. For one, although the *Hoodia* market seemed to have experienced a serious breakdown, it was nonetheless regarded as a best practice example by which to set new precedents. The *Hoodia* case is actually the only known case where an ABS agreement was developed in the South African context. The case created increasing awareness for an integrated system to protect and promote traditional knowledge (Chennels 2010). Moreover, in discussing *Hoodia*, a so far marginalized group of indigenous people, the San community, was brought into the public and political discourse[26]. Without the *Hoodia* case, the San community would probably not have started articulating their needs and objectives in public. *Hoodia*, as an example for other (potential) medicinal plants of South (and southern) Africa, thus stands not only for economic expansion, but also for new (indigenous) agency, one positive side effect of bioprospecting.

Conclusion and Outlook

As the *Hoodia gordonii* case outlined at the beginning, the many workshops, open discussions and solution finding missions in between and the *Hoodia* Task Force Meeting at the end of the chapter revealed, the path towards a fair and appropriate ABS is like a gravel road, bumpy and uneven. On this road, the pursued aim, benefits that can be shared, is hardly ever reached. Even the *Hoodia* example, the only current 'best case example' in South Africa, has not really achieved its goal, namely the regular sharing of benefits with the San Council. Strenuous ABS regulations largely complicate bioprospecting, at least from the view of bioprospectors. The fundamental problem remains how to estimate the value of the intangible property with cultural value of indigenous communities. The complicated illustration of Dr. Matsabisa quite clearly illustrates the complexity of sharing in a facts and

---

25   Two other meetings were scheduled for 2009. One was held in October 2009 to discuss the future potential of the *Hoodia* market. The meeting was attended by members of the regional *Hoodia* working group and by Vital Solutions (a German-based phyto-business), Phytopharm and Phytotrade Africa. The real challenges and opportunities for a future *Hoodia* market were identified and practical solutions were sought (from email, Robby Gass, October 2009). The second meeting, which was set to take place in December 2009, was cancelled for not further explained reasons.

26   For more information, see: www.san.org.za.

figures scheme that does not yet deal with the socio-cultural background and emotional value of knowledge. His earlier statement cited in the previous chapter – "I am not interested in the spirit, I am only interested in the molecule" – suggests that his interest in finding a culturally adequate solution is low. In fact, finding a solution is difficult, as it would demand stepping back from Westernized ideas of property and commercialization.

Often, however, ABS negotiations reach a dead-end before any benefits can be negotiated, either because no product is developed, as was the case in the plant exchange in Thulamahashe, or because a community cannot be detected or is too scattered and widespread (maybe over different countries) to constitute a 'community' with whom to discuss an ABS agreement according to national ABS legislation. For the latter problem, this is a significant hurdle, since cross-national legislation has not yet been implemented for ABS. Even when an ABS agreement is finally negotiated and implemented, as was the case in the *Hoodia* example, it still does not guarantee benefits, at least not in monetary terms. But beyond all of these failings and disadvantages of ABS legislation and to be (or not to be) negotiated ABS agreements, this ABS coin does have another side. ABS entails a clear definition of the owner of traditional knowledge. The owner, mostly indigenous communities, may claim new rights over their knowledge. To quote Marilyn Strathern:

> At no moment in history have we seen the world shrinking in terms of actual resources, and yet expanding in terms of new candidates for ownership. New kinds of entities are being created and new claims for property made (...) and never more so than in the world of biological knowledge or resources (Strathern 2000, cited in Reddy 2006: 165).

This quote leads directly to the other side of the coin of ABS, and knowledge protection or claims of ownership. Different concepts of property in international property law would give more space and rights to those who manage and govern ecosystems – namely indigenous communities – and could ensure the effective conservation and sustainable use of these ecosystems. These rights would not only support sustainable development but would also consolidate the stewardship of indigenous people over their tangible and intangible property. By developing a biocultural community protocol (BCP), for instance, communities may find a stronger voice in their own locales and beyond, be able to demonstrate their biocultural rights, and manage and control their own resources. The following chapter will give space to further engage with this line of thought.

Chapter VII
Partial Solution: The Biocultural Community Protocol

> I don't believe in the commercializa-
> tion of plants. The important thing is
> to strengthen the healers in their cul-
> tural capacity as part of the community,
> to strengthen their own values, not the
> commercial idea that proposes financial
> benefits.
>
> Marie-Tinka Uys, Hoedspruit, April 2013

Introduction

As Marilyn Strathern has argued, "The market thus disembeds what is usable, whe-
reas the thrust of the indigenous IPR [intellectual property rights] movement is to
re-embed, re-contextualize, indigenous ownership in indigenous traditional culture. Tradition, we may remark, is an embedding concept" (Strathern 1999b: 167).
I begin with this quote to unfold the synopsis of this final chapter. After chapter
VI, which dealt with the challenges that ABS bestows on the actors involved, this
chapter analyzes the extent to which the notion of "cultural property" (Coombe
2009), here culturally embedded medicinal plants and associated knowledge, creates new value (beyond and yet related to commercial value), expressed in newly
emerging forms of intellectual property and environmental governance. Holders
of intangible cultural heritage are making distinctive claims under the auspices of
international treaties, conventions, international customary law and human rights
norms (Coombe 2011: 79), which is releasing new "cultural agencies" (ibid.). I argue that the translation process of cultural property from a (local) relational entity to a legal instrument of national and global scale may encourage indigenous
peoples' "cultural agency" and induce the valorization of their cultural heritage and
identity. The process may also lead to financial revenues if appropriately harnessed
(though so far, this has only happened to a limited extent, as the previous chapter
has shown). This approach therefore demands critical reflection. Is the enactment
of indigenous communities in legal and political language and practices motivated

by support for indigenous peoples, biodiversity and cultural heritage? Or is it driven by more elaborate schemes to gain economic value out of "cultural property" (Takeshita 2001; Yudice 2003)? Or is it a combination of both?

This chapter cannot present a complete answer to these questions that takes into account all variables. What I do aim to do, however, is to provide a situational analysis of the Kukula Healers of Bushbuckridge Municipality in the context of these questions. The largely rural area of Bushbuckridge is currently facing modernization processes and a concomitantly gradually declining biodiversity. In this context, traditional healers can and do play a vital role in the preservation of cultural traditions and biodiversity. At the same time, they must continuously defend their traditions and reposition themselves in a rapidly changing society. Aware of these challenges, the Kukula Healers, in cooperation with local and national NGOs, developed a biocultural community protocol (BCP) to define and govern their cultural property, summarize their core values, strengthen their position in society and ensure their ability to negotiate their needs with external stakeholders. In the process of developing the BCP, the healers had to discuss and develop (new) ways of sharing and protecting their traditional knowledge, aligned to new external conditions. As was described in chapter IV, the sharing and protection of knowledge in healers' traditions is subject to a set of rules and regulations inscribed in customary law. Through the BCP, this existing system was expanded into a new system, a 'traditional knowledge commons pool' (Abrell 2009; Hess & Ostrom 2006), with 'commons' being "a particular form of structuring the rights to access, use and control resources" (Benkler 2006: 24; Ostrom 1990).

This chapter illustrates the transformation and expansion process of one system of knowledge governance into another by asking a set of questions: How did the relations of the Kukula Healers to their property change with the developmen of a BCP? Which actors were involved in establishing the new system? In what contexts are these systems embedded? And what has been the outcome of these processes? Systems of knowledge governance entail provisions for knowledge protection. These systems, when involved in economic exchange, stand in contrast to current intellectual property law, which tries to integrate cultural properties into its established laws. This can be read as the imposition of Western intellectual property law on indigenous communities and their customary laws. Understanding established as well as re-established structures of knowledge governance could help to find new *sui generis* solutions for knowledge protection.

The following celebration of the Kukula Healers, illustrates the intense level of cooperation between the Kukula Healers and several local and national NGOs as well as the government, local tribal authorities, and other local actors such as the management of Kruger National Park, and represents the reorganization of cultural property protection through the development of a BCP.

Interim Celebration in Share

The huge festivity tent sparkled red and blue against the green fields and the high mid-autumn sun in Share, a small village in Bushbuckridge Municipality. The tent was filled with about 300 traditional health practitioners and a number of other distinguished guests. The male healers and the guests were seated on chairs, the women sat gathered in groups on the floor. From time to time, one of the healers jumped up to dance energetically, supported by the clapping hands and drums of the other healers. In this area, a tent of this size would normally indicate either a wedding or a funeral. This gathering, however, was exceptional. It was the interim function of the Kukula Healers celebrating the acknowledgement of a three-year long process that had involved negotiating a non-disclosure agreement (NDA) with a local small-scale cosmetics company on shared plant material and associated traditional knowledge, the development of a BCP, and the creation of a constitution and a code of conduct/ethics for the healers' association. It was also a celebration that signified the custody of the healers over their traditional knowledge of healing and of the biodiversity in which they live, and their role in their communities as well as in conserving the natural resources and knowledge on which they rely.

It was a unique celebration in post-Apartheid South Africa. It was initiated to signify a process of self-determination and integration for a marginalized group that for a long time had been the target of political repression and exclusion. Among the many guests was a representative of the Kruger National Park management, the Kruger to Canyons (K2C) Biosphere Region committee, the Department of Environmental Affairs and Tourism, the Share Community Council, a nurse of the Hluvukane Community Health Center, visiting North American students residing and studying in the nearby Southern African Wildlife College, and a camera team from one of Germany's main TV stations. The CEO of the Kukula Healers, Rodney Sibuyi, officially opened the function with a speech, beginning with the introduction of all of the invited guests. He also mentioned those who were unfortunately unable to attend, most importantly the local chief Philip Mnisi and his cabinet, some local church members and their leaders, and traditional healers from other organizations in the region. He finished his long list of greetings with "*thokozane bayethi ndunankulu*" (may the Lord God be with you at all times). Rodney thereafter continued his speech, passionately recounting the process that the Kukula Healers had gone through to get where they were today:

> My speech will come from what we have developed within our organization, the Kukula Traditional Health Practitioners. In cooperation with Natural Justice in Cape Town and the K2C committee, we managed to develop a biocultural [community] protocol. The reason why we came to develop this protocol is because of the ongoing history that has destroyed our ancestors and the knowledge that was

taken away by researchers without any access and benefit sharing. Also, we realized that we as healers are not fully recognized by the government. We therefore decided to develop this protocol as a sustainable tool and a public voice that will give us direction at all times. This will also be inherited by the new generation. (...) Our objectives with the protocol are to protect our culture and traditional knowledge, to ensure the sustainable use of biodiversity, to also raise awareness of the above by giving education. We also want to organize ourselves to be respected by society and want us to be linked to the formal health system. Additionally, we want to develop strategies to supplement income and to ensure quality assurance performance. (...) We hope this function will earn [us] more credibility to different stakeholders and the government departments as well.

As he finished, Rodney firmly and self-confidently raised his head, supported by the dancing and clapping hands of his fellow healers. Subsequently, the other guests delivered their speeches, tracked by the camera team that filmed the event for a spot on the German news channel to be shown the next day. Particularly significant was the speech of the representative of Kruger National Park, Soli Themba. He made clear that future cooperation between the park and the healers was both wished for and crucial, particularly with regard to preventing the "pandemic of rhino poaching," as well as engaging in the environmental monitoring of plant species. Given the fact that traditional healers had been denied free access to the many nature and game reserves in the area during Apartheid times, this was a groundbreaking statement. The representative of the Department of Environmental Affairs and Tourism, in turn, promised financial and ideological support for the Kukula Healers in the future. Whether this will ever materialize was at that moment of less importance than the mere presence of a representative from the department, a concession of respect and acknowledgment for the healers. Eventually, after all of the speeches had been held, the printed and laminated copies of the Kukula Healers' code of conduct/ethics and name tags were distributed to every healer, an important step in identifying affiliation to the group and self-recognition as healers.

Finally, it was time to eat. A cow had been collectively chosen through a selection process that had lasted many months. It had been slaughtered in the early morning hours and prepared and cooked throughout the day. Together with a huge amount of pap (maize meal), the meat was served to the visitors. The ceremony continued into the night, with intense drumming, singing and dancing, and the drinking of *umqombothi*, traditionally brewed beer. It was the largest celebration the healers had ever had since their establishment in 2009, and probably one of the largest and most representative celebrations held by healers in a region where healers still struggle for integrity and acceptance.

A Willful Cow and the Dialogic Path to Empowerment

The Kukula Healers had prepared the interim celebration over a period of five months, including planning the huge tent, choosing and purchasing the cow to be slaughtered, and preparing the food for the celebration. This process had included allocating and distributing the money that had been provided by Natural Justice for the Kukula Healers; this was the responsibility of Marie-Tinka of the K2C committee. The money was largely received from the ABS Capacity Development Initiative of the Deutsche Gesellschaft für International Zusammenarbeit (GIZ) and was given to the healers on the basis of a "to-do work plan"[1].

Of the 46,600 Rand given for the time frame July 2011 to March 2012, the 8,000 Rand spent for the cow was at first regarded by Marie-Tinka as an inappropriately large expenditure, and it caused a financial debate between her and the healers. For the healers, the cow was imperative for the ceremony, signifying their strength and willpower in the process of developing a BCP. Symbolically, the chosen cow revealed itself to have quite a willful character. The day she was brought from the *kraal* of the original owner, the *induna* (sub-chief) of Share, to the *kraal* of Rodney Sibuyi, she seemed to have felt her destiny. It took four men to pull the bullheaded cow out of the *kraal* to bind her to a tree, where she was supposed to be slaughtered. She managed to escape, however, and run back to the *induna*'s *kraal*. After being captured and brought back once again, her ordeal ended in a torturous death, with her head being chopped off with a simple axe. The small dispute about the purchase of the cow significantly illustrates the differences in perceptions of the K2C committee member Marie-Tinka, a white, Afrikaans-speaking woman from Hoedpruit, and the needs of the Kukula Healers. Holding a huge celebration without offering adequate food would have been unthinkable for the healers and would have been regarded as disrespectful to the honorable visitors in attendance.

The ambitious speech of Rodney representing the healers was the result of the intense process that the healers had gone through in developing the BCP and subsequent legal tools from 2009 until 2012. Without the development of the BCP, Rodney's relatively self-confident speech would never have happened. During Apartheid, the Witchcraft Suppression Act, originally from 1957, was reinvigorated particularly strongly, and traditional healers had to be careful about what they revealed in public for fear of persecution (mostly related to witchcraft accusations). With the advent of democracy in 1994, this situation has slowly begun to change, though this history still has a lasting effect until today (Ashforth 2005; Comaroff & Comaroff 1993; Geschiere 1997; Niehaus 1993, 2012). With new political amendments, the reputation of traditional healers has slowly begun to improve. Today, healers practice

---

1   The workplan was developed by Natural Justice, also get funding for the collaboration with the Kukula Healers by funding institutions, the GIZ among them.

their services in a less secretive and cautious manner, although both their practices and knowledge system are threatened by prevailing disbelief, as well as by churches and biomedical health institutions competing for believers and patients. With the BCP, the Kukula Healers constituted and stabilized themselves as a group and negotiated a new form of knowledge pooling, sharing and exchange that differed from traditional forms of sharing and exchanging knowledge. This new form provisionally enabled the healers to negotiate their property with interested parties, such as researchers, research institutions and companies.

The BCP is a tool promoted and implemented by the NGO Natural Justice. The hope is that it may bring about new forms of "dialogic democracy" between healers and their communities, the government, civil society and the private sector, and thus lead to more "rights based development" (Coombe 1998b, 2003, 2009, together with Alywin 2014), as well as to collectivities making possessive claims to act as market actors for economic purposes (Comaroff & Comaroff 2009). Building on Foucault's notions of governmentality (Foucault 1991), Cori Hayden proposes the term 'environmentality' as a "provocative terrain of investigation" in this field (Hayden 2003: 83; Gupta 1998; Argawal 2005). As Foucault explained:

> This word government must be allowed the very broad meaning it had in the sixteenth century. Government did not refer only to political structures or to the management of states, rather, it designated the way in which the conduct of individuals or of groups might be directed – the government of children, of souls, of communities, of the sick (...) To govern, in this sense, is to control the possible field of action of others (Foucault 2002: 341).

With 'environmentality', some scholars (Agrawal 1995, Hayden 2003) have suggested, governance has come to serve in a new international form that changes (and controls) the lives of local people of the Global North as much as the industries and scientific institutions of the Global South. It is not only the environment that the global community and nation states aim to protect and control in order to prevent future threats imposed by climate change or biodiversity degradation, for instance, but also the people who live in this environment.

In addition, intellectual property law is a governance tool that legally forces nation states as well as local communities to adjust to market needs when they engage in the trade of resources. Environmentality together with intellectual property law may suggest new rights-based approaches to citizenship (Coombe 2011: 82) and a new valuation of biological diversity and heritage regimes (Harvey 2002; Watts 1999). Against this background, it can be said, "all ecological projects (and arguments) are simultaneously political-economic projects (and arguments) and vice versa. Ecological arguments are never socially neutral any more than sociopolitical arguments are never ecologically neutral" (Harvey 1993: 23).

In the context of bioprospecting, new relations, hopes and aspirations may be engendered by intellectual property leverage, instigated by global politics, the state and influential companies. Differently expressed, "Government designates not just the activities of the state and its institutions but more broadly any rational effort to influence or guide the conduct of human beings through acting upon their hopes, desires, circumstances, or environment" (Inda 2005: 1). The web of relations between people, plants, knowledge, politics, law and the economy "creates value, labor, monetary transactions, and capital accumulation, but just as important, is a site of promise, hope, fear, and speculation that itself sets new relationships in motion" (Hayden 2003: 75). As Foucault purported:

> What government has to do with is not territory but, rather, a sort of complex composed relation of men and things. The things, in this sense, with which government is to be concerned are in fact men, but men in their relations, their links, their imbrications with those things that are wealth, resources, means of substance, the territory with its specific qualities, climate, irrigation, fertility, and so on; men in their relation to those other things that are customs, habits, ways of acting and thinking, and so on; and finally men in relation to those still other things that might be accidents and misfortunes such as famine, epidemics, death, and so on (Foucault 2000: 208f.).

Environmentality in the field of bioprospecting of medicinal plants in local communities in the Global South is an interplay between NGOs, which have often become powerful political actors in the context of weak state governments (Oomen 2005), indigenous communities, which ought to be trained in understanding legal and political frameworks, and (intellectual) property, here plants and knowledge. Therein, NGOs act as lawyers and mediators between different stakeholders, interests and emotions, as well as political advocates who encourage actors' compliance with rights, innovation and capacity building (Fowler 2000). Their agency in environmental governance also forges new forms of knowledge held by newly empowered subjects and collectivities, as well as the NGOs themselves. Intellectual property law and the adjustment of communities to these laws are vital for the installment of new approaches to rights.

In addition, environmental governance is dependent on the environment as such. The K2C Biosphere Region plays a vital role in the context of developing a BCP. The region was already introduced in chapter II, but the interview with Marie-Tinka Uys (MT) of the K2C committee in Hoedspruit in May 2012 reflects on the role of the region in environmental governance as well as community development and capacity building. Marie-Tinka was initially hesitant to be interviewed, but did eventually willingly agree to speak to me and be recorded. She included a brief history of the K2C Biosphere Region:

BR: What is K2C, when did it start and what is its purpose?

MT: The K2C has been adopted, or accepted, in the world biospheres network[2] in 2001. Prior to the adoption, we are up now for a 10 years review of UNESCO. The process to get registered was a big stakeholder consultation process. UNESCO takes areas in the world, special areas, next to protected areas where there can be a demonstration of the reconciliation of biodiversity conservation and sustainable development. Illustration-demonstration sites, and they link them to a network. So, in South Africa, we have at the moment six biosphere reserves (...) Now, eh, the process before was (...) eh, in the early 90s, we started a what we call a community development forum, which was the first time that white people and [black] communities started to talk to one another. Because we lived very apart and even today, 18 years after [the end of Apartheid], we are still having very much issues around land being separate. So, at this forum we started to work on issues. We were concerned because conservation is such a huge land use reduction sector in our area that is expanding since the early 90s by thousands and thousands of hectares; that is not going to be sustainable in the future. Here is a new dispensation. It was very exciting to have this interaction between leadership from both sides. It was quite a transformation in terms of who are our leaders in the white community. The white male became suddenly, is, you know, terrible. But maybe some of the white female[s] had a better chance to communicate.

BR: But did the white female[s] become the new leaders?

MT: No, not really. Ya, but in a sense they do. Ehm, the issue here, then in 1998, I wrote a proposal to the World Bank. And they had a sub-program called Melissa, which stands for: Managing the Environment Locally In Sub-Saharan Africa. That program doesn't exist anymore, but they gave me a little money. I was still working at theSouth African wildlife college (I was working there for 8 years). And from there we had driven a consultation process, put the agitation together and then we became a biosphere reserve. We had very little support from the government. The purpose is in the mission and [the] vision is mainly demonstrating the reconciliation of biodiversity conservation [with sustainable development]. When I look at the map and see all these conservation areas and the communities living there, it doesn't look like a sustainable picture to me. What needs to happen, I will tell you (...) we are going to do big projects, there is a big global environmental fund process.

BR: Ya, after the COP 17.

MT: South Africa gets a total of 90 Million USD. Now there are two main objectives. The one is protected areas expansion. They want to expand protected areas

---

2   UNESCO World Network of Biosphere Reserves (WNBR) (see: www.
unesco.org/new/en/natural-sciences/environment/ecological-sciences/biosphere-re-
serves/world-network-wnbr).

further for biodiversity species conservation. And the other one is what we call mainstreaming of biodiversity. You know, green economy jobs creation, making sure that the municipalities are doing waste management in line, including the landscape. That can still grow and create an understanding of [the] importance of ecosystems.

The main objectives of the K2C Biosphere Region, according to Marie-Tinka, are therefore biodiversity reconciliation and job creation in the green economy. To get there, the K2C area started bringing black and white leaders of the communities together to establish a functioning cooperation structure. This was in the 1990^s after the end of the Apartheid regime. The cooperation between the K2C committee and the Kukula Healers is only one of many such examples where local communities have been encouraged to participate in environmental protection and sustainable biodiversity programs that at the same time (may) generate new green economy jobs. This is an ambitious enterprise, especially in the still highly segregated areas of Mpumalanga and Limpopo Province, where white landowners and black employees have little else in common than an employer-employee relationship. In this context black communities are playing an increasingly important role in the process of sustaining local biodiversity and cultural heritage. The K2C committee fosters the mobilization of communities to claim their rights to resources and traditional knowledge.

In this context, the call of the NGO Natural Justcie to implement a biocultural community protocol was more than welcome, as biocultural community protocols foster the objectives of the K2C biosphere region and it scommittee. As a politically accepted tool it also enforces dialogue with local communities, strengthens community's rights and envision the sustainable protection of the environment. Whether all these so well sounding objectives were put into reality will be scrutinized in the course of the neyt sections, starting with describing biocultural community protocol of the Kukula Healers, its significance for environmental governace as the protection if medicinal plants and traditional knowledge.

The Biocultural Community Protocol: Vision and Reality

In the previous chapter, databases were presented as one solution, albeit limited and not fully satisfying, for the question of how to protect the knowledge used in or generated for medicinal plant products. Databases help to contain already existing knowledge or to document newly discovered knowledge. But they cut out most of the socio-cultural and spiritual aspects of the respective knowledge. They basically cut out the lifeworld of the knowledge holders (Laplante 2009, 2014, 2015).

The BCP is thought of as an alternative for knowledge protection. It tries to affirm indigenous peoples' rights as presented in the Declaration of Indigenous Peoples' Rights to Genetic Resources and Indigenous Knowledge (2007)[3], which begins with the words:

> [We are] Reaffirming our spiritual and cultural relationship with all life forms existing in our traditional territories; Reaffirming our fundamental role and responsibility as the guardians of our territories, lands and natural resources; Recognizing that we are the guardians of the indigenous knowledge passed down from our ancestors from generation to generation and we reaffirm our responsibility to protect and perpetuate this knowledge for the benefit of our peoples and our future generations.

Against this background, a BCP may improve healers' abilities to communicate and cooperate with other stakeholders such as government agencies, researchers and NGOs, in terms of bringing about a better understanding of communities' biocultural values and customary laws related to the management of natural resources and the challenges faced[4].

The NGO Natural Justice is a 'global player' that collaborates with international donor agencies (e.g. GIZ, UNEP) and the South African government (e.g. Department of Science and Technology, Department of Environmental Affairs and Tourism), and acts as a legal broker in the transformation of legal language into comprehensive models. Specifically, it partners with indigenous peoples in the community to assist them to understand the laws that regulate the most important aspects of their lives – their land, biodiversity and culture – by implementing BCPs. Such a protocol is designed as a means to protect communities against biopiracy, to secure (intellectual) property protection and enable communities to speak for themselves in negotiation processes with third parties. A BCP is, therefore, supposed to be a community-led *sui generis* instrument that "promotes participatory advocacy for the recognition of and support for ways of life that are based on the customary sustainable use of biodiversity, according to standards and procedures set out in customary, national and international laws and policies" (Jonas, Bavikatte & Shrumm 2010: 102ff.). In this context "it is important to look not just at the forms of collective and individual identity promoted by practices of government, but also at how particular agents negotiate these forms – how they embrace, adapt, or refuse them" (Inda 2005: 11).

The development of the BCP and the agreed upon 'traditional knowledge commons pool' (hereon TK commons pool) with the Kukula Healers will be described

---

3   See: www.ipcb.org/resolutions/htmls/Decl_GR&IK.html.
4   See: www.unep.org/communityprotocols/PDF/communityprotocols.pdf (last accessed February 16, 2016).

as a new system of knowledge protection, as compared to the traditional way of protecting knowledge taught in the *izimpande*. The TK commons pool was initiated to react to conflicts that arose in the interaction of healers with third parties and intellectual property law. In the development process, the healers adjusted their traditional ways of governing their resources to a system that enables market openness and control at the same time. While the BCP may seem to be a rights-based solution intended to cope with the demands of intellectual property law by giving space to the collective protection of collectively held property, it does nevertheless have its shadow sides. The BCP is, first and foremost, only provisional and supportive, and is not a legally binding tool. Furthermore, its long-term effects and continuation without the support of donor agencies are not yet identifiable. What then, after all, are the pursued aims of the BCP?

"It is About the Process": BCP Promotion

The NGO Natural Justice, which started implementing BCPs in 2007, is – understandably – convinced of their power and possibilities. Natural Justice was initiated by two law students from the University of Cape Town, Kabir Bavikatte and Harry Jonas, as 'Natural Justice – Lawyers for Communities and the Environment'. According to their website, Natural Justice's vision is "the conservation and sustainable use of biodiversity through the self-determination of Indigenous peoples and local communities"[5], and their mission is "to facilitate the full and effective participation of Indigenous peoples and local communities in the development and implementation of laws and policies related to the conservation and customary uses of biodiversity and the protection of associated cultural heritage"[6]. To fulfill this mission, one of their objectives soon became the implementation of BCPs, not only in South Africa but in many other countries worldwide and not only with traditional healers but with various indigenous communities (including the camel pastoralists of Kachchh, India and the Gunis; Medicinal Plant Conservation Farmers of Rajastan and the Samburu Livestock Breedes).

According to Natural Justice, BCPs are global efforts to integrate and educate indigenous communities about their rights, provide communication and negotiation skills, and to learn about the value of their own tangible and intangible property. In an interview with Gino Cocchiaro, one of the core members of Natural Justice, that I conducted in June 2012 in Cape Town, he articulately promoted BCPs and described their advantages, while continually, though maybe unintentionally, glossing over their disadvantages:

---

5   http://naturaljustice.org.
6   http://naturaljustice.org/representative-work/legal-research/.

BR: What do you think are the strengths and the weaknesses of the BCP?

GC: Developing a BCP is a process of dialog and communication. A BCP really supports indigenous development. So looking at a community, I mean, what are the fundamental principles and values each community has and looking at visions of the future of the community, what do they want to achieve, how do they define themselves? All these things. This is the way to start. That is really the idea. Working with what is already there. The community principles should be the pillar of indigenous development. Using their processes and visions of the future. That's the way they want to go. That might be, for example, to engage with an external actor, you need to form an association, and they decide if they want to do so, that is how they go on. (...)

BR: What do you see as the weaknesses of a BCP?

GC: If you view a BCP as a piece of paper, then I can understand the weakness. (...) But the actual strength for the community is the process of developing a BCP. And what I mean by that is that, ehm, say we've got a community that comes together. They want a facilitator usually. The process of reflection and internal dialog is one of the positives immediately. Because all these communities, if they are living their lives normally, there is no interaction with external agents, but there's got to be some sort of trigger to develop the BCP. And so discussing the trigger, the interests, that is always a positive process. And so they can discuss. Historically, we have always had principles in line with the foundation of our societies. But how do we address this? And that requires a reflection. I mean, the BCP supports such a process by opening it up, by suggesting opening it up to the community. And it also highlights possibly some of the problems in the community. So if that process brings it to the surface, then this is very positive. And then the community can say: We can always decide to interact with this community, with this project, with the government. That makes them strong. So, that trigger supported a process of the BCP, developed a process where the community grew together. In terms of the Kukula Healers, it brought them to discuss. With communication between government, support from K2C, legal rights were explained, capacity is built, it will just grow. So the BCP might just be a piece of paper, but these guys together have a lot more power.

In the above interview excerpt, Gino Cocchiaro reflects on the influence of a BCP on communities. According to him, the BCP supposedly brings a community together to discuss its needs and wishes, usually in cooperation with a facilitator. The moment of bringing a community together is triggered by particular circumstances. In the case of the Kukula Healers, the trigger was not just one but a conglomeration of many different coincidental developments. According to Gino, the healers' community would have had more difficulties in coming together to discuss their needs without the BCP. This may be true from the perspective of an NGO member embedded in development rhetoric and interested in promoting the BCP. But communities do speak and negotiate a lot, even without a BCP. However, the legal and written authority of a BCP might have had an influence on the perception of the healers, who otherwise would have perhaps 'only' discussed their issues in more private circles.

In the second half of the interview, I insisted again on a reflection on the weaknesses of BCPs. Again, Gino Cocchiaro swerved, but came then to a central problem of many developmental interventions:

> **BR:** But how to keep that [the process of the BCP] a sustainable space?
>
> **GC:** Ya, well, that needs a lot of work with each community. For the lack of anything else, they need support, financial support, capacity. But I mean that, at least we can try to bring that capacity to a certain level. I mean, there might always be the need for support. That is the reality of a certain situation. But I don't think anything will be lost.
>
> **BR:** Yes, but what if, for example, Rodney is not the leading figure who pushes everything?
>
> **GC:** Hmm, ya, these are issues that will come up at a time and they are very true. So the answer to that will be that plans have to be made in terms of succession, building capacity. Of course the BCP has weaknesses. Financial support is one of them. And of course it does not solve all problems. And that people might not, like the government might not pay attention to it. That a BCP can be produced the wrong way and lead into a bad process. But [it] is really about the process, about a BCP not just being a piece of paper.

Gino repeatedly referred to the words (financial) *support, process* and *capacity building*, and the difficulties of keeping the processes of self-empowerment and self-sustainability that are initiated by the BCP going. In particular, the dependency on the financial, administrative and legal support of donor agencies like Natural Justice, as well as on the administrative support of the K2C committee, might always remain an issue for the community in question. Natural Justice financed many of the activities of the Kukula Healers, such as larger meetings with the excecutive committee and workshops. The moment finances stop flowing; activities may also come to an end. The communities would then have to build their own projects to sustain their livelihood, which may prove to be an ongoing (perhaps insurmountable) challenge, as will be shown in the course of this chapter. This does not suggest that BCPs are not framed by success, but every coin has two sides. The story of the BCP of the Kukula Healers is a story of success, but also one of subtle frictions that has an unpredictable and fragile future.

The Kukula Healers Coming into Being

Over the six months I spent with the Kukula Healers and intermittently with members of Natural Justice, I learned, through bits and pieces of conversation and in-between stories, to know to history of the Kukula Healers association. It was, in fact, a number of coincidental developments that all came together to bring about the founding of the Kukula Healers in 2009. The NGO Natural Justice, which was founded in 2007, was interested in implementing a BCP in South Africa. At the same time, the K2C committee, the regional organization in charge of taking care of the Kruger to Canyons Biosphere Region, was, among others, interested in initiating sustainable biodiversity conservation and low carbon emission projects in order to fulfill the requirements of being a UNESCO biosphere reserve. In parallel, the core team of the not yet established Kukula Healers had just detached from the larger Bushbuckridge Healers organization to form their own association. Furthermore, the local cosmetic company Godding & Godding was interested in expanding their line of products. Finally, the government, in line with the National Biodiversity Act (2004), was encouraging ABS as a means of poverty reduction and protecting indigenous knowledge as human rights justice. ABS in this sense was seen as a gateway for local development, community empowerment, the sustainable conservation of biodiversity and economic growth.

The key event in the foundation of the Kukula Healers was the fact that, as a result of mistrust, internal quarrels and lack of future visions, a small group of healers from Hluvukane had decided to separate from the largest healers' association in the area, the Bushbuckridge Healers, which was seated close to the municipal capital Bushbuckridge. "The leader of this organization," explained Rodney Sibuyi, "was an uneducated man who never went to school [impande], took the membership fees [70 to 140 Rand], but never had any plans or visions for the organization. He only puts all the money in his own pocket." Together with his friends Adah Mabunda and Charles Mthetwa, the three healers decided to leave the group and start their own organization. Rodney applied for funding at Bushbuckridge Municipality, but was rejected on the basis of not having a bank account. He suggested that the money could be transferred to the bank account of the Nyanga Traditional Healers Organization for Africa based in Johannesburg[7], and then sent back to Rodney. This request was also rejected because money used for activities in Bushbuckridge

---

7   Many healers in the Bushbuckridge area were, at the time, also members of the Nyanga Traditional Healers Organization for Africa. Being a member of the organization is a guarantee that the healer is capable of healing patients in an ethical, efficient, safe and hygienic way. The organization also works with the government to ensure the good work of traditional health practitioners (www. traditionalhealth.org.za/t/aboutus.html, last accessed January 5, 2015).

Municipality is strictly meant for local activities, and cannot be transferred to an organization in another region. Rodney and his fellow healers thus decided to create their own organization, which they called the Traditional Health Practitioners of Bushbuckridge (THPB), with an independent bank account, and from 2009 onwards they started meeting at Vukuzenzele Medicinal Plant Nursery.

Vukuzenzele is a small medicinal plant nursery in Role, a suburb of Thulamahashe. It was initiated in 1998 under the guidance of Mama Rose, a vivid and ambitious healer in her early sixties. During a visit to Vukuzenzele, Mama Rose told me: I have been working as the deputy director of an umbrella organization at Bushbuckridge, which managed development and income generating projects in the Bushbuckridge area. I then attended a bee keeping course in Cambridge, United Kingdom, and a plant conservation course in Greenglen, Durban (informal conversation, Vukuzenzele, December 2010). Building on her acquired knowledge, she set up Vukuzenzele as a local development project to supply healers with medicinal plants and the government with medicinally valuable tree seedlings (of pepper bark tree, for instance) to sustain the rapidly degrading biodiversity of the area by means of reforestation. Interestingly, Mama Rose also revealed, "You know, Britta, we black people, we know nothing about plants." Was this an idea she had gained in the courses she had attended, I wondered? But Mama Rose did not continue elaborating on this statement.

Later, in 2009, the Department of Water Affairs and Forestry acknowledged the work of Mama Rose and her co-workers by financing a pump to bring water from the nearby river to the nursery. They also sponsored a fence to protect the seedlings and plants from cattle and goats grazing on the adjacent common land. The project continued to grow, and a couple of years later, in 2008, the Department of Social Development offered financial support to the Vukuzenzele project to build two stone buildings: one to serve as an education and conference center and the other from which to sell medicinal plants. When I visited Vukuzenzele in December 2011, the buildings were still under construction, and the finances had basically come to an end. However, Mama Rose remained determined: "I want these additional traditional *rondavel* [southern African-style round huts] as an education center for tourists and school classes." This was, nevertheless, more of an imagined future than a reality. Although the government buys 600 tree and other medicinal plant seedlings every September for the reforestation of biodiversity poor areas, Vukuzenzele was at the time still struggling to survive financially. Mama Rose was hoping that after the COP 17 meeting in Durban in 2011[8], she would be allocating

---

8   The seventeenth session of the Conference of the Parties (COP 17) conference on climate change was held in Durban in 2011. The K2C Biosphere Region area is affected by climate change (more – and more violent – storms, hotter summers, colder winters), which was an issue discussed at the COP 17.

more funding. Until then, she would put all her personal time and strength into Vukuzenzele.

Figure 13 Plant seedlings watered by healers

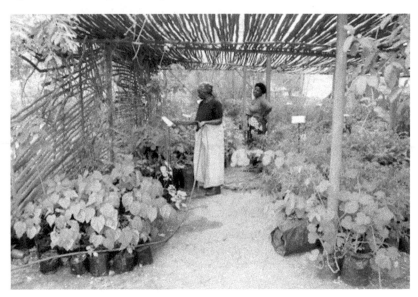

© B. Rutert.

The K2C management committee is responsible for tourism, community development and sustainable biodiversity protection in the K2C Biosphere Region. In her function as a K2C committee member, Marie-Tinka was very active in setting up community and biodiversity protection projects in the larger area. Coincidently, the Cape Town-based NGO Natural Justice was interested in cooperating with communities to develop BCPs. To pursue this aim, Natural Justice, under the lead of the African ABS Initiative, first connected with Wayne Twine of the Wits Rural Facility of the University of Witwatersrand[9], who connected them with Marie-Tinka, who then connected them with Mama Rose. Because of her background as a healer as well as her knowledge of beekeeping, her experience with the plant nursery and her extended network of healers in Thulamahashe, Mama Rose was an obvious person to approach to bring healers together to engage in the development of a BCP.

In June 2009, 20 healers of Mama Rose's circle were brought together with the NGO Natural Justice, members of the K2C committee and the Mpumalanga Rural Development Program. This group of different stakeholders discussed issues regarding access to natural resources and medicinal plants and the protection

---

9   The Wits Rural Facility lies at the road to Orpen Gate, about 30 km away from Hluvukane.

of traditional knowledge. A number of consecutive meetings were held to discuss these issues further. After this first kick-start meeting, the as yet unstructured and unorganized group of 20 healers grew in the second meeting to 80 healers; this included Rodney Sibuyi, Adah Mabunda and Charles Mthetwa, who had not attended the first meeting but had heard of it through their own gatherings of their new healers organization at Vukuzenzele . Due to their rapid growth, the association changed their name from the initial name Traditional Health Practitioners of Bushbuckridge (BHPB) to Kukula Traditional Health Practitioners Association, in short Kukula Healers (Kukula means "we will grow"). It was an impressive start for an association that did not exist before 2009. The rapid growth of the Kukula Healers might have had its roots in the density of the population living in the small villages spreading between the larger trading towns of Acornhoek and Thulamahashe. Intense cell phone communication and mouth-to-mouth propaganda among the traditional healers of the area easily spread the word of the formation of the Kukula Healers as a new group. The lack of any other, similarly successful associations might additionally have contributed to its quick success.

Rodney was already known in the area for being a strong healer, as well as for his wise leadership in the community development council (CDC) of Share/Hluvukane and for his eloquent English. He was therefore immediately elected CEO of the new association. Rodney's fluency in English was invaluable for communication with the K2C committee members as well as with Natural Justice. Furthermore, Rodney was not only the elected spokesperson, but was also the best person in taking the lead.

Since the members of the Kukula Healers were spread across Thulamahashe, Acornhoek and Hluvukane, transportation between the villages was difficult and expensive, which sometimes posed a problem for the regular meeting of all members. The association therefore formed a management committee of 26 healers. These 26 healers would, in turn, be represented by six executive committee members: the CEO Rodney Sibuyi, the chairman Adah Mabunda, the second chairman Charles Mthetwa, the third chairman Lion Thethe, the secretary Singulo Kumalo and the treasurer Lethea Olifant. For meetings with Marie-Tinka, for instance, or for decisions made in the name of the Kukula Healers, the six representatives would meet first. But even this was not always easy; Adah lived in a remote community called Gottenburg next to the entrance gate to Mayeleti Game Reserve, and Lion Thethe lived in the Welverdiend community, both of which are about 30 minutes' drive away from Hluvukane, where the executive committee met (shifted from Vukuzenzele Medicinal Plant Nursery). Furthermore, meetings were often hindered by money or weather constraints; Adah, for instance, was intermittently unable to come after heavy rains flushed away the road to Gottenburg. Nevertheless, in the monthly meetings, in which every Kukula Healer could participate, the activities and decisions of the executive committee would be discussed with the larger group.

While Rodney managed the Kukula Healers with success, Mama Rose felt usurped and resentfully started to take a distance from the healers, ending in the separation of the Vukuzenzele Medicinal Plant Nursery project from the Kukula Healers. Mama Rose later claimed defensively, "I left the Kukula because of all the work at Vukuzenzele." Rumors said that Mama Rose had 'power issues' and that because of her bossiness, other Vukuzenzele members had also parted from the nursery. For her part, Mama Rose claimed that they had left due to having to do too much work for too little pay: "They don't want to know about plants, they only want to make fast money. After some time, they get lazy. So it is a problem to keep the garden going. You know, Britta, it is much easier to work in a family than in a cooperative" (conversation at Vukuzenzele, December 2011).

At a workshop on the Traditional Knowledge Commons in Cape Town in March 2012, where Mama Rose and Rodney were both invited, some major misunderstandings and personal sensitivities could eventually be resolved. Mama Rose was also able to see that cooperation leads to more (financial) support than smaller solitary projects. The Vukuzenzele project and the Kukula Healers had very similar future plans, including the idea of building an education center on medicinal plants. The work plan for 2013 for the Kukula Healers developed by Natural Justice as a provision for funding also included "the formalization of project cooperation between Vukuzenzele and the Kukula Healers." Nevertheless, Mama Rose remained distant to the Kukula Healers. She still participated in meetings, workshops and celebrations, but mainly kept to herself in Vukuzenzele.

The development of the Kukula Healers would probably not have been so successful without the funding of Natural Justice. The NGO had initiated the first meetings at Vukuzenzele, paid for transportation and food, and provided continuous finances for the development process of the BCP, including several overnight workshops where the management committee of 26 healers was accommodated at the Wits (Witswatersrand University) Rural Facility, as well as for the translation of the BCP into different languages and the printing costs. The financial dependency of the healers on the NGO remained until the point at which I left the area in May 2010, continued until the end of 2015, and may indeed continue further.

The Biocultural Community Protocol

The BCP that was developed between the Kukula Healers and Natural Justice did eventually manifest in August 2010 as a 23 page printed color document, translated into Shangaan, Sesotho and English. It entails detailed information about the needs of the healers, their position and responsibilities within their communities, and their ways of dealing with requests from outside parties interested in their knowledge[10]. The core of the protocol describes the close relationship of the healers with their communities and the surrounding environment, including "How we connect our communities via our culture to our biodiversity"[11]:

> Our harvesting of medicinal plants is guided by our spiritual values and is regulated by our customary laws that promote the sustainability of our natural resources. For example, we ask our ancestors as we harvest to ensure that the medicines will have their full effect, and believe that only harvested leaves or bark that are taken in ways that ensure the survival of the plant or tree will heal the patient. This means that we take only strips of bark, selected leaves of stems of plants, and always cover the roots of trees or plants after we have collected what we require. Also, we have rules linked to the seasons in which we can collect various plants, with severe consequences such as jeopardizing rains if they are transgressed. Because we harvest for immediate use, we never collect large scale amounts of any particular resource, tending to collect a variety of small samples. This inhibits over-harvesting[12].

This excerpt of the Kukula Healers' BCP expresses ecologically-based customary laws that protect the environment and relate the healers to the health needs of their communities. It outlines the values and moral norms of the healers. Certainly, not all of these normative rules are met in everyday life. I actually saw a number of breaches. But documenting these rules enshrines their importance and is an effort to ensure the ongoing respect for threatened cultural tradition and degrading biodiversity. The Nagoya Protocol, which states that parties shall "take into consideration indigenous and local communities' customary laws, community protocols and procedures (Art. 12, Sect. 1), and support the development of [c]ommunity protocols in relation to access to traditional knowledge associated with genetic resources and the fair and equitable sharing of benefits arising out of the utilization" (Art. 12, Sec. 3 (a)) is the stepstone for developing a BCP. According to Kabir Bavikatte, one of the founders of Natural Justice:

> The value of a community protocol lies in their ability to act as the glue that holds together the total mosaic of a community life that is fragmented under different laws and policies, with the understanding that the conservation of nature is a result of a holistic way of life (Bavikatte 2011: 23).

---

10   Biocultural Protocol of The Traditional Health Practitioners of Bushbuckridge, 2010 (http://community-protocols.org/wp-content/uploads/documents/South_Africa-Bushbuckridge_Biocultural_Protocol.pdf).

11   (ibid.: 1).

12   (ibid.: 2); see also: http://naturaljustice.org/video/photo-story-bcp-traditional-health-practitioners-bushbuckridge/ (last accessed October 16, 2016).

The fundament behind the promotion of BCPs is all well and good. In everyday reality, however, they are not so easily applicable and ratified and are rather an ongoing process, also framed by failure and delay. These challenges also faced the BCP of the Kukula Healers; for instance, the tribal authority Chief Mnisi was, at first, not interested in communicating or cooperating with the healers about the protocol. Other community members and organizations, like local churches, did also not take cognizance of the new developments of the healers. Nevertheless, the Kukula Healers were eventually successful in completing the BCP, and with it they have implemented a tool to reaffirm their importance in their communities, that enables self-governance, promotes them as stewards over their local resources, and includes them in the preservation of biodiversity and hence of the land and environment in which they live. The BCP as a primarily non-market approach (Brush 1994) is, however, also a means to cope with economic market demands. It provides for legal requirements such as prior informed consent and ABS from "researchers who (in the past) provided us with few details of who they are working for and what our knowledge will be used for"[13]

Another key aspect of the BCP is its push for access to nature reserves, namely Mariepskop, a mountain on the edge of the Drakensberg Escarpment, a biodiverse and fertile area with rare medicinal plants. Over-harvesting by *muthi* hunters and firewood collectors in the communal areas has led to medicinal plants vanishing or being harder to find, and hence to the lack of these plants for healing practices. Accessing nature and game reserves is a strong concern of the healers in order to be able to maintain their customary use of regional plants. The K2C biosphere region, however, is dominated by privately or governmentally owned nature and game reserves. These reserves are inaccessible to the local population and collecting plants is strictly forbidden. The wish to gain access to Mariepskop was documented in the BCP and was discussed with the area's manager Gwyneth Depport at the workshop to develop a Code of Conduct/Ethics, with positive results: the Kukula Healers may enter the nature reserve if led by a knowledgeable guide. Accordingly, the BCP provides a strong call for cooperation and dialog with local authorities, the government, the K2C committee, local health facilities like Hluvukane Health Clinic, the South African Wildlife College as well as Kruger National Park and other game and nature reserves. Cooperation and dialog will hopefully strengthen the healers' position in their communities as well as their integration in sustainable environmental protection programs.[14]

---

13   See: Biocultural Protocol of The Traditional Health Practitioners of Bushbuckridge, 2010 (http://community-protocols.org/wp-content/uploads/docu ments/South_Africa-Bushbuckridge_Biocultural_Protocol.pdf).

14   In one example, Rodney Sibuyi and other Kukula Healers were trained as environmental monitors at the South African Wildlife College. In 2014, the Kukula Healers were approached to support Kruger National Park in the fight against rhino poaching, as many poachers were

When reading the BCP, however, it soon becomes obvious that the ideas have been strongly guided by external actors such as Natural Justice. This is legible in the prevalence of the language of policies and law. Although the content of the BCP is based on the ideas and needs of the healers, Natural Justice has clearly guided these formulations. But what exactly motivated the healers to develop a BCP, aside from the influence of Natural Justice? How exactly does the local situation of the healers look in everyday life? Why did they agree to develop the BCP? What concerns and motivates the traditional healers most in their everyday lives? And how has the BCP been embedded in their personal lives as well as in the lives of their communities?

"Our Knowledge Is Threatened":
Traditional Healers in a Changing Society

Besides the rich and deep collection of knowledge of many traditional healers, and the many customary laws that protect knowledge, knowledge transference faces many constraints. Even before the development of the BCP, the healers were aware of the fact that the society in which they live has changed through the influences of modern technology and work migration, and with these changes they felt the pressure to adjust their tradition to meet current demands. In interviews with Kukula Healers members, they recounted challenges that they found threatening to their traditions, like the advent of a modernizing society[15], modern technologies, young people seeking higher education or at least better paid, "clean jobs," the lack of interest of the younger generation in the "old tradition," the tendency towards short training periods for traditional healers with a consequent deterioration in quality of the transferred knowledge, economic, environmental and political changes, as well as subliminal jealousy and envy. When I spoke to Rodney's or Adah's children, they preferred well paid jobs such as working in an office, in the IT sector or in tourism, and they often had a dismissive attitude towards traditional healing, claiming instead to be Christians; going to church was declared as incompatible with traditional healing. Indeed, Adah himself explained that the younger generation is no longer interested in traditional healing and customary laws: "They prefer partying," she said, hinting at the *sheebeen* (local pub) opposite her house, "and jobs in the IT sector."

This perceived stance of younger people being against traditional healing stands in contrast to the supposedly increasing number of people who train as traditional

---

supposed to live in communities next to the park (http://kruger2canyon.linmedia.co.za/articles/news/13173/2012-05-25/traditional-healers-take-a-stand-against-rhino-poaching, last accessed October 30, 2015).

15   Modernization processes in African societies have been largely discussed in i.e. Geschiere 1997 and Geschiere et al. 2008. For more generall discussion on „modernity" see also Giddens 1991, 1994.

healers. One explanation for this is the fact that in today's money-based economy, becoming a healer is (also) a means of economic survival (Dietzel 2013). Normally, a consultation fee is 100 Rand. For additional services, depending on the treatment and the applied and prescribed *muthi*, patients pay supplementary fees. The motivation to train as a healer may also derive from the idea of getting fees for training other healers. Economic incentives, amongst others, motivate people to train as healers, regardless of whether they have had the calling or not. Though while some healers can sustain their livelihoods through the consultation of patients, not all healers are in the position to have many patients, especially in a densely populated area like Bushbuckridge Municipality, with its estimated 8000 traditional healers (estimation from informal conversation with Remember Mathebula, regional politician and former member of the K2C committee). Many healers thus had to rely on other income sources, such as breeding cows, donkeys, goats and chickens, renting out donkeys, running a sheebeen or even leading a church. Many of the Kukula Healers also claimed in interviews that people today prefer to go to the health clinics. Others seek support and spiritual guidance from churches, including the Zionist Christian Church or private churches such as those established by Nigerian migrants. The priests of these churches regularly defame traditional healers and often speak out against people visiting traditional healers at all, based on the accusation that they are manipulative and only want to take people's money. Lion Thethe (LT) explained the influence that the church has had on traditional healing and customary laws.

> **LT:** Customary laws are for the whole [of] Africa. They were the custodians of the moral attitude of the community. That is where the community puts belief and trust. But with the church, the change started from there. But the children who grow up from the church, they are experiencing to live with the church and with modernization. And so, today, people believe only in the clinic, even though the African healers know a lot about disease. Let's say, maybe a child gets sick, because of his or her ancestors. She will die. Before, I remember when a child gets sick. It's critical and when the parents go to the inyanga and he throws the bones and he says there is that person from long ago and you find that problem and when you get home, you will be amazed because the child runs and it [is] healed. Even from the Bible we know, it says: 'Your belief will make you get up and walk'. We believe in our ancestors. The Bible says, 'How can you love God, whom you cannot see, but fail to love your brother?'
>
> **BR:** Why do people feel threatened by the healers?
>
> **LT:** No, they put it in a different way. The Bible says: 'Respect your mother and your father'. (...) But today, the preacher comes and says, 'Your forefathers are demons'. (...) Even when your father or mother can let you down, God cannot let you down.

Lion Thethe above illustrates the difficulties between traditional healing and "the churches"[16]: traditional healers believe in the ancestors, while the churches preach belief in God and diminish the power of the elders (ancestors) to substitute for the power of God. He pointedly questioned this stance by asking, "How can you love God, whom you cannot see, but fail to love your brother"?

Against the background, it was nevertheless the case that most of the healers whom I spoke to were members of one of the churches in the area. They had no issue with combining a belief in God with their belief in and work with the ancestors. Rodney, for instance, told me that it was a Zionist Christian Church priest who had suggested that he should train as a healer. Rodney himself had also opened his own "church," located on a spot under a tree next to his house, where people of Share community would gather for a congregation every Sunday. He had never trained as a priest, but he had had the vision that he should "pray with and for his people." Another member of the Kukula Healers, Mr. Ntala (MN), explained in an interview in December 2011 that he did not see any problem with being a traditional healer and a priest of his own church. Even the ancestors seemed tolerant of the combination:

BR: So, you are a priest and a healer?

MN: Ya, I have gone for training [as a healer].

BR: First you were a healer and then a priest? Is there no conflict?

MN: No, not according to the ancestors. I can still give the medicine to the patients.

BR: Was it like a calling to become a priest?

MN: No, I was a healer before, so in the long run, I had a dream that I must change, become a priest. So, I went to someone who was a healer and then a priest. Then I had a dream that I must build a church; I had the dream four times. I heard like a voice like God say that I must build my church here. This is a Zion Church here. Lots of traditional healers, they go to Zion, because they allow them to be healers.

BR: And is your church full?

MN: Yes, it's always full, but a lot of them are healers.

This ambivalent stance of the healers toward the churches, and vice versa, was repeatedly mentioned in other interviews. Ambivalent positions were also noticeable in other realms of the everyday lives of the Kukula Healers and others. Jealousy and suspicion, for instance, were often mentioned as a major factor negatively impacting the process of knowledge transference, which led some healers to not share their knowledge with others. The traditional healer Andaleti Nkomo in the Eastern Cape had this to say on the subject in March 2009:

---

16   There are innumerable churches in this multi-ethnic region. Additional research would be required to understand the contradictory relationship between traditional healers and local churches in the area.

> **BR:** And do you talk about your knowledge in the community? Do you share your knowledge with others?
>
> **AK:** Oh, that is a problem, because all traditional healers are jealous. They don't like to share the knowledge. But eh, I am not like this. I started to go to church first. I am open. So, I like to share, I do tell others.
>
> **BR:** What are people jealous about?
>
> **AK:** It is like a competition. Because they always will think that patients and clients will come to me and not to the others, when I tell them what I use and people only come to you and not to me.

Andaleti Nkomo thus ambivalently regarded knowledge sharing. She said that she herself did not have any issues with sharing her knowledge, but the fear of envy and jealousy of her fellow healers did hold her back.

Jealousy and suspicion were more often pronounced in interviews in the Eastern Cape than in Bushbuckridge Municipality. The fact that it was mentioned less by the Kukula Healers is presumably because I approached them at a point in time when they had already extensively discussed knowledge sharing in the process of developing the BCP. They were so well versed in the rhetoric of sharing that the idea of not sharing was only pronounced as a means of protecting specialized knowledge, and not motivated by jealousy. This is not to say that jealousy is not a common motivation for secrecy in the Bushbuckridge area. Indeed, jealousy is often associated with witchcraft accusations, which in Apartheid times, but also in the post-Apartheid era (Ashforth 2001, 2005), have made healers particularly vigilant when it comes to knowledge sharing. As Adam Ashforth (2001: 5) has explained:

> Witchcraft in the South African context typically means the manipulation by malicious individuals of powers inherent in persons, spiritual entities, and substances to cause harm to others (...) the motive of witchcraft is typically said to be "jealousy" (which in ordinary usage here encompasses envy).

Comaroff and Comaroff (1991, 1993) argue that jealousy in the context of traditional healing and witchcraft accusation is bound to economic competition. Being an expert of particular knowledge makes one economically superior to other healers, which creates a mixture of desire and despair, ending in jealousy in times when healers have to struggle for economic survival in a context in which their livelihoods are primarily based on monetary income[17].

---

17   For the scope of this thesis, it would go too far to engage deeply with notions of witchcraft. This has been done elsewhere. Isak Niehaus, for instance, claimed that in Green Valley in the Homeland *Lebowa*, witchcraft and witch hunting is a political occurrence, which represents social changes in society (Niehaus 1993, 2012). He also wrote extensively about the fear of witchcraft in Bushbuckridge/Impalahoek, which he suggests is not only a consequence of a new form of capital accumulation (cf. Geschiere 1997) or the consequences of economic glo-

With the integration of traditional healers into the legislation and the attempt
to professionalize traditional healing (see also Last & Chavunduka 1986; Zenker
2010, 2015) through the registration of all healers at the Department of Health, the
attitude towards knowledge sharing has slowly changed in the healers' minds. Lion
Thethe, in an interview in January 2012, explained why sharing knowledge has become so important today, and why the Kukula Healers decided to share knowledge
with one another, as well as with actors outside of traditional healing:

BR: And does sacred knowledge exist?

LT: We have sacred knowledge, but not in that way, because everything should
be in [the] public. If maybe you used to keep knowledge secret, you will find that
maybe if you put it out, you can get help. But if you keep your knowledge you make
it too confidential. You can't get assistance. People will never know what is your
problem. All in all, you have to be open. What is the secret there? It can be a secret
among the members. Because maybe I come to her [a healer], I need a treatment,
it is maybe her secret because she knows something about this treatment. She
may keep that part secret because this is how she can make money. But if I want
to know about that secret, I have to go through that training, because this is the
only way. But beyond that, with the inyangas [in this context, inyanga are divin-
ers/sangomas], we must share. Because you find that today the government says
the doctors must share with the inyangas. Because you find that another person
comes to the hospital and the disease the person is carrying needs the inyanga. So
the doctors must be free to let him go and then he comes back. Even the inyanga,
they mustn't treat the patient until he dies. If maybe you find that our inyanga
doesn't have the machine like adding blood or the water [transfusion], so then
you take that person to the hospital. And don't be proud or jealous. Bring the person to the hospital. And then you carry on with the treatment. So, if you keep that
secret, many people will die.

BR. So, you also don't mind sharing with the public? With the community?

LT: Yes, we must share, so that people don't hide the diseases that they are having.
People, they used to stay quiet sometimes. But you need to be open.

BR: And was it always like that?

LT: No, not always. Before it was really a secret. They were not talking to each
other. Maybe you happen to have a problem or a disease you happen to keep se-

---

balization with the formation of "occult economies" (a means to employ magical means for
material ends; Comaroff & Comaroff 1998, 1999). It is, he argues, "also about other things, i.e.
the re-invention of tradition (Sanders 2003), the accumulation of wealth beyond economic
wealth, i.e. accumulation of people and the wealth of people (i.e. accumulation of zomies).
Those who were accused of being witches "keeping zombies" were poor in possession and
people (Niehaus 2005: 199f.).

cret, only speak to one inyanga. But today, inyanga share and they know which inyanga knows about this and this disease. He can help you then.

Lion Thethe insisted that the sharing of knowledge, especially because of diseases like HIV/AIDS or tuberculosis, is vital. Sharing provides help for people in need and strengthens communication between the different health institutions, an often contested and not always integrative space (Wreford 2008, 2009). Learning "Western ways of healing" (Zenker 2010: 229; Decocteau 2008) broadens knowledge in fighting prevalent diseases like HIV/AIDS. If you do not share, you will not be helped in the challenge of treating these diseases. If knowledge is not shared, mistrust is more likely, which is more threatening to healers than the sharing of knowledge. Openness has, therefore, to some degree been exchanged for the previously highly valued secrecy. "In earlier times," Rodney explained, referring to the times during Apartheid, "we didn't share our knowledge. The knowledge holder owned the knowledge. But now, we [the healers] realized that we need to share knowledge, otherwise this knowledge is going to die" (informal conversation, Share, December 2011).

This new position of knowledge sharing came not least with the awareness that their knowledge has an increased value in the knowledge economy. In an interview conducted in Hluvukane, Rodney (RS), Charles Mthetwa (CM) and Charles's cousin, Pitso Mthetwa (PM), revealed the new stance of the healers with regard to their knowledge and the sharing of this knowledge. I asked about their ideas on revealing knowledge to an external research institution:

BR: (...) If the IKS Lead Program or another research institution would come to ask you for knowledge, would you mind sharing?

RS: Yes, we want to share our knowledge, but only if we come together and come to an agreement, because many people come and take our knowledge. The researchers come and go away with our knowledge.

CM: And make a lot of money.

BR: And the agreement must then be with the healer or with all Kukula Healers?

CM: It must be within the organization. We have the rule: If someone comes, we need to ask him [the following]: What is it exactly that you want to do and what is the amount of medicinal plants you want to have? After we give you this, what are we going to get? What are our benefits? We can't just give. That's why we came to an agreement with Sue from Godding and Godding. If the research comes right, we need to know exactly what are the profits, because it is our knowledge. Sue does not have the knowledge. She might have the knowledge on how to do the products, but the knowledge comes from us. It is us who know what to use against this and this disease.

PM: Because sharing is good, because you learn (...).

I cannot draw on interviews from the time before the Kukula Healers had started developing their BCP, since I only arrived in the area at the end of 2011. Nevertheless, the idea that knowledge has been taken away by outsiders (in the above quote, by researchers) was probably common to many traditional healers both before and after developing the BCP, and indeed it was often expressed in the many conversations and interviews that I held with them. Realizations of biopiracy were often expressed in sentences like " It is us who know what to use against a disease" or "It is our knowledge", indicating on the value of their knowledge and the threat when someone wants to take "our knowledge" away. At the same time, the realization that the sharing of knowledge may be vital for the future of their profession was also mentioned repeatedly.

This ambivalent stance towards sharing was also reflected in the ambivalent position of traditional healers with regard to the churches or local health clinics and the community. In both the Eastern Cape and Bushbuckridge, many lay people I spoke to outwardly claimed, that they would never consult a traditional healer, though they actually did consult healers – often secretly – for spiritual guidance, as well as for family, job or health related issues. Even Philip Mnisi, the 78-year-old chief of the area between Acornhoek, Thulamahashe and Hluvukane, explained in an interview in April 2012 that he endorses the developments of the Kukula Healers and that he and many others consult traditional healers. Indeed, at no point in the interview, which had up to that point seemed to have been specially formulated for me, the 'white researcher', did he speak negatively about traditional healers:

BR: And have you heard about the BCP? The document that the healers set up?
PM: I have heard about it and also gave [them] permission to dig roots, and now it is officially announced that the healers can dig the roots [on common land].
BR: What is the most important role the healers have in the community?
PM: It is to heal the ailment diseases, because there are diseases even the hospitals cannot heal. But the healers can do that.
BR: Do you yourself consult sangomas?
PM: Definitely.
BR: And the indunas [sub-chiefs], do they also go?
PM: Yes, everybody.
BR: And is there something to support traditional healers to save medicinal plants or knowledge?
PM: Ya, there is such a policy that is there. But you know, most of the people are bypassing, and get access to the land. They perform biopiracy. Like that one who cut the tree yesterday there, and then got fined.
BR: Do you think that your children will go to traditional healers? How will children perceive the future of customary laws and traditional healers?

PM: Ya, the government of today is going back to our cultures, so after some years they are going back to the roots. So, there will not be many changes.

The chief not only acknowledged the healers as important for the communities and their cultural life, but also permitted them to access common land to dig roots and collect medicinal plants. This exception is significant, because the chief is the official in control of administering common land. He is not the owner, as common land belongs to the state, but the organizer and distributor of tenure. He has control over the land titles and is responsible for the allocation of the 'permission to occupy' for residents. In regulating access to common land, he may fine the trespassing of access rules with high penalties. So-called illegal *muthi* hunters, for instance, can be fined by the chief for illegal harvesting, which is a big problem because it leads to the rapid extinction of plants and to traditional healers having to buy medicinal plants elsewhere (mostly from traders from Mozambique).

One day in April 2012, for instance, Rodney's father called him to tell him he had seen *muthi* hunters leaving the commons area, carrying bags loaded with plants. At the time, Rodney and I were not far from the location that Rodney's father described. We jumped into the car and rushed over. As we approached, we saw a white Toyota pick-up truck packed with seven people and seven bags full of plant material heading towards Acornhoek. We passed the Toyota and Rodney indicated for them to stop. The surprised driver stopped immediately. Rodney explained that they were not allowed to collect medicinal plants on the commons without the permission of the chief. He requested that they come to the tribal authority's office on the road to Acornhoek. At the office, they were told to hand over the collected plant material and pay a fine of 3000 Rand. They vigorously defended themselves. "We did not know about the law, that collecting plants on common land is no longer allowed. We never needed permission [before]," they claimed. They continued, "We come from further away and were instructed to collect medicinal plants for Johannesburg *muthi* market." The whole incident made Rodney very agitated. "*Muthi* hunters are threatening our tradition", he exclaimed, "but it is not easy to prevent them from collecting". But now, under the provision of the Biodiversity Act, at least *muthi* hunters can be caught and punished more easily, so "that they know," [not to continue to illegally connect medicinal plants] as Rodney suggested.

The above description of the 'capture' of these *muthi* hunters is an example of the contestation over natural resources in an area where the local biodiversity is under progressive threat. The extinction of plants leads to the extinction of particular knowledge associated with these plants, which is just one of the many threats that the healers experience. In sum, the ambivalence between the denial and acceptance of traditional healing in healers' communities, as well as the urgency to protect indigenous knowledge and medicinal plants, brought the healers eventually to the conclusion that a BCP may be a useful tool in helping to improve their situation.

Reorganizing Knowledge Protection:
The TK Commons Pool

As has been shown so far, traditional healing is not a static system. On the contrary, indigenous knowledge is in flux and adaptable, and influenced by other knowledge systems, even though it might retain a nucleus of accumulated knowledge that always remains stable. While secrecy may remain the safest way to protect knowledge, this does not exclude the aspiration to share knowledge with third parties. Accordingly, traditional knowledge systems are subject to both internal and external adaptations and changes. Traditional healers are capable of adapting to changing politics and integrating the transformations of a modernizing society with new demands with regard to public health care[18].

Lion Thethe, in the interview cited above, quite frankly said that traditional healers should share knowledge to combat diseases like HIV/AIDS, as well as to overcome the general mistrust against healers. He suggested that openness creates more trust. Among the Kukula Healers, the sharing of knowledge was seen as commonsense; this had been extensively discussed during the group's establishing phase. The healers had realized that in order to enable negotiations with third parties, neither secrecy nor their traditional way of sharing and protecting knowledge would provide a way forward. Therefore, the relatively strict rules of not sharing knowledge with outside parties were redefined and reorganized. In a process of "re-inventing their tradition" (cf. Hobsbawm & Ranger 1992; Prickett 2009), the Kukula Healers sat together to formulate and define this new form of sharing, pooling and distributing knowledge. The result, the 'traditional knowledge commons pool' (TK commons pool), came about as a response to these challenges, epitomizing flexible adaptation rather than fatalism, helplessness and capitulation. This flexibility speaks against the often-reproduced notion that indigenous knowledge is closed, non-systematic, holistic and advances on the basis of experience (Banuri & Apffel-Marglin 1993; see also Howes & Chambers 1980; Sillitoe 2002). Instead of looking at indigenous knowledge and traditional medicine as static systems only used for healing, they can be viewed as a strategic resource (Knipper 2010: 205; Meier zu Biesen, Meier zu Biesen et al. 2012; Langwick 2011) to increase the bearer's social and political status and position within society, or as a tool to gain additional "secondary income" (Unschuld 1975) beyond mere healing. In the context of the Kukula Healers, their traditional system of knowledge sharing and protection was transformed into a system adapted to the market, which they used strategically to gain more political power, as well as, in the best case, to generate a secondary income.

---

18   On the relationship between the public health sector and traditional healers, see Freeman and Motsei (1992); Wreford (2008) for South Africa; Meier zu Biesen (2012) for Zanzibar; Langwick (2011) for Tanzania.

The idea for the TK commons pool did not come from the healers themselves, but was introduced by Natural Justice, who suggested that they establish a knowledge commons pool to assemble knowledge on medicinal plants in order to strengthen the healers as knowledge holders and create awareness of their rights to their property. The creation of the TK commons pool required the community of knowledge holders to develop, in accordance with their customary laws, the terms and conditions for access to their knowledge. To enter into such a process, Natural Justice supported them with questions pertaining to legal and administrative rules and regulations, as well as financially with a budget allocated from other funding agencies (in this case the Gesellschaft für Internationale Zusammenarbeit, GTZ). The legal aspect comprised making the language of politics and instruments that commonly protect knowledge in the world of intellectual property law legible and approachable to those who have never been involved with it before. So what does this mean with regard to the TK commons pool of the Kukula Healers?

"We Want to Share Our Knowledge": The TK Commons Pool

"We want to share our knowledge, but only if we come together and come to an agreement," expressed Rodney assertively in a short TV spot on one of the largest German television news channels, the ARD Tagesthemen (daily news). He most probably would not have been able to make this assertive statement without having gone through a number of workshops, trainings and discussions in the course of developing the BCP. The statement indeed had a taste of learned development rhetoric. But how can traditional healers share knowledge that is protected by customary laws and the moral guidelines set out by the ancestors, and protect it against the pressure of commercial interests from outside entities? And at the same time, how can they claim their own economic interests with regard to the disclosed knowledge? As was said in chapter IV, traditionally, knowledge is organized along distinct forms of knowledge transference. It is gained during healer training in a particular *impande*, received from the ancestors and is extended through experience, communication with the ancestors and the sharing of knowledge with other healers. During the training, it is restricted by specific rules of transfer; the knowledge is embedded in a 'bounded community', guarded by the ancestors, and there are strict prohibitions on sharing knowledge with people outside of the *impande*.

According to the rules and the fact that knowledge is restricted to a particular group of knowledge carriers, traditional knowledge can be viewed as a commons, i.e. "a particular form of structuring the rights to access, use and control [of common] resources" (Benkler 2006: 24; Ostrom 1990). The commons refers to "the great variety of natural, physical, social, intellectual, and cultural resources that human beings hold in common or in trust to use on behalf of themselves, on other humans

beings (…) and which are essential to their biological, cultural, and social reproduction" (Nonini 2007: 1). In addition, it is "a resource shared by a group of people
that is subject to social dilemmas" (Hess & Ostrom 2007: 3). In her book 'Governing
the Commons' (1990), the political economist Elinor Ostrom defined eight 'design
principles' for effective common pool resources (CPR) management:

1   Define clear group boundaries.
2   Match rules governing use of common goods to local needs and conditions.
3   Ensure that those affected by the rules can participate in modifying the rules.
4   Make sure that rulemaking rights of community members are respected by
    outside authorities.
5   Develop a system, carried out by community members, for monitoring mem-
    bers' behavior.
6   Use graduated sanctions for rule violators.
7   Provide accessible, low-cost means to dispute resolution.
8   Build responsibility for governing the common resource in nested tiers from
    the lowest level up to the entire interconnected system (Ostrom 1990: 90).

A commons has many rules and sanctions that need to be kept alive in order to
restrain abuse. Abuse of the commons is, at least in bioprospecting today, also dependent on the forces that come with the demands of the economic market. As
Donald Nonini claims, "all commons are functioning arrangements that connect
people to the material and social things they share and use to survive and operate outside – but most frequently alongside – capitalist markets" (Nonini 2007: 6).
However, he continues, "the functional webs of interdependence that people who
organize their lives around a commons have created cannot be reduced to market
valuations" (ibid.). Although the market does have an enormous influence on the
knowledge commons, it is not totally dependent on market forces. It has and continues to exist independently of the economic market, though some adaptation of
knowledge sharing to capitalist market needs does occur.

When knowledge is inappropriately shared outside of the bounded (or secret) community of traditional healers, especially when the knowledge leaves
the boundaries of the *impande*, it is subject to social dilemmas (Hess & Ostrim
2007: 3). All major aspects of the healers' practice are in danger of losing their
purity, and hence power, when not guarded closely (cf. Douglas 1966). Interviews
with Kukula Healers revealed that knowledge that is shared without previously
requesting permission from the ancestors and/or informing other healers may
lead to punishment by the ancestral powers, possibly even the death of the person
responsible. I could not definitively determine whether this was mere rhetoric
or an actual practice. The narrative went that when the ancestors are ignored,
such as when a calling is not followed or knowledge is illegitimately disclosed,

the ancestors will punish with illness, social rupture and even death (cf. Ashforth 2005b). This comes into conflict with the call for disclosure made by the CBD and the National Biodiversity Act, a conflict that encourages the "probability of betrayal" (Simmel 1906) through the seductive prospect of potential monetary and/or non-monetary benefits.

To resolve this tension, the Kukula Healers finally decided to reconstitute their original traditional knowledge commons, which prohibited the sharing of knowledge outside of the *impande*, into a TK commons pool – a pool of knowledge that is shared among all members of the association. The TK commons pool that was established has a "commons structure" (Ostrom & Hess 2007), though it is nevertheless different from the original traditional knowledge commons. This pool consists of all knowledge that each individual member is willing to add, as well as all collectively known knowledge that the healers are willing to share with the public. Disclosure to the public can, however, still only occur under specific restricted conditions, to some extent guided by rules manifest in the CBD and the National Biodiversity Act, including notions of prior informed consent, non-disclosure, ABS agreements and co-patenting.

The TK commons pool has blurred boundaries. Rodney told me that when the TK commons pool was discussed, the Kukula Healer members agreed that all knowledge that would help healers to improve their services to their communities and help them to enter into negotiations with outside stakeholders could be shared. A general consensus was also reached that knowledge could not be shared with people outside of the healers' community, unless all members of the community agreed to it. Knowledge, however, is not a fixed entity. It is lived experience and everyday practice. Knowledge lives within every healer and within his or her family and community, and is thus already partially shared in everyday life. One healer told me in an interview, while sitting next to her husband, "You know, I don't share my knowledge with anyone." She then smiled and looked at her husband. "Also not with him." I could see that she was speaking 'officially' here in the interview; personally, I had the impression that she might share some knowledge and/or practices with her husband. Keeping knowledge fully secret in an orally oriented society, where living closely together is a common rule, is difficult. Healers might talk with their spouses or other relatives about plants, as they are often prepared in the communal living areas. Children may also be sent to collect plants, or at least join in on plant collections. Family members thus habitually get to know about medicinal plants and the preparation of *muthi*, when it is prepared in the healers' homesteads. Knowledge as lived experience, embedded in everyday practices, can thus only be partially kept secret.

Notably, not all members of the group share *all* of their knowledge, because this could lead to the weakening of their individual healing specialization. In interviews, this was articulated in partially contradictory statements. On the one hand, it was claimed, "I don't mind sharing all my knowledge." On the other hand, some healers revealed, "I would keep some knowledge for myself, as it strengthens my position as an expert." This sense of individual ownership over particular knowledge was valued as more important than the collective ownership of the association. From what I gathered in the interviews, it remained vague to me what knowledge exactly had been opened up for sharing and what was kept secret for private and professional purposes. I had the impression that this was a flexible decision made by each individual healer.

As a result, not all knowledge was fed into the newly established TK commons pool. Healers retained knowledge for their own (economic) protection. Therefore, while the TK commons pool can be described as a pool of knowledge shared among a group of people, it has its limitations, which are mostly built, to refer back to Donald Nonini, "alongside the capitalist market" (2007: 6). It is, first of all, built to be able to engage with the demands of the global economic market, i.e. to control knowledge in the global knowledge economy, which is governed by intellectual property law. Second, it has internal limitations due to the fact that nobody knew exactly what knowledge this TK commons pool contained. When I asked about the content, the answers I received were usually somewhat diffuse, ranging from "I share everything" to "I agreed on sharing when someone wants specific knowledge from me" to "I don't share everything." No answer ever revealed what exactly the pool contained, whether knowledge on plants or practices, and who exactly contributed to it. It seemed to be more of a common agreement *that knowledge may be shared*, but not about *what knowledge exactly* is shared.

In the process of sharing their knowledge with the company Godding & Godding, the Kukula Healers thus accepted that their knowledge on the "soapy plant" and the "oily *muthi* mixture" that were involved in the plant exchange in Thulamahashe was open to be shared. The original knowledge of the oily extract, for instance, came from an elderly healer who had migrated from Mozambique and had lived for 20 years in Hluvukane. The form in which this extract was presented at the plant exchange, as a crude oily mixture, was not, however, applicable for the economic market. It demanded further processing, to be done by Godding & Godding. The company did not ultimately find any viable cosmetic value in the mixture, but in the event that it had, the healer would have had to incorporate a line of collective knowledge holders (i.e. her ancestors from Mozambique as well as the other living healers in the area) into further ownership negotiations. Being part of the Kukula Healers association would have helped in negotiating ownership rights, providing stronger group coherence and a stronger (legal) partner in ABS negotiations.

The healers may come together again to agree on the sharing of other knowledge, if another third party (other than Godding & Godding) were to approach them for knowledge sharing. In this case, the same rules would be valid: first, the agreement of all Kukula Healers members would be required before the knowledge could be shared; second, there would have to be a trust relationship between all healers. Trust overrides jealousy and fosters the trustful sharing of knowledge and of any benefits that may materialize. The latter did not transpire during the time that I was staying in the area, and of course its likelihood in the future is not guaranteed. Financial benefits did not emanate from the knowledge exchanged with Godding & Godding, since the company did not continue to work with the exchanged plant material. And though the TK commons pool had been helpful in the case of the plant exchange in Thulamahashe, to me it remains unclear whether it will have a lasting effect.

The TK commons pool remains a blurred entity, which is built on the *inclusion* of knowledge, the *expansion* of people, *setting boundaries* of controlled sharing as well as *limitations* of what is shared and how. It upholds the relations that are attached to knowledge, but allows for an expansion of this web of relations as well as their strengthening. It basically brings people together to discuss the value of their property, knowledge and medicinal plants. This supports Gino Cocchiaro's earlier argument that BCPs, and with them the development of a TK commons pool, brings dispersed and unorganized communities together to discuss their needs, which inevitably leads to them taking a stronger stance with regard to their needs. Knowledge, in an agreed upon TK commons pool, is a binder of social cohesion. In addition, the negotiation process enables healers to engage in a new deep effort of introspection into their values, norms and communities. Lewis Hyde summarized his thoughts on this in his book 'The Gift' (1983):

> When 'knowledge' passes from hand to hand in this spirit, it becomes a binder of many wills. What gathers in it is not only the sentiment of generosity but the affirmation of individual goodwill, making those separate parts a spiritus mundi, a unanimous heart, a band whose wills are focused through the lens of the 'shared knowledge'. Thus the knowledge becomes an agent of social cohesion, and this again leads to the feeling that its passage increases its worth, for the social life; at least, the whole really is greater than the sum of its parts. It brings the group together, the 'knowledge' increases in worth immediately upon its first circulation, and then like a faithful lover, continues to grow through constancy (Hyde 1983: 35).

The following graph illustrates the sharing of knowledge outside of the boundaries of an individual *impande*, but still within the boundaries of all involved *izimpande*. The TK commons pool, through its innovative combination of knowledge sharing and protection, supports the Kukula Healers' ability to govern and further develop their knowledge, while at the same time enabling a coherent group identity, which also strengthens their cultural heritage. This new tool of governing intangible property may, however, lead to legal clashes, as it will be confronted with the legal demands of intellectual property protection.

Figure 14 The TK commons pool

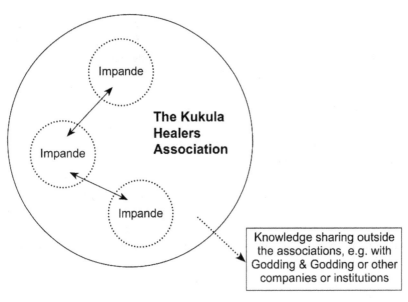

© B. Rutert.

Legal Implications: When Intellectual Property Meets the TK Commons Pool

The Kukula Healers' TK commons pool was established in order for them to have a commonly agreed upon tool to defend their knowledge as intangible property against those who seek to control knowledge within the boundaries of intellectual property rights and law, in particular research institutions such as the IKS Lead Program and the company Godding & Godding. In the event that a research institution or company approaches the healers for information on medicinal plants, such a request could lead to clashes between the two systems, namely customary law and intellectual property law. The former is a system that protects and governs collectively held knowledge, while the latter protects the inventions and innovations of individual knowledge holders, mostly within larger companies or institutions. When these two systems meet, a battle over rights and law is almost guaranteed.

Historically, the battle of rights and law in South Africa has its origin in the beginning of colonialism in the 17th century. With the invasion of the Dutch settlers it was 'Roman-Dutch law', and with the arrival of British settlers it was 'English law', and these systems were slowly established in the Cape area and gradually forced upon the indigenous population. In colonial South Africa, the state legal system was guided by a positivist approach that ignored the social origin of laws and defined local Africans as having no law at all (Bennett 2004). But customary laws had and continue to exist, and they were/are imbued with socio-cultural values, ethics and traditions (ibid.; Oomen 2005) that were/are lived beyond the legal forces of colonial and later Apartheid and then also post-Apartheid powers. Nevertheless, they "have been treated as inferior, scarcely deserving recognition as true laws" (Bennett 2011: 30) and were never fully integrated into either the colonial or Apartheid constitutions. For highly specialized systems such as state law, the mutability of customary law was regarded as unreliable and incompatible. With the new democratic constitution of 1993, amended and finalized in 1996, customary law was integrated for the first time and "the perception of customary law as inferior to the common legal system slowly reversed" (ibid.: 31).

Intellectual property and indigenous knowledge are concepts that for a long time traveled separate historical pathways. Intellectual property is a generic term for systems of positive law, some of which, such as patent law, have medieval origins (Drahos & Frankel 2012: 1; see also Drahos 1996; Mgbeoji 2006). These ideas underlined property securitization in early, middle and late capitalism (Drahos & Frankel 2012: 3). Indigenous knowledge has much older roots, though it was only recently brought into the legal debate (cf. Brush 1996), and with little acknowledgement of its innovative qualities. Innovation is legally designated to new products only. As a predominantly market-oriented tool, developed in the context of industrialized nations, intellectual property law testifies its inability to deal with traditional knowledge. For example, one requirement of patentability is that an invention has to be novel and documented. Copyright protection, with its requirements of 'originality' and its limitations to what is actually recorded, is thus unsuitable for the traditional songs and melodies of indigenous peoples that often only exist in oral form. "Geographical indication," another prerequisite of intellectual property law, also does not apply to knowledge that is habitually used beyond a specific region, often with ownership that cannot be located, as was the case with *Hoodia gordonii*. Concurrently, intellectual property law is unable to integrate traditional knowledge since it is non-inventory, collectively held and inalienable.

Nevertheless, customary laws in themselves have been acknowledged as a form of knowledge protection, most recently with the Nagoya Protocol, which in Article 12 (1) says:

> In implementing their obligations under this [Biocultural Community] Protocol, Parties shall in accordance with domestic law take into consideration indigenous and local communities' customary laws, community protocols and procedures, as applicable, with respect to traditional knowledge associated with genetic resources.

Article 12 (1) of the Nagoya Protocol suggests integrating customary law in accordance with domestic law (which is state law of South Africa). The vagueness of the definition of the Nagoya Protocol may therefore enforce the ambivalent position whereby at state's domestic law eventually overrides customary law (Vermeylen 2013: 190). Putting down customary law in a documented, and thus provable, form may help to balance out this legal power battle; a battle that is not new. Jacques Derrida argued that the continued use of the oral/written distinction is always haunted by the underlying racist distinction of the colonial project (Derrida 1976)[19]. The distinction between state law and local customary laws, which stems from colonial times and where the written word is still regarded as more stable and trustworthy than the oral word (Vermeylen 2013: 192), continues until today. In accordance with the notion of *lawfare* (Comaroff & Comaroff 2009: 53), the healers, with their BCP, conformed to the requirements of a legal system that still insists on provable, written documentation. Narratives such as myths, origin stories and oral customary law are, from a legal point of view, less relevant. But the BCP is also an attempt to put customary laws into a legal form, applicable to the (legal) requirements of the National Biodiversity Act (PIC, NDA, ABS and co-patenting) and intellectual property law, yet with the aim of moving beyond the so far dominant idea of individually held innovations of intellectual property law.

A Sui Generis (Partial) Solution: A Legal Trust

As was indicated above, the manifestation of customary law in a semi-legal tool like the BCP, which is not an official legal tool but may be used in legal negotiations, can be read as an imposition of legal categories and of the written word on oral cultures. Nevertheless, the BCP brings intellectual property law, which demands written documents as legal proof, together with what is important to the healers. The BCP is thus an intermediary between two different legal systems.

In the discussion on how to make use of the Kukula Healers' BCP with regard to knowledge protection under current intellectual property law, Gino Cocchiaro of Natural Justice and Bernard Maister of the intellectual property unit at the University of Cape Town Law School developed a 'legal trust' model. The legal trust is a model whereby the Kukula Healers, as a legal entity, may decide about their knowledge and knowledge protection schemes as well as about how to share the possible benefits that may derive from their knowledge. It deals with questions such as how to share benefits appropriately in the community and who should take responsibility for this process. The trust model is a legal mechanism with a long history in Western legal regimes, and in South Africa it is recognized and governed by the Trust Property Control Act 57 of 1988. This act defines a trust as "the arrangement through which the ownership in property of one person is by virtue of a trust

---

19   For further details about the interface between the written and the oral, see also Goody
      (1986).

instrument" (ibid.) placed under the control of another, namely the trustee. The trustee then administers or disposes of the property "according to the provisions of the trust instrument for the benefit of the person or class of persons designated in the trust instrument for the achievement of the object stated in the trust instrument" (ibid.).

Theoretically, in the case of the plant exchange in Thulamahashe between the Kukula Healers and Godding & Godding, the *trust* was based on the property that the healers provided to the company, comprising the plant material itself and the associated knowledge. The *trustee*, as the person or class of persons who can legally administer the trust property, could have been an outside entity, i.e. a lawyer or a K2C committee member, but also a designated group defined within the Kukula Healers association, such as the six executive committee members. The trustee would eventually control and organize the potential benefits arising from the trust and delegate them to the beneficiaries. The *beneficiary* could in this case have been, for instance, children of Kukula Healers members. A legal trust model thus extends the traditional understanding of reciprocity, and even the reciprocity that is implied in the TK commons pool, as it may potentially lead beyond the boundaries of the healers association and reach into the communities or families of the healers.

Practically, the legal trust model only comes into being in the event that benefits actually materialize. In the case of the Kukula Healers and Godding & Godding, this has, so far, not happened. In January 2012, Sue Godding explained in an interview that I conducted with her in the presence of Rodney Sibuyi at the small cosmetics factory situated between Hoedspruit and Acornhoek that "The soapy leaves and the oily liquid have not been analyzed yet. The Christmas business in December had not left any spare time for further research. And, ehm, unfortunately, the leaves have gotten rotten by now, so we cannot use them for investigation anymore." She apologized for the "bad timing of the plant exchange in December" and reassured us many times that she "still believe[d] in these natural products." "My [black] employees," she added, "do not believe at all in this rubbish. And I, personally, would also prefer to buy nicely packed soaps and creams" (information from interview with Sue Godding, February 2012). To be applicable for the market, the products exchanged by the healers would obviously require some commercial as well as aesthetic upgrading. The Godding & Godding cosmetic silk products, for instance, which are supplemented with 'African additives' such as Marula and Baobab tree essence, are styled with sophisticated white packaging with the G & G initials printed in silver[20]. It is marketed as an expensive product line, mainly for wealthy tourists on their way to Kruger National Park or customers who buy the products in up market shopping malls.

---

20   http://goddingandgodding.com.

In April 2013, when I went back to Bushbuckridge Municipality for a private visit, I learned that Godding & Godding had still not considered conducting any further research on the offered plant material. Next to their problems with the gioverment for not having complied with the Biodiversity Act regarding some of their products, the company had, in addition, gone through a recession. Even new plant material, which the Kukula Healers had iven to someone in the company, had never reached Sue Godding (personal communication with Sue Godding, March 2013). The company was basically uninterested in further developing anything from the plant material. Marie-Tinka, who had also been part of the plant exchange in Thulamahashe, said:

> Honestly, I don't believe in the commercial path. It is much more important for the healers to stabilize their own position in their communities as social and therapeutic workers and as stewards over environmental knowledge. It was Debby who much more pushed the commercial path (from personal communication with Marie-Tinka, March 2013).

The healers, in contrast to Marie-Tinka's opinion – which to me sounded slightly paternalistic, and also reflected her position as administrator of the financial support that the healers received from Natural Justice – had hoped for the successful development of a cosmetic product, though they adapted to the situation with the motivation to continue with other projects. Rodney repeatedly held, "We must make money, Britta, but how? We must develop our own business." The accusations, pronounced by Kukula Healers, that Debby had taken some of the exchanged material to give it to a German company did not turn out to be true; they were possibly based on the lack of direct communication between the Kukula Healers, Marie-Tinka, Debby and Godding & Godding. Most communication was supposed to be held via Marie-Tinka, but as Rodney told me in December 2013, she had stopped working with the healers and left the entire communication to another K2C member.

Against this background of the plant material and knowledge of the healers never ending up in a product and hence never materializing any benefits to be shared – a situation that is not uncommon in bioprospecting activities – the legal trust remains a mere theoretical concept. The idea of a trust model therefore can, for now, only stand as a hypothetical 'best case scenario' (also for other communities) and as one further step in the quest for solutions for the fair sharing of benefits arising from bioprospecting. Nevertheless, establishing a BCP, and with it the TK commons pool, helped the healers of Bushbuckridge Municipality to identify their needs, manifest their position in society and understand parts of the often highly sophisticated legal language implied in knowledge protection and ABS agreements, through the many workshops they attended in their cooperation with Natural Justice.

The BCP thus remains a partial solution. The healers had hoped for financial benefits, but were flexible in terms of adapting and reconsidering their original objectives, and remained dependent on the financial support of Natural Justice. Without this support, the healers association would not be able to meet regularly to discuss their objectives and future perspectives. At the time of my stay with them, they had no businesses or projects that offered them any sort of financial income, besides their own individual incomes from traditional healing and/or other small-scale businesses or family support. In this sense, the BCP remained what the World Intellectual Property Organization has defined as a *defensive mode of protection*. The TK commons pool contributed to this defensive mode of protection, as well as to the politicization of the healers, by helping them to view their knowledge as a "strategic resource" (Knipper 2010). It was intended not only to protect their knowledge and claim ownership and governance over their resources, but also to potentially make financial use of their property in the future. The TK commons pool may help the healers, as it enabled them to bundle their knowledge into a pool under their own sovereignty. In adition, the TK commons pool as a new concept was also discussed beyond the boundaries of the Kukula Healers in Bushbuckridge Municipality – i.e. during a workshop in Cape Town in March 2012, which I describe in the section below.

A Traditional Knowledge Commons Workshop (March 2012)

The workshop on the traditional knowledge commons was initiated under the umbrella of the Open A.I.R Network and the GIZ ABS Capacity Developmentz Initiative, and facilitated by Natural Justice, the workshop was entitled 'Non-traditional users of traditional knowledge: Opportunities and challenges around compliance'. Together with Mama Rose and Rodney, I joined the workshop. There were also four Natural Justice members and three researchers and intellectual property experts from Ghana, Kenya and South Africa. Together, we discussed questions such as "What is a traditional knowledge commons?" "How is a commons possible in a space of multiple cultural backgrounds?" and "How can we make use of the knowledge commons in knowledge protection schemes?"

In the discussions about the traditional knowledge commons, Mama Rose and Rodney explained the cultural and spiritual values of traditional healers in Bushbuckridge Municipality to the other participants, who were mainly legal experts working in NGOs or at the university. Mama Rose explained, "We look at their [the ancestors'] knowledge in a very different way than just a commodity to be bought and sold. We want to be involved in the use of our knowledge and be recognized for our contribution." Mama Rose and Rodney placed emphasis on the cultural and spiritual values of traditional knowledge in the context of an intellectual property law system focused on economic values. The discussions went on in the search for answers to the question of how to protect traditional knowledge in the age of the global knowledge economy. The TK commons pool can define the ownership of knowledge included in potential upcoming products by giving credit to the spiritual and cultural background of indigenous knowledge, though it cannot protect the knowledge when it gets involved in commercialization processes. The discussions were further concerned with the question of how to protect collectively held knowledge under intellectual property law. The inclusion of the ancestors as an entity similar to a legal person could not be (legally) integrated. But it is also possible that their full integration is not necessary or even aspired to in this context. More important may be for academically and legally minded persons to understand the lifeworld of the healers, their epistemology and ontology, in order to support them in governing themselves and the environment they live in.

What I noticed in this regard was an ongoing switch between understanding and misunderstanding between the healers and the other participants. Oftentimes, when one of the legal participants spoke, Rodney or Mama Rose had to come to me for clarification. Since I had lived with the healers for four months at that point, I was somewhat able to translate the highly sophisticated language of the mainly academically and legally trained participants. The convoluted technical language assumed a prefabricated legal language, a knowledge consensus, or a sort of universal truth – and power designation – that Richard Rottenburg has defined as "metacode" (Rottenburg 2009: xxix). The two healers had acquired some understanding of the language and meaning of these metacodes in the many meetings they had had with Natural Justice. They could engage in "code switching" between essentially epistemologically heterogeneous worlds, a process whereby practitioners "develop a specific form of meta-knowledge that enables them to move back and forth between different forms of knowing that become labeled as culturally specific knowledge and globalized knowledge" (Rottenburg 2012). However, even this ability of code switching did not mean that the healers could fully comprehend all of the language used in the workshop. In turn, when Rodney tried to explain the role of the ancestors in knowledge production, for instance, the academically trained workshop participants also came to me for understanding, as I, after the months spent with the healers, was also regularly engaged in code switching. Even though Rodney's English was good, he nevertheless did not find the right words of the legal language. In attempting to explain the ancestors, he was basically trying to explain something that is non-codifiable in terms of legal languag

The Pursuit of Integration by Law

In their own right, as well as supported – or pushed – by national and international policies and NGOs, the Kukula Healers, by developing a BCP, discovered their potential as environmental entrepreneurs and stewards of their knowledge and the environment in which they live. They developed the BCP and the TK commons pool for their own means, though both were probably instigated (as well as possibly indoctrinated) by the advances of the NGO Natural Justice. Some scholars have noted that not only legal systems but also neoliberal governmentality seeks to empower local communities to recognize traditions as a source of social capital (Bebbington 2004; Coombe 2011; Perreault 2003) and encourage people to adopt a possessive and entrepreneurial attitude toward their culture and the social relations of reproduction that have traditionally sustained them (Coombe 2009: 399; Greene 2004; Lowrey 2008). Comaroff and Comaroff (2009: 56) framed the new entrepreneurial endeavors of indigenous peoples as *ethno-preneurial*. Furthermore, supported by legal tools, mechanisms and institutions, through *lawfare* local communities are pushed into presenting and promoting themselves and to "render cultural identity into the language of copyright, sovereignty, and patent" (Comaroff and Comaroff 2009: 30f.; Comarof 2001), as well as to "forum shop" (Benda Beckman 1981) for the most advantageous jurisdictions and legal institutions both within and beyond the nation state in which to pursue their collective interests (Comaroff and Comaroff 2009: 56–57). The Comaroffs further propose:

> For one thing legal instruments appear – we stress – appear – to offer a means of commensuration: a repertoire of standardized signs and practices that, like money in the realm of economics, permit the negotiation of values and interests across otherwise intransitive lines of difference (2009: 37).

Developing the BCP may be regarded in terms of such "standardized signs and practices" that enable the negotiation of values and interests. In addition, "Law making is power making," as Walter Benjamin (1978: 295) asserted, and hence the intensive quest, or the external demand, that indigenous communities govern themselves in a system of legal sovereignty also means drawing on their own legal claims and systems. An internal jurisdiction, in short, creates new sovereignty for communities. "Unlike liberal conceptions of rights that emanate from a conceptualization of the individual as the fundamental agent of social activity, a biocultural approach to rights takes as its primary focus the community and the myriad relationships that bind it together" (Abrell et al. 2009b: 5).

The Kukula Healers took this biocultural approach and formed it into tools that allowed them to negotiate within a predetermined system; for instance, the non-disclosure agreement that they made with Godding & Godding was a legal obligation enforced by the National Biodiversity Act. Without an adjustment to these legal tools, the exchange of plant material and further negotiations would not have been possible. A BCP can thus be framed as a tool of *ethno-preneurship*, which encourages communities to claim their rights to their property, and a tool of *lawfare*, the adjustment to legal requirements (see also chapter VI). The legal securitization

of the Kukula Healers continued with the manifestation of their own constitution and subsequently a code of conduct/ethics. Gino Cocchiaro, who supported the
healers in this process, explained that as "all companies and institutions have a
constitution and a code of conduct/ethics, so the healers too sould have such legal
manifestations" (from interview, Cape Town, June 2016).

The Kukula Healers Constitution and Code of Conduct/Ethics

For the Kukula Healers to develop a constitution, the process basically required the
participation of two parties: the healers themselves as a newly founded association,
and the NGO Natural Justice. The former was the executing and receiving party,
while the latter was the delivering and supporting party. The healers' lack of a legal
education made it necessary for them to receive legal support in formulating the
constitution.

The role of NGOs as actors in the field of global policy making and local implementation has been discussed widely (i.e. Escobar 1994; Ferguson 1990; Fassin
2007; Ticktin 2014). Generally, NGOs act as important players in humanitarian and
human rights interventions by merging and interacting between the state and local
communities (Fassin 2007; Rottenburg 2009; Dilger 2011). NGOs have become the
"favored child" of official development agencies (Fischer 1997: 442) in the wake of
weakening states in the Global South. They form a wide range of formal and informal linkages with one another, and with government agencies, social movements,
international development agencies and communities. These relationships have a
profound impact on how globalization, or the implementation of globally accepted efforts like the Millennium Development Goals (MDGs) or intellectual property
rights, actually take place and how they are enacted and experienced in local lives
(Fischer 1997).

In the case of the Kukula Healers, it was mostly Natural Justice who took the
lead in developing the relevant documents. Representatives of the government were at times present, but during the period that I observed, between December 2011
and May 2012, it was only the NGO that worked with the healers. The NGO also suggested that in order to solidify and professionalize the association, a constitution
and code of conduct/ethics would be vital. The constitution was developed before I
began my research. In a four-page long text, the objectives of the association were outlined, among them: the protection of cultural practices; the sustainable use
of biodiversity resources, income and property ideas; rules for the management
committee; and the financial responsibilities of the treasurer (to name but a few).

The code of conduct/ethics was then developed in a two-day workshop at Wits
(Witwatersrand University) Rural Facility. The workshop was initiated as part of
the "to-do work plan" funded by Natural Justice. The participants consisted of the

larger management committee of 26 members of the Kukula Healers, Mama Rose, Gino Cocchiaro and Johan Lorenzen of Natural Justice, Marie-Tinka of the K2C committee, Gwyneth Depport of Mariepskop and myself. Equipped with flipcharts and cards, and coffee and tea for the breaks, the workshop was then steered by Gino Cocchiaro and Johan Lorenzen, though Rodney was the main facilitator and translator.

The workshop began with a Christian prayer and continued with intermittent dancing in the coffee breaks, which livened up the focused and target-oriented atmosphere. The objectives of the workshop were, next to developing a code of conduct/ethics, to decide on "signs of identity" such as nametags, a uniform, a logo and, most importantly, a certificate to signify membership, as well as the identification of a "way forward" for the future. According to the healers, having a code of conduct/ethics generally ensures "more power to knock on the door of the government." The two days were filled with intense discussions about customary laws, the ethical rules of the healers and their position in society. The discussions were held in smaller groups that were then brought together in the larger panel. Like many other meetings I attended of the Kukula Healers, I was impressed by the progressive and organized way in which they held their meetings. During the entire six months I spent with the healers, I never witnessed any sort of argument or disagreement, at least not openly. The only conflict was between Mama Rose and the Kukula Healers, and even this seemed vaguely resolved after Mama Rose and Rodney had reconciled at the traditional knowledge commons workshop in Cape Town. Mama Rose participated in the workshop with equal enthusiasm as the others.

The preamble of the code of conduct/ethics underlines the wish of the healers to be trusted and regarded as credible in their communities and by other stakeholders. It also puts forward the code of conduct/ethics as a means of knowledge protection and sustainable use of resources. Representing trustworthiness, integrity and honesty were the core imperatives of the healers, also to counteract still prevailing witchcraft accusations and other preconceptions that exist against them. Subjects like honesty and responsibility, relationships with other healers, patients and apprentices, and consultation fees were also intensively discussed, to ensure the credibility of traditional healers in their communities and to adjust to the requirements of the Traditional Health Practitioners Act (2007), which proposes the professionalization of traditional healers in South Africa with the registration of all healers nationwide. The code of conduct/ethics is a moral and ethical index, especially with regard to healers' behavior, with aspects of the value of reciprocity in knowledge sharing as well as referring patients on: to another healer in case he/she is an expert in a specific field, or to a health clinic in case the healer cannot treat the problem sufficiently. Next to relationships with patients and other healers, the relationship with the environment was also a central point for the healers (probably also pushed by Natural Justice and the K2C committee). The sustainable harvesting of plant material and the prohibition on over-harvesting were expressed as important.

The strong emphasis on the moral and ethical behavior of the healers displays their wish to be accepted and acknowledged in their own communities and beyond. This may also be seen as a sign of the general professionalization efforts regarding traditional healing in South Africa, an endeavor that started at the beginning of the last century already with the establishment of first healers associations.[21] The Traditional Healers Council that is suggested in the Traditional Health Practitioners Act, for instance, only accepts members of an organization and not individual healers. In addition, the Department of Health registers all healers individually. The general idea is that as a registered and certified association, the Kukula Healers have much more negotiating power with regard to other stakeholders such as the government, NGOs, companies, researchers and nature reserve owner.

Apart from attempts to professionalize themselves, neither the BCP nor the constitution or code of conduct/ethics provide a means for financially self-sustaining projects that could help the healers to attain independence from NGOs like Natural Justice. The question of capacity building is, next to local community empowerment, one of the core interests of Natural Justice in their support of such communities. Capacity building was therefore on the agenda for the years 2013/2014. But to what extent did the healers think of their own independence and future plans for self-sustaining development?

Future Scenarios: Self-Sustaining Entrepreneurs?

For the entire time that I was in Bushbuckridge, it struck me how engaged the Kukula Healers were in the association. They always managed to get the management committee of 26 healers together for a workshop or other events. In particular, the four core executive committee members Rodney, Adah, Charles and Thethe were always ready to meet, organize and discuss activities and coming projects. Whenever something was on the agenda, such as speaking to the local *induna* about getting the permission to occupy a piece of land close to Welverdiend community, all four

---

21   The foundation of healers associations in Natal in 1930 demarcated first efforts to professionlize traditional healing. The Natal Native Medical Association, for instance, was founded in the 1920th. The association "hired lawyers, lobbied the national and provincial governments, wrote a constitution, held public meetings, and issued certificates to its members" (Flint 2008: 151). Those healers, who were accepted as members, were regarded as being in a powerful position against those, mostly rural and secluded healers Being a member of an association implied being in a superior position to those who are not included as well as showed a demarcation line to white biomedical physicians. Members of a healers association had "formal education" of a formal training program (ibid.153).

managed to get together. They were deeply engaged in keeping the association going and finding future tasks that may, at some stage, enable them to sustain themselves. Their activities were very much self-motivated. The financial and structural support of the K2C committee or Natural Justice were invaluable, but not the only driving force; though of course having the NGO as a supporter increased their motivation as well as opportunities to move forward.

Consequently, I wondered what would happen to the Kukula Healers once the support and funding stopped, i.e. when Natural Justice decided to close this 'case' to invest in other 'cases', or when the German government stopped supporting ABS as a means of local development. What will happen when the sources that feed these "tales of development" (Escobar 1995), in this case the tale of indigenous entrepreneurship and custody over resources and environmental protection, run dry? Will they remain, in the end, just another tale? Additionally, although the BCP evokes the impression of a positive development for the Kukula Healers, and may stand as a role model for other communities, it does have a questionable downside. The BCP is not an official legal document, and does not have any binding implications. It is, first and foremost, a shiny 23-page long document that can be distributed in the surrounding communities, and at national and international workshops and conferences. But that may be it. Other communities may also want to develop such a protocol, which might be good for Natural Justice, as the NGO is largely supported by donor agencies to implement BCPs. But what, in the end, does the BCP really provide for the Kukula Healers, besides greater recognition and an improved self-image? I can only offer partial answers here, as the protocol had only just been developed and further outcomes will only reveal themselves in the future. However, the long-term effects of the BCP may turn out to have similar implications as many other development efforts: it may simply fizzle out.

The following section is concerned with these questions. Developing the BCP is not just a process of short-term engagement, leading to a document. It should also be a step towards taking responsibility for the governance of collectively held cultural property. It is an attempt to take over public stewardship of these resources and therewith an attempt to engage in public political life and in sustainable environmental protection. But here again, dependency on external factors comes into play. Would the Kukula Healers be in the position to define themselves as custodians over their knowledge and stewards of biodiversity without the support of Natural Justice? How can they provide for their own future?

Capacity Building for an Independent Future

In interviews, many Kukula Healers members expressed the wish to frame options for future cooperation. Some pronounced that they wished that the government would support them more to build up future projects. Others claimed that they "wanted to continue cooperating with the local health clinic to share information on prevalent disease like HIV/AIDS and tuberculosis". The Kukula Healers and the Hluvukane Health Clinic held monthly meetings to share information, but this, some argued, "could be intensified and could even lead to the establishment of a traditional health clinic", where healers would provide health information and cooperate closely with the Hluvukane Health Clinic. Others again wished "to receive additional training from the nearby South African Wildlife College (SAWC) on how to protect medicinal plants and how to plant medicinal plants in gardens or larger plantation projects". These wishes were not unrealistic and could build up cooperation between the healers and other local stakeholders. It would involve the dissemination of indigenous knowledge on healing to local institutions, and in turn the healers would receive knowledge. Many of these visions had already been put into practice. There was regular cooperation between the Hluvukane Health Clinic and the Kukula Healers, some of the healers had received training from the SAWC, and at Vukuzenzele Medicinal Plant Nursery plants were being bred (though the latter was only partially attached to the Kukula Healers). None of these cooperations, however, were income-generating projects for the Kukula Healers.

On one of our many rides on the way to organize activities or conduct interviews, I asked Rodney about the future plans of the Kukula Healers. On these rides, Rodney often fell asleep, and would then wake up and start, while still drowsy, deep ethical and philosophical discussions about leadership ("As a leader you must always be transparent, put things on the table so that your people know what you are doing"), relationships ("No, you cannot cheat on your wife, it is disrespectful") and life ("You must always have a plan in life"). The future of the Kukula Healers, however, was a core subject that concerned him deeply and we regularly discussed chances, opportunities and ways forward. His ideas ranged from eco tourism projects to traditional healing educational centers for the younger generation and for tourists, to a health clinic and a plant nursery. Rodney's 'future philosophies' were probably one of the motivations that drove him to spend a very large amount of unpaid time and work in the management of the Kukula Healers. Almost every week, we discussed how the Kukula Healers should proceed in the future. But two things were even more pertinent to Rodney than tourism and the environment: it was the survival of the traditional healers' knowledge and practices, in short their cultural identity and heritage and the education of the future generation about these knowledge and practices. A subject close to his heart seemed to be the education of a society that is increasingly losing touch with the environment in which they live and the traditions they have grown up with. Biodiversity is created through interactions between human communities and local ecosystems (Coombe 2001).

The Kukula Healers were pushed by the NGO Natural Justice, which is itself an 'invention' of a particular global political situation of interests in sustaining biodiversity and cultural heritage, the association soon established itself as an environmental agent, standing as an important local steward for sustaining the environment, based on their trans-generational knowledge on plants and the environment. Pushed by this sudden attention, financial support, their new position in society and the remarkable efforts of all healers to keep the association going, they started developing future plans, with two future projects in mind.

First, in cooperation with the K2C committee (the project initiators) and Gwyneth of Mariepskop, the healers assessed a project that combined agro-forestry with the creation of an education center. The project was thought of both in terms of maintaining sustainable biodiversity in the K2C Biosphere Region as well as ensuring local community development, including capacity building and income generation. The main focus of the project was agro-forestry, which was linked to the K2C committee's strong interests in carbon-offset projects (e.g. cultivating plants that take a maximum of carbon from the air) to fulfill its obligations as a UNESCO declared biosphere reserve. But the plan also included the planting of Marula trees and the cultivation of cash crops like maize, organic vegetables and medicinal plants.

The initial project site under consideration was a huge plot of land between Welverdiend and Orpen Gate leading into Kruger National Park, southeast of Hluvukane in the arid area of the Lowveld. The vast, dry plot of land had just a few bushes and trees and very little water; a small streamlet of water flowed through the middle of the property during the rainy season, but in the winter season basically dried up. Making this former patch of bushland into arable land would have required a lot of commitment on the part of the healers. Each member of the Kukula Healers had one or two additional jobs, as well as families and animals to care for. For Rodney, Adah and Charles, reaching the plot would take 40 minutes. Only for the healers who lived in Welverdiend or Clare, the closest villages, would it be possible to regularly work on the land without requiring a significant amount of time to reach the plot. In addition, the healers alone could hardly sustain the costs of cultivating the land, and hence their dependency on a donor agency would remain inevitable. After seeing the property and evaluating these issues, the proposal seemed unsustainable.

Another idea was to build the project in the even further away Mariepskop, a mountainous yet more fertile area. Getting there would cause even more transportation problems for the healers, not only in terms of time but also financial costs. But on the other hand, getting into Mariepskop, cooperating with the management of the nature reserve and working there would accomplish one of the targets of the healers, namely gaining access to so far inaccessible and closed off nature reserve areas with their valuable medicinal plants. After decades of restricted access to areas that were originally part of their plant collecting grounds, this was quite motivating for the healers, also because communal land is generally over-harvested by firewood collectors (fulfilling a daily living need) and *muthi* hunters.

My fieldwork in this area ended before this (or any other) project had come into being, and still in 2012 and 2013, when I revisited the area, the project ideas had not developed further. Indeed, it might simply be one of those 'future scenarios' that are developed in the enthusiastic wake of emerging activism, but which come to an end the moment the support of the donors ends. I can only hypothesize here. I know that some Kukula Healers members had been invited by the management of Kruger National Park to help in anti-rhino poaching activities, while other were involved in the environmental monitoring of medicinal plants[22]. An independent future may yet not be provided with the establishment of the BCP and the traditional knowledge commons pool. Furthermore, Bushbuckridge Municipality remains an impoverished area. Even if a few jobs are created in the green economy sector, they will probably not provide a sustainable future for all Kukula Healers members. But as Marie-Tinka said, this was not the idea of the process. The main idea was the empowerment of local communities. Empowerment is not only about economic stability or future perspectives, but is also about developing a new position in society. And this objective was reached in case of the Kukula Healers, who began cooperating with different local organizations, the Kruger National Park and Mariepskop, the Mnisi tribal authority as well as the NGO Natural Justice. This can be regarded as a first step towards gaining a voice, where marginalization and disregard had once been prevalent. The story of the Kukula Healers continues. Natural Justice continues to financially and legally support them. In 2015, Natural Justice applied for funding from the Open A.I.R. Network to conduct a case study of the Kukula Healers as social entrepreneurs, who continue, in cooperation with local stakeholders, to contribute to the sustainability of the biodiversity and cultural diversity of the region.

Conclusion

Notably, solutions for ABS and knowledge protection remain partial, local and fragile. The development of a BCP as a procedural, group formation tool seemed to have helped the Kukula Healers to create a group identity, which was grounded on the wish to protect their 'cultural property'. This process was supported by NGOs, Natural Justice and the K2C committee in particular, and was pushed further by the Kukula Healers themselves. The cultural value of their property made them aware of their own value: in their communities, as cultural and environmental stewards, as representatives of a new post-Apartheid South African community that

---

22   http://natural-justice.blogspot.de/2015/11/the-kukula-traditional-health.html (last accessed October 16, 2016).

engages in political, legal and economic discourses about rights-based, democratic empowerment.

Despite these positive developments, the process does also, inevitably, have a shadow side. Hardly anything of what the healers had hoped for – financial benefits and the sustainability of their cultural property – had yet come to fruition. It almost felt as if it really was more about the *process* as such and the *capacity* to deal with such a process, as Gino Cocchiaro suggested in my interview with him, than about the protection of cultural property per se. The Kukula Healers had gained recognition in their communities and made an effort to stand up against witchcraft accusations and marginalization. They also managed to cooperate with important, powerful stakeholders, such as tribal authorities, the South African Wildlife College, Kruger National Park and the Kruger to Canyons (K2C) Biosphere Region, and had brought attention to their cultural property as a legally and politically discussed matter.

In this sense, the development of the BCP and of the TK commons pool did have some effects. Whether these effects will have a long-term influence remains to be seen. Tangible outcomes, such as monetary benefits or even non-monetary benefits like a traditional healing education center, were not in sight as of December 2013. *Ethno-preneurial* results were, likewise, only visible in as far as the healers had becom politically and leally more sound (as suggested by the term *lawfare*). The value of the process of developing a BCP is thus less monetary and more political and legal, and oriented fundamentally towards identity and cultural heritage. Reducing the 'value' of bioprospecting to mere economic terms would not do justice to a more complex process. These processes are different in every local context, but they are guided by national and international politics, which in the process of "studying through" cause a different effect each time they are applied. Further research would further contribute to the evaluation of their effects. ABS agreements seem important, and a driving factor behind such processes, but might also be the last outcome that can realistically be expected.

Chapter VIII
Closing Pandora's Box: Conclusion

Introduction

At this point, the trajectory of (the value of) medicinal plants and associated knowledge through the different sites and situations of this research comes to an end. The trajectory led from nature to healers' communities in the Eastern Cape and Mpumalanga/Limpopo Provinces, through the fabric of the biochemical analysis of medicinal plants and into access and benefit sharing (ABS) and intellectual property rights (IPR) politics and (indigenous) knowledge protection. What did this trajectory reveal? What are the results of this long journey through many diverse sites across South Africa, with their many actors and their different interests and motivations? What did this trajectory tell us about the value of medicinal plants and (indigenous) knowledge? What values were we actually talking about when we looked at the values of *muthi* and (indigenous) knowledge? And why are these values so strongly contested in democratic post-Apartheid South Africa?

To answer these questions, this book looked at the specific configurations, or assemblages (Deleuze & Guattari 1997), that emerged in the *contact zones* (Pratt 1992) and sites of research. By following medicinal plants and knowledge through different sites – healers communities in the Eastern Cape and Mpumalanga/Limpopo Province and the Indigenous Knowledge Systems (IKS) Lead Program in Cape Town – this book looked at the discourses and values that emerged from the interaction of different human actors – traditional healers, scientists, members of the government and NGOs – and non-human actors – different medicinal plants (i.e. *Hoodia gordonii* and *Sutherlandia frutescens*) as well as the technologies and devices of laboratories and healers.

At first, the trajectory revealed that bioprospecting, by definition, is a scientific and economic project, with the stakes corresponding accordingly. But soon other values and interests started to play a vital role as well. To grasp all of the values, I unraveled the entanglement of tangible (medicinal plants) and intangible ([indigenous] knowledge) property at each site as well as across sites. I demonstrated that the emerging values were built according to economic, legal and political interests, but at the same time were interrelated with national and local claims of cultural identity and heritage. In short, the book showed that medicinal plants and knowledge are highly contested. This contestation began with the landing of Jan van Riebeck at the Cape in 1652, and has continued until today.

Historical Contestation

This book unraveled the enormous challenges in which medicinal plants as tangible property, but even more so (indigenous) knowledge as intangible property, were and are situated in South Africa. Due to the lack of documented information on the relationship between plants and people *before* the colonial invasion of the Cape in 1652, the contestation between property, people and politics could only be examined from the beginning of (colonial) documentation, which, as has been pointed out, was mostly written by white men (Pratt 1992). These first written records and diaries reveal the ambivalent interactions between early researchers and adventurous travelers and the local population of South Africa, ranging from astonished curiosity and respect for the knowledgeable 'natives' to a totally dehumanizing and dissecting gaze cast on nature and people (ibid.). Driven by the vision of exploring and conquering this *terra incognita* or *terra nullius*, the invading imperial forces thought that natural resources could ultimately be taken without giving anything in return, beyond small material goods such as tobacco or alcohol. Early plant taxonomies and the growing collections of flora and fauna gathered by European universities and botanical gardens are some of the most obvious examples of early biopiracy (Makay 1996). These colonial, mostly non-reciprocal, encounters also reflect the early exposure of local indigenous populations to Western notions of property, an external concept brought to South Africa through the imposition of Roman-Dutch law that forwarded the notion that property is individually owned, an idea that stood in contrast to the views among the local population that property was/is embedded within the relational negotiations of collectively owned possessions such as cattle (Gluckman 1965: 36ff.; Bennett 2011).

The first meetings between researchers and travelers and the local population were individual encounters during the former's journeys into the interior of the Cape and later to the rest of the country (Flint 2008: 96). These encounters were embedded in a "complex space where, despite their highly unequal powers, practitioners from all different knowledge traditions have exercised agency – none of the systems had been hermetically sealed with respect to culture and practice, and none has remained unchanging or static" (Augusto 2008: 193). The exchange of knowledge and resources was thus in constant flux. Over time, medicinal plants "became an important means of establishing dialogue and trust, as well as a means of physical survival" (Flint 2008: 95). Remedies and cures were included in the pharmacopoeia of both sides; white settlers used local remedies to treat local diseases, while local healers integrated the medicine of white health practitioners into their practices. However, with the ongoing establishment of colonial power, politics and law, this increasingly influenced the power struggle between the colonial rulers and the local people, chiefs and traditional healers, with the latter "representing the existence of a judicial and political system that strengthened chiefs and interfered with the implementation of white rules" (ibid. 109). This 'resistance' to colonial rule was reacted to with yet more restrictive laws and punishments, including the criminalization of traditional healers, mostly out of fear of witchcraft. The ongoing project of replacing traditional medicine with biomedical medicine and practitioners represents the power struggle between the two systems that continues to this day. The principle of taking without giving was expanded during the Apartheid years, with the dispossession of local black (indigenous) populations from their lands and regions and the diminishing of their legal rights, including the right to practice traditional healing, which was prohibited under the Witchcraft Suppression Act of 1957. These restrictions were only slowly reversed following the end of the Apartheid regime in 1994, with South Africa becoming a signatory of the Convention on Biological Diversity (CBD) in 1995, with the promulgation of the new national constitution in 1996, and in 2004 with the adoption of two policies dealing with indigenous knowledge systems, namely the Traditional Health Practitioners (THP) Act (amended in 2007) and the National Environmental Management: Biodiversity Act (NEMBA).

In order to understand the contestation over knowledge in the realm of bioprospecting today, it is important to understand the relationship between knowledge, plants, people and politics in South Africa's history of colonial invasion and Apartheid. As has been shown, plants and knowledge were never 'just' resources, but were strongly linked to territories, politics and the law, and were from the beginning entities in interaction, which rendered biopiracy an issue from the very beginning.

Ambivalent Relations: Secrecy Versus Disclosure in the Global Knowledge Economy

To understand the value of plants and knowledge in the context of bioprospecting in contemporary South Africa, I also had to reflect on my own position as a researcher from the Global North; an issue that was strongly linked to the central point of this book, namely the ambivalent relationship between *secrecy* as a means of protecting knowledge as well as traditional culture and values, and knowledge *disclosure* as a means of making (potential) economic, socio-political or humanitarian gains. My position as a researcher ranged from my being angrily chased away to being warmly welcomed and integrated into healers communities. I never asked for knowledge on plants, but I was nevertheless put in the position of being an alleged biopirate who could potentially sell the plants and knowledge of my interlocutors to pharmaceutical or other companies. On the other hand, I was regarded as someone who would bring information about the healers to the rest of the world, i.e. in the form of a published book, as well as other forms of 'speaking for' traditional healers[1]. No less ambivalent was my position at the IKS Laboratory, where I was easily integrated, yet most of the knowledge and meetings remained closed to me, the inquiring ethnographer, perhaps as a result of the information feudalism of the global knowledge economy (Drahos 2002). Disclosing scientific knowledge to outside persons or scientific entities could mean losing the rights to that knowledge, usually claimed in the form of a patent. Hence my position as an ethnographic researcher was as ambivalent in the biochemical laboratory as it was in the realm of traditional healing.

As an inquiring researcher, I was thus subjected to the politics of bioprospecting, which nowhere were more salient than in the ambivalent incongruity of knowledge protection versus knowledge disclosure. Some knowledge was disclosed to me, but most was kept secret. Secrecy and customary rules of knowledge protection are still valid and effective today, but they are partially disrupted by the seduction of knowledge disclosure, which is transported with the message of the global knowledge economy and manifested in the idea that when disclosing valuable knowledge, the knowledge discloser might be able to reap certain benefits, ensured through the settling of an ABS agreement. This message came with the ratification of the CBD and the National Biodiversity Act, as well as the agreement on Bioprospecting and Access and Benefit Sharing (BABS 2008), which was slowly disseminated to rural areas and local (healers) communities via word-of-mouth, transferred from healer to healer, within healers associations as well as in trainings and workshops held by NGOs and the government. Some healers communities that received and understood the message of ABS and the opportunities that supposedly came along with it considered it worth taking the chance of disclosing previously secret knowledge.

The IKS Lead Program, for instance, was one institution where knowledge on medicinal plants or plant mixtures could be disclosed by traditional healers and other citizens. Disclosure was only possible following specific rules and guidelines, which stated, for instance, that a prior meeting had to be held with IKS staff members in order to share information about the claim and to create a trust relationship. These meetings were not intended for the in-depth sharing of cultural information, but for the sharing of information that would be crucial for the consequent scientific analysis. In the case of the medicinal plant claim of *Rohelia* made

---

1   I gave, for instance, a one-hour radio interview about the research to a German audience on RBB Kulturradio (July 8, 2010), and contributed information to an online article (also in German) for the Berliner Tagesspiegel (July 10, 2010): http://m.tagesspiegel.de/von-heilern-und-heilpflanzen/1878480.html.

by Mrs. Dihara in Beaufort West (see chapter V), the cultural background of the claim (and claimant) was not at all important; the information of interest to the IKS Lead Program was related to the disease that was being treated by the claim and how successful the claim had been so far, both of which had to be proven with patient records. The vital information obtained in relation to the claim of the Mdehle Inyanga Healers Association, a more 'indigenous claim', was about the disease it treated (diabetes), its dosage and that there was a successful record of treated patients. Deeper cultural or spiritual knowledge was not discussed in the meeting.

However, the Mdehle Inyanga healers had, prior to the meeting, discussed among themselves whether they wanted to share the knowledge, and had likely consulted the ancestors for approval to disclose it to the IKS Lead Program. Knowledge held by healers communities is not supposed to be shared without the agreement of the ancestors, as Ntate Ndeni explained to me. It was repeatedly said by various healers that those who disclosed knowledge without the ancestors' permission could be punished with disease and even death. Though I personally never came across an example of a healer whose death was said to have resulted from the improper disclosure of knowledge, I nevertheless understood the ancestors here as a moral entity controlling and protecting the dissemination of knowledge. Losing control over knowledge also means losing control over cultural being, social cohesion and well-being in communities. Therefore, knowledge requires comprehensive protection, which was traditionally provided by the traditional knowledge protection system of sharing knowledge only within the boundaries of the *impande*, a hierarchically structured body with elder healers (*magobela*) training the younger healers-to-be (*thwasa*) before they can be initiated. Knowledge sharing beyond the boundaries of the *impande* is well guarded, both by the healers themselves and by the ancestors.

This generations-old traditional knowledge protection system does not, however, provide sufficient security in the global knowledge economy, where knowledge, once subject to commercialization in the form of a product, is commonly protected under intellectual property law. When indigenous knowledge is disclosed to a third party, such as the IKS Lead Program or the company Godding & Godding, the knowledge leaves the secured space of traditional knowledge protection and enters a new unprotected realm that is governed by economic market-oriented tools of intellectual property law. In this unprotected space in the interstices between customary protection and intellectual property protection, knowledge is vulnerable and subject to easy abuse. In recognition of this issue, alternative means of knowledge protection have been sought that can maintain the traditional knowledge protection system, and is at the same time capable of adapting to intellectual property law.

Bioprospecting Trapped: Torn Between the Commons and the Anti-Commons

In chapter I, the *tragedy of the commons* (Hardin 1968) – the over-utilization of common resources – was contrasted with the *tragedy of the anti-commons* (Heller 1998) – the under-utilization and overprotection of common resources, which disturbs the continuation of research and development. As has been shown throughout this book, in the activity of bioprospecting both 'tragedies' play a fundamental yet contradictory role. Indigenous peoples have long been subject to the tragedy of the commons: their resources have been (over-)utilized by outsiders over the course of many centuries of biopiracy, but also by their own over-use, i.e. through firewood collection and the over-harvesting of certain plant species. The politics of the CBD and the National Biodiversity Act restricted access to natural resources and (indigenous) knowledge and prohibited the free collection of plant material both by and for the use of healers as well as by and for companies and research institutions. Furthermore, in their quest for new drug leads, some companies began simply to screen random plant samples collected directly in nature, without including indigenous communities, traditional healers or their knowledge.

Uli Feiter, the owner and director of the medicinal plants and pharmaceutical company Parceval, for instance, expressed his resentment over the National Biodiversity Act, mostly because it infinitely complicated his business with medicinal plants. He nevertheless ultimately decided not to give up altogether and endeavored to work more closely with local communities in the Eastern Cape (in part because he was already fully occupied with the Pelargonium trade). Being sued for biopiracy would most probably have doomed his company, so collaboration was the best way forward. The company Godding & Godding, in contrast, eventually dropped out of further cooperation with the Kukula Healers, basically due to the problems that arose over being charged for not having appropriately complied with the National Biodiversity Act. Therefore, the new biodiversity legislation, while it enables the protection of medicinal plants and indigenous knowledge, is also a threat to those who are engaged in bioprospecting.

Here I want to come back to the question of whether and how it is possible to make economic use of medicinal plants and the indigenous – partially sacred and spiritual – knowledge attached to them, while simultaneously protecting knowledge and plants against inappropriate (ab)use by 'outside' companies, research institutions and/or individual researchers. Chapter VI displayed how ABS politics seem to provide more obstacles than opportunities. I described how companies (such as Godding & Godding), businessmen (like Robby Gass, Uli Feiter and Nigel Gericke) and scientific institutions (such as the IKS Lead Program) had to figure out how to share benefits, and frequently came up against the mostly unresolved questions of what to share and with whom. I examined biocultural community protocols (BCPs) as a proposed integrative community approach to circumvent or at least deal with the obstacles that ABS and IPR politics induce. Before any form of ABS agreements can be negotiated, however, medicinal plants and associated knowledge first have to go through a translation process, from plant and knowledge embedded in the cultural context of healers' communities to a pharmaceutical or cosmetic product of use in the commercial market. The first step in this translation process, which in itself is not easy to reach, is that a plant must find its way into a biochemical laboratory for analysis.

From Indigenous Knowledge to Scientific Knowledge to Economic and Scientific Value

The IKS Lead Program in Cape Town, a governmentally owned scientific program aimed at supporting and promoting indigenous knowledge systems, had the task of scientifically advancing indigenous knowledge systems and medicinal plants. Medicinal plants reach the laboratory – if it all – in manifold, non-linear ways. Either plants that are already known are re-screened for new valuable compounds, or promising new plants or plant combinations are disclosed to the laboratory in the form of medicinal plant claims made by traditional healers and other citizens. Once a plant or plant combination has entered the laboratory, it traverses a process of *particularization, abstraction* and *validation* (Agrawal 2002) aimed at detecting the smallest possible unit of the plant material, a new chemical compound. The knowledge that comes with the plant material is already filtered out during the medicinal plant claim meeting. Only information valuable for detecting new drug leads is of interest.

Nikolas Rose (2007) describes the process of extracting life – here, the social and cultural life that comes with medicinal plants – out of living beings – here, medicinal plants – as the "molecularization of life" (cf. Laplante 2014). This "molecularization of life" is part of the twenty-first century politics of "life itself" (Rose 2007: 3), which involves the translation of the "situated [local] knowledge(s)" (Antweiler 1998; Haraway 1988; Geertz 1983) of various ethnic groups, communities and individual knowledge holders into global pharmaceuticals, which leads to distinct forms of (bio)value and power regimes of global biocapital in the capitalist market (Waldby 2000, 2002; see also Foucault ([1978]/1990). In effect, the disclosed plants and knowledge are reduced to the mere scientific value of a chemical compound in order to secure "scientific facts" (Adams 2002), "efficacy" (Waldram 2000) and safety for later users; mostly, but not only, consumers of pharmaceutical products in the Global North. The food company Unilever, for instance, dropped out of further research and development of *Hoodia* products due to safety issues that were allegedly detected in products containing the chemical compound P57 extracted from the plant.

Medicinal plant material and associated knowledge are, aside from being subjected to the attempt to fuse indigenous and scientific knowledge, forced into a
procedure of standardization marked by clinical trials. This procedure, which will
eventually lead to the commercialization of products valuable for the global pharmaceutical market, reduces all possible values to mere biologically valuable and
scientifically and economically usable facts. The production of biovalue is a scientific attempt to control the 'lack of safety' that comes with 'raw' medicine, without
acknowledging the already existing knowledge of traditional healers and their epistemological and ontological background.

On the other hand, the IKS Lead Program had the task to "support and promote indigenous knowledge systems". This was primarily practiced by following up
medicinal plant claims (though these did not come only from traditional healers),
by inviting healers to training courses on tuberculosis, for instance, and by including them in the educational curriculum of the IKS Lead Program, e.g. as teachers
for visiting school children during National Science Week. These endeavors of *integration*, however, seemed more a measure of *including* traditional healing and its
practitioners into the scientific realm, of making use of them, and less about acknowledging and integrating their knowledge systems. Indeed, the cultural value
of indigenous knowledge systems only played a limited a role in the scientific assignment. This was pointedly summarized by the IKS Lead Program Director, Dr.
Matsabisa, when he stated "I am not interested in the spirit, I am only interested
in the molecule."

The impetus behind indigenous knowledge systems being seen as having merely economic and scientific value was also politically manifested at the national
level in the IKS Policy of 2004, with its aim of strengthening the contribution of
indigenous knowledge to social and economic development. With the IKS Lead
Program's further engagement in poverty reduction and local development projects, including the La Serena *Sutherlandia frutescens* plantation site in De Doorns, it
did also contribute to rural economic development. In these projects too, however,
indigenous knowledge systems only played a side role. The *Sutherlandia* plantation
site, for instance, did not have much to do with indigenous knowledge systems;
Sutherlandia is a well-known plant in South Africa and information on it can be
found in commonly available botanical books and databases. George, the plantation site manager, was also not interested in indigenous knowledge; *Sutherlandia*
for him was "the global solution" to health issues. Indigenous knowledge systems
hardly played a role here, at least not in a deep cultural sense. The promotion of
knowledge holders – traditional healers – was thus ultimately linked solely to the
agendas, results and endeavors of the scientifically- and economically-aligned program.

This economic notion of (bio)value thus "overdetermines all alternative forma-
tions, as well as non-economic strata of social life" (Žižek 2004, cited in Sunder

Rajan 2006: 6). The ancestors, for instance, cannot be utilized or capitalized in a biotechnological system specialized on the extraction of commercially exploitable goods, unless a sales strategy can find a way to merchandize the spirit. The spiritu-al-cultural component, which is basically carved out at the laboratory door, may, for instance, be later added by a company – to a limited, marketable degree – to under-line the authentic character of a pharmaceutical (i.e. *Umckaloabo*), a cosmetic (i.e. a hair shampoo with *Marula* essence) or a food supplementary product (i.e. *Hoodia* powder for dietary products). The marketing strategy for *Umckaloabo*, for instance, employs a stereotype of Africa and its ethnic groups. The webpage as well as the products are promoted with the image of people equipped with spears and shields standing under an Arcadia tree against the background of an orange-red sunset. Playing with such 'authentic' African images may provide a good marketing strate-gy – in the *Umckaloabo*® case, it suggests the warmth and strength of rural Africa – but this strategy does not, in the end, provide any information about the cultural background and value of the original knowledge used to make the product.

Understandably, the main interest of pharmaceutical companies or scienti-fic research is to produce scientifically valuable results and to sell their produc-ts. Uli Feiter of Parceval frankly summarized this interest with the words, "I am a businessman, not a social worker." Both Dr. Matsabisa and Uli Feiter were open about their aspirations with regard to medicinal plants and indigenous knowledge. However, they had to conform to the (inter)national legislation of the CBD, Natio-nal Biodiversity Act and the BABS regulations, and were thus forced, aside from all economic interests, into cooperations with indigenous knowledge holders. Uli Fei-ter in particular was deeply involved in interactions, negotiations and cooperations with local communities. These negotiations and cooperation increased his sense of understanding of the cultural and emotional value comprised in bioprospecting, which also forced them to look beyond the veil of economic interests alone.

The Comaroffs have claimed "ethno-commodities and the value they accrue re-main subject in many ways to the whims of capital and the preconditions of tho-se who profit from its circulation" (Comaroff & Comaroff 2009: 27). This may be true, "But this is much too simple" (ibid.). The 'commoditization only' suggesti-on sounds perhaps too much like a deterministic reduction to mere economic va-lue. The negotiations and cooperations with healers and healers communities that Uli Feiter as well as Dr. Matsabisa evoked under the pretense of ABS agreements ultimately showed that indigenous communities, when properly included, do not have to be the mere victims of commercially-interested companies or scientifically-oriented research institutions, but, as "ethno-preneurs" with "indigenous agency" (ibid), they can also make use of the commercial interest in their tangible and in-tangible cultural properties. The Comaroffs hold that "ethno-preneurialism frames identity as a mode of finding selfhood through vernacular objects" (ibid.: 28). The-rein "identity is increasingly claimed as property by its living heirs, who proceed to manage it by palpably corporate means: to brand it and to sell it, even to anthropologists, in self-consciously consumable forms" (ibid.: 29).

I suggest, therefore, that economic interest may certainly be a driving motivation, but to my mind the analysis should not become trapped in reducing bioprospecting to economic and scientific interests alone. This is difficult, given that almost everything in bioprospecting, from its defined objectives – the scientific and economic utilization of genetic and biological resources – to the politics in which it is embedded – the CBD and National Biodiversity Act – propose economic incentives to be the main motivation. Therefore, the next section returns to the question posed in chapter I about how much of the suggested 'empowerment politics' transported in ABS and IPR is in fact created with the intention of making indigenous peoples ally with bioprospectors in order to ultimately feed the economic market (Takeshita 2001).

Bioporspceting: A Paradigm Beyond Mere Scientific and Economic Value

Politics may to some degree be created to make indigenous peoples ally with bioprospectors in order to feed the economic market, but this leaves out the agency that arises from the opportunities that bioprospecting politics also encompass. Leaving out indigenous peoples' agency puts them back into the colonized, marginalized and disempowered corner under the pretense of neoliberal market regimes. And indeed, indigenous peoples may be the 'victims' of economic market interests. The Masakhane community in Alice in the Eastern Cape, for instance, had to fight for their rights to continue to use the extraction method that they, and other communities in the area, had been using for centuries. If the German company Schwabe had sustained the patent on the method, the communities would have officially no longer been allowed to use it. Although dependent on the market, the community nevertheless showed forms of resistance and agency against it.

The Kukula Healers of Bushbuckridge Municipality also expressed forms of empowerment and agency that were linked to the ABS and IPR politics with which they worked, though they also had the momentum of a group of people and individuals who had deliberately decided to work for the sustainable future of their communities, independent of such external politics. Indeed, in the case of the Kukula Healers, some members were, before the association's establishment, already actively involved in environmental protection projects. Mama Rose, her husband David and some other healers had established the Vukuzenzele Medicinal Plant Nursery, while Rodney Sibuyi, Adah Mabunda and Charles Mthetwa had established a new association of healers. Political interests might have motivated their activities, but first and foremost they were interested in actively contributing to the life of their communities and the surrounding environment. Mama Rose was interested in medicinal plants and had realized that environmental protection is inevitably linked to traditional healing practices and the plants she needed for her practice. Hence, she established Vukuzenzele Medicinal Plant Nursery *before* the NGO Natural Justice came to know about her. Similarly active were Rodney Sibuyi, Adah Mabunda and Charles Mthethwa both dedicated healers and active members of their communities. They had also decided to form their own healers' association *before* their involvement with Natural Justice. It was only later that Natural Justice and the K2C committee introduced the idea of the BCP.

Traditional healers may appear to be disempowered in the larger, national political context, although I hold that this may be a very limited understanding of disempowerment. Most recently with the implementation of the THP Act and the IKS Policy, traditional healers have started to be active participants in national politics (Zenker 2010, 2015; Laplante 2015). In addition, local communities have their own structures and local hierarchies (Oomen 2005), in which traditional healers play an important role (Flint 2008). Healers are not per se disempowered, and yet they are still at the margins in terms of political and legal rights, power and economic influence, and still they must fight against witchcraft accusations, competition from churches and biomedical health clinics, and a young generation deeply in doubt about traditional ways of living.

Natural Justice thus encountered a group of healers who were integrated in their communities. This integration had an ambivalent connotation, however, because on the one hand they were fully accepted and active members of their communities like every other member, but on the other hand the healers were also subject to resentment, threats and witchcraft accusations, which were also expressed in the diminishing number of consulting patients over the years. Developing a BCP was therefore not only an idea imposed by Natural Justice, but also an opportunity to improve their situation as traditional healers by receiving political attention and recognition as well as local credit for cooperating with the NGO, the K2C committee, Kruger National Park or Mariepskop. The seeming decline in the healers' reputation in their communities could thus be upgraded with the impact of their cooperation with such external entities and stakeholders. This cooperation will perhaps not lead to financial income (although the cooperation with Natural Justice brought about moderate financial support for the association), but could encourage their stronger position within society. This scenario was, however, strongly linked to ABS and IPR politics and laws.

The Opportunities and Challenges of Law

The legal concept of ABS is defined in terms of the success of a product. Without a product and benefits, there can be no ABS agreement. However, ABS entails a whole set of negotiations and discussions that must take place *before* the actual benefits

can arise. In the case of the Kukula Healers and Godding and Godding, prior informed consent (PIC) and a non-disclosure agreement (NDA) were negotiated before
the exchange of plant material and associated knowledge occurred. These negotiations encompassed the development of a trust relationship between the knowledge
providers – the Kukula Healers – and the knowledge users – Godding & Godding
and their representatives, the K2C committee.

In what the Comaroff's (2009, 2006) have defined as *lawfare* – the use of legal means for political and economic ends (Comaroff & Comraroff 2006: 30f.; see
also J.L. Comaroff 2001) – communities are forced into the rhetoric of ABS and
IPR politics by means of legal tools (such as PIC, NDA, MTA). Natural Justice, for
instance, supported the Kukula Healers by providing legal 'education' in the form
of introducing the healers to international and national ABS and IPR politics. The
formation of an association as a legally accepted group, and the development of a
constitution and a code of conduct/ethics, enabled the healers to structure their so
far unstructured group and to access the corresponding legal rights. As an official
association, which cooperated with Natural Justice and the government, the Kukula Healers also managed to gain more local recognition within their own communities, as well as from other stakeholders like Godding & Godding, Kruger National
Park, the Mariepskop Nature Reserve, as well as outside groups such as the Open
A.I.R. Network, the latter of which published an academic article and produced a
YouTube video with and about the healers[2]. Many meetings and discussions with
the healers and Natural Justice and the K2C committee brought about a deepener
understanding of their political and legal requirements as a group, a group that had
had little previous contact with such formal, legal structures. The PIC and NDA that
they negotiated with Godding & Godding were new forms of collaboration intended as a securitization of their rights to their property. Also, as an association,
ownership rights are much easier to defend within the realm of intellectual property law; the traditional knowledge (TK) commons pool that the healers developed
enabled the association to hold rights over their collectively gathered knowledge,
with the legal rights holder being the association. In negotiations over knowledge
exchange, the healers can therefore protect their collectively held knowledge as a
legally, and emotionally, united group.

As the Comaroffs wrote in *Law and Disorder in the Postcolony* (2006), *lawfare*
"might also be a weapon of the weak, turning authority back on itself by com-
missioning courts to make claims for resources, recognition, voice, integrity,
sovereignty" (Comaroff & Comaroff 2006: 145). In this sense, *lawfare* thus applies a
double standard. In the case of ABS, on the one hand it replaces local customary
laws of knowledge protection with enforced legal structures, while on the other it
enables communities to learn about these legal structures, adapt to them and make

---

2   www.youtube.com/watch?v=Ve8i-akzCOk (last accessed February 15, 2019).

use of them. Law making, to cite Walter Benjamin, is power making (Benjamin 1978: 295). And thus indigenous communities may connect their identities to the legal rights attached to their property and thus accept the law as an instrument of political and legal leverage and local empowerment, brought about by NGOs such as Natural Justice and governmental institutions and departments.

In addition, in ABS negotiations and the quest for knowledge protection, customary rules of knowledge protection and new legal structures to adapt to the economic market rules of intellectual property law co-exist. The Kukula Healers did not give up their old structures of knowledge protection, and they still applied them in their daily practice as healers. However, with the TK commons pool they developed a scheme that integrated the new system, which allowed for the opening up of protected knowledge in order to pursue economic interests, into the old system, which protected knowledge against outside influences. Although neither the TK commons pool nor the BCP were legally binding tools, the knowledge held by different healers was brought within a legal framework – i.e. an "assemblage of legal practices, legal institutions, statutes, legal codes, authorities, discourses, texts, norms and forms of judgment" (Rose & Valverde 1998: 542; see also Strathern 1999) – which did the work of "interpellation in fields where rights are negotiated and collective subjects are recognized and invested with new responsibilities for managing cultural goods" (Coombe 2011: 81).

The support of NGOs to help indigenous communities understand and make use of legal tools may help them to define their rights and thus also to rise up from their politically marginalized position in society to a position where negotiation at eye level is possible in the larger community, for instance with tribal authorities like Chief Philip Mnisi, other stakeholders in the region and with external entities like national and international companies. In addition, with an association like the Kukula Healers, a new cultural subject was created, which could act and react as an agent engaged in the sustainable use of biological resources and resource management (Brosius, Tsing & Zerner 1998, 2005).

Looking at indigenous communities simply as a new entity through which to apply the messages of the CBD and other environmental and indigenous policies like the National Biodiversity Act and the IKS Policy could easily fall into the trap of romanticism, essentialism and reductionism: communities are not *per se* the 'new' solution to combat environmental degradation and cultural loss. Furthermore, they must still struggle to claim their rights to property. The example of the Kukula Healers may be an overly positive one, also because I entered into their process during a peak of positive feedback and cooperation; future perspectives had still to be developed. Additionally, a BCP does not automatically make a community independent and strong, so that it can sustain itself economically and emotionally. Breaches may happen, as occurred in other development projects (cf. Escobar 1998). Their processes may fail, or lead 'only' to 'minor successes' beyond economic benefits; for example, a stronger political voice and the protection of the cultural identity and heritage of their communities.

Examples like that of the Kukula Healers may indeed contribute to solutions, or at least pathways, towards the preservation of cultural heritage and biodiversity, if they are not only regarded as 'close-to-nature natives' but rather as equally strong participants in political processes. The reduction of indigenous actors to 'the good native' who is passively awaiting global and national politics fails to acknowledge the movements, interests and motivations of indigenous communities beyond politically and legally imposed structures. Communities like the Kukula Healers do have economic interests, but they also have additional interests in local empowerment as well as future visions for the next generation, such as sustaining the environment and livelihood they live in. However, they are also not so naïve as to believe that their society does not change. In contrast, developing a BCP is a sign of adaptation to the changes within society, and to their positioning themselves anew within this society.

Bioprospecting as a Means of Hope

Bioprospecting evokes hopes of participating in the economic benefits that may – yet hardly ever do – result from such activities. These hopes lie not only in indigenous communities, but among other non-indigenous citizens as well. It is a somewhat "vague hope" (Crapanzano 2003: 6), which also includes disappointment and frustration. All efforts put into bioprospecting are primarily endeavors towards an (imagined) 'better future'. But on the way to this better future, a lot of activities, emotions, new configurations and assemblages come together, which may either lead to a success story or to one of the many dead-end roads of bioprospecting. Cases like the *Dicoma anomal* patent, whereby the IKS Lead Program under Dr. Matsabisa had submitted a patent claim on an antimalarial property of the plant, do occur; new associations like the Kukula Healers are formed; NGOs such as Natural Justice, the BCPs and the Nagoya Conference in 2010 have influenced international politics; and notions of property – like the exchanged plant material and associated knowledge of the Kukula Healers – have become more emotionally contested.

This positive assessment does not ignore the more negative aspects of bioprospecting, namely the ongoing yet subtler forms of biopiracy occurring among still disempowered communities. In effect, the voice of the Kukula Healers might have been heard in international, national and local forums, and yet their actual daily life situation did not change much. But, as Gino Cocchiaro from Natural Justice and Marie-Tinka Uys from the K2C committee rightly proposed, bioprospecting is about the process and the later capacity building, not about selling 'culture' to the capitalist market. In this sense, I suggest that the capitalist market may be the initiator, the spark that lights the fire of hope, but it is not the driving factor that leads to a continuation of activities (especially when no benefits have been realized). The Kukula Healers, for instance, continued to meet and be involved in activities with local stakeholders, including representatives from Kruger National Park, until now, January 2016, as I heard from Rodney Sibuyi during a recent phone call. In the end, capacity building and the learning process of democratic and political negotiation processes might even be more important than economic benefits. Or as Coombe (2011: 93) has suggested, "the communities 'empowered' by recognition of their traditional knowledge, their tangible and cultural heritage, or their traditional cultural expression may sometimes be artifactual, but they are still emphatically real and have material and political consequences."

Future Perspectives

This book provides a new approach to the complexity of politics, economy, science, law and socio-cultural perspectives on medicinal plants and (indigenous) knowledge, which were all assembled in the field of bioprospecting in the years 2009 to 2012. By bringing together actor-network theory (ANT) with a trajectory of property and values in multiple sites and contact zones, this book offers a valuable analysis of the contestation of medicinal plants and (indigenous) knowledge in post-Apartheid South Africa. This was done less to continue building on the existing demarcation between traditional knowledge(s) and healing practices on the one hand, and scientific knowledge(s) and practices on the other, and more to highlight both the demarcation as well as the mutual dependency and interaction between the two. It has also been shown how much the production (or lack of production) of a pharmaceutical product from medicinal plants is dependent on a number of often-coincidental factors. The trajectory from nature to healers to product is disrupted by political, legal and socio-cultural constraints, which are partially annulled – or used – for new dialogues, cooperation, agency and future perspectives (such as indigenous communities becoming indigenous entrepreneurs or 'ethno-preneurs'). This is not to say that these interactions are not driven by past and present power imbalances, but that the focus shifts to a more holistic view on the mutuality and interdependence of the different human and non-human actors in the field of bioprospecting. Bioprospecting is, without question, a scientific and economic enterprise, but it would not exist without natural resources, the people using these resources, and the politics and laws that bring these resources and people together, or conversely that separate them.

The unique contribution of the present book lies in the provision of an example of how to assemble the many disrupted and yet associated human and non-human actors in the field of bioprospecting in post-Apartheid South Africa. This book could thus stand as an exemplar for similarly embedded future anthropological research projects. Understanding the complexity and complicity of local communities, their knowledge systems, practices and materials in interaction with local, national and global institutions and organizations and their knowledge systems and practices, as well as with overarching political, economic and legal implications, may help to deal with prevalent (global and local) challenges such as climate change or health crises. Against the often repeated critique of ANT that it lacks an analytical integration of power, I rather suggest that the way in which I have used ANT in this book contributes to a better understanding of the interrelations, but also the tensions and conflicts, that accrue when human and non-human actors assemble in innovative configurations, and where 'new' and 'old' technologies, laws, politics, the economy and different actors meet.

Hence, this book may provide a methodological and theoretical framework for coming projects, where "old" and "new" technologies meet, e.g. projects like a recently promoted project at the Central University of Technology in Free State, South Africa, where engineers working on software that "mixes modern and ancient [i.e. tribal] knowledge to predict the onset of droughts"[3].

This is only one example of cooperative ventures, which seek for innovative future solutions for prevalent local, national and global environmental and/or health problems. Innovation and creativity therefore cannot and should not be viewed as a monopoly of countries of the Global North, who bring new technologies to the Global South (though intellectual property law fortifies this stance); instead, it is a question of collaborative cooperation. Questions of fair and appropriate ABS and knowledge protection beyond – or within – current intellectual property law may play an ongoing role. This book granted a first step towards understanding the correlations, interrelations and interactions of the human and non-human actors involved in the process, whereby values are produced, whose differentiation – as provided in this book– may flow into further considerations about the fair and appropriate sharing of benefits and the integration of customary rules of knowledge protection in – or beyond – intellectual property law.

---

3   For further information on the project, see: http://motherboard.vice.com/read/south-african-scientists-think-software-and-tribal-knowledge-can-predict-drought (last accessed February 5, 2016).

Bibliography

Abrell, E. (2009a): Implementing a Traditional Knowledge Commons. Opportunities and Challenges, Cape Town: Natural Justice.

Abrell, E. (2009b): Imagining a Traditional Knowledge Commons, Cape Town: Natural Justice.

Adams, V. (2002): "Randomized Controlled Crime: Postcolonial Sciences in Alternative Medicine Research." In: Social Studies of Science, Vol. 32(5–6), pp. 659–690.

Andrew, M. (2007): "Case Against 'Muthi Murders' Postponed" (http://beta.iol.co.za/news/south-africa/case-against-muthi-murderers-postponed-322766).

Antweiler, C. (1999): "Local Knowledge and Local Knowing. An Anthropological Analysis of Contested 'Cultural Products' in the Context of Development." In: Anthropos, Vol. 93(4–6), pp. 469–494.

Agrawal, A. (1995): "Dismantling the Divide Between Indigenous and Scientific Knowledge." In: Development and Change, Vol. 26, pp. 423–439.

Agrawal, A. (2002): "Indigenous Knowledge and the Politics of Classification." In: International Social Science Journal, Vol. 173, pp. 287–297.

Agrawal, A. (2005a): Environmentalility: Technologies of Government and the Making of Subjects, Durham: Duke University Press.

Agrawal, A. (2005b): "Environmentality, Community, Intimate Government, and the Making of Environmental Subjects in Kumaon, India." In: Current Anthropology, Vol. 46(2), pp. 161–190.

Anderson, J. E. (2009): Law, Knowledge, Culture. The Production of Indigenous Knowledge in Intellectual Property Law, Cheltham & Northampton: Edward Elgar.

Appadurai, A. (1986): The Social Live of Things. Commodities in Cultural Perspectives, Cambridge: Cambridge University Press.

Arundel, A. (2001): "The Relative Effectiveness of Patents and Secrecy for Appropriation." In: Research Policy, Vol. 30, pp. 611–624.

Ashforth, A. (1998): "Witchcraft, Violence and Democracy in the New South Africa." In: Cahiers d'Etudes africaines, Vol. 150–152 (VIII 2–4), pp. 505–532.

Ashforth, A. (2000): Madumo. A Man Bewitched, Chicago: University of Chicago Press.

Ashforth, A. (2005a): Witchcraft, Violence and Democracy in the New South Africa, Chicago: University of Chicago Press.

Ashforth, A. (2005b): "Muthi, Medicine and Science. Regulating 'African Science' in Post-Apartheid South Africa." In: Social Dynamics, Vol. 31(2), pp. 211–242.

Asdal, K. / Brenna B. / Moser, I. (2007): Technoscience. The Politics of Inventions, Oslo: Unipub.

Ball, S. J. (1990): Foucault and Education, London: Routledge.

Banuri, T. / Apffel-Marglin, F. (eds.) (1993): Who Will Save the Forest? Resistance, Knowledge, and the Environmental Crisis, London: Zed Books.

Barnard, A. (2006): History and Theory in Anthropology, Cambridge: Cambridge University Press.

Bavikatte, K. S. (2011): Stewarding the Earth: Rethinking Property and the Emergence of Biocultural Rights. PhD thesis, Department of Law, University of Cape Town.

Bavikatte, K. S. / Robinson, D. F. (2011): "Towards a People's History of the Law: Biocultural Jurisprudence and the Nagoya Protocol on Access and Benefit Sharing." In: Law, Environment and Development Journal, Vol 7 (1): p. 35 (www.lead-journal.org/content/11035.pdf).

Bavikatte, K. / Jonas, H. / von Braun, J. (2010): "Traditional Knowledge and Economic Development: The Biocultural Dimension." In: S. M. Subramania / P. Balakrishna, Traditional Knowledge in Policy and Practice: Approaches to Development and Human Well-Being, Tokio, New York and Paris: United Nations University Press.

Bebbington, A. (2005): "Social Capital and Development Studies 1: Critique, Debate, Progress?" In: Progressive Development Studies, Vol. 4, pp. 343–349.

Berger, P. (2010): "Assessing the Relevance and Effects of 'Key Emotional Episodes' for the Field Work Process." In: J. Davies / D. Spencer (eds.), Emotions in the Field. The Psychology and Anthropology of Fieldwork Experience, London and Basingstoke: Stanford University Press, pp. 119–143.

Beinart, W. (1998): "Men, Science, Travel and Nature in the Eighteenth and Nineteenth-Century Cape." In: Journal of Southern African Studies, Vol. 24(4), pp. 775–799.

Benkler, Y. (2006): The Wealth of Networks, New Haven, London: Yale University Press.

Biehl, J. / Locke, P. (2012): "Deleuze and the Anthropology of Becoming." In: Current Anthropology, Vol. 53(3), pp. 317–351.

Bennett, T. W. (2011): "Ubuntu: An African Equity." In: Potchefstroom Electronic Law Journal, Vol. 14(4), pp. 30–61.

Bennett, T. W. (2004): Customary Law in South Africa, Landown, Cape Town: Juta.

Bennett, T. W. / Patrick J. (2011): "Ubuntu, the Ethics of Traditional Religion." In: T. W. Bennett, Traditional African Religions in South African Law, Cape Town: University of Cape Town Press.

Beinart, W. (1998): "Man, Science, Travel and Nature in the Eighteenth and Nineteenth Century Cape." In: Journal of Southern African Studies, Vol. 24(4), pp. 775–799.

Beinart, W. / MecGregor, J. (2003): "Introduction." In: W. Beinart & J. MecGregor (eds.), Social History and African Environments, Oxford, Cape Town: James Currey / David Philip, pp. 1–24.

Bell, C. / Paterson, R. (eds.). (2008): Protection of First Nations Cultural Heritage: Laws, Policy, and Reform, Vancouver: University of British Columbia.

Benjamin, W. (2008[1936]): The Work of Art in the Age of Mechanical Reproduction, London: Penguin Books.

Berglund, A. I. (1976): Zulu Thought Patterns and Symbolism, London: Hurst & Co.

Berlin, B. (1992): Ethnobiological Classification: Principles of Categorization of Plants and Animals in Traditional Societies, Princeton: Princeton University Press.

Berlin, B. / Berlin, E. A. (2004): "Community Autonomy and the Maya ICBG Project in Chiapas, Mexica: How a Bioprsopecting Project That Should Have Succeeded Failed." In: Human Organization, Vol. 63(4), pp. 472–486.

Bhat, R. B. / Jacobs, T. V. (1995): "Traditional Herbal Medicine in Transkei." In: Journal of Ethnopharmacology, Vol. 48(1), pp. 7–12.

Biehl, J. / Lock, P. (2010): "Deleuze and the Anthropology of Becoming." In: Current Anthropology, Vol. 51(3), pp. 317–351.

Birch, K. / Tyfield, D. (2012): "Theorizing the Bioeconomy: Biovalue, Biocapital, Bioeconomics or ... what?" In: Science, Technology & Human Values, pp. 1–29.

Bladt, S. / Wagner, H. (2007): "From Zulu Medicine to the European Phytomedicine Umckaloabo." In: Phytomedicine, Vol. 14 (1), pp. 2–4.

Blaser, M. / de Costa, R. / McGregor, D. / Coleman, W. D. (2010): Reconfiguring the WebLife: Indigenous Peoples, Relationality, and Globalization, in Indigenous Peoples and Autonomy: Insights for a Global Age, Vancouver: UBC Press.

Bloch, M. / Parry, J. (1989): "Introduction: Money and the Morality of Exchange." In: M. Bloch / J. Parry (eds.), Money and the Morality of Exchange, Cambridge: Cambridge University Press.

Bloor, D. (1999): "Anti-Latour." In: Studies in History and Philosophy of Science, 30(1), pp. 81–112.

Boas, F. (1938[1911]): The Mind of Primitive Man, New York: The Macmillan Company.

Bok, S. (1983): Secrets. On the Ethics of Concealment and Revelation, New York: Vintage Books.

Bourdieu, P. (1986): "The Forms of Capital." In: L. Richardson (ed.), Handbook of Theory and Research for the Sociology of Education, New York: Greenwood, pp. 241–258.

Bourdieu, P. (2000): Pascalian Meditations, Cambridge: Polity Press.

Bowker, G. (2008): Memory Practices in the Sciences, Cambridge and MA: MIT Press.

Bowker, G. / Star, S. L. (2000): Sorting Things Out. Classification and its Consequences, Cambridge, MA: MIT Press.

Braid, M. (1998): "Africa: Witchcraft Returns to Haunt New South Africa." (www.independent.co.uk/news/africa-witchcraft-returns-to-haunt-new-south-africa-1139937.html).

Brendler, T. / van Wyk, B-E. (2008): "A Historical, Scientific and Commercial Perspective on the Medicinal Use of Pelargonium Sidoides (Geraniceae)." In: Journal of Ethnopharmacology, Vol. 119(3), pp. 420–433.

Brink, A. (2006): Praying Matris, Secker Warburg.

Broodryk, J. (2002): Ubuntu: Life Lessons from Africa, Ubuntu School of Philosophy.

Brosius, P. / Lowenhaupt-Tsing, A. / Zerner, C. (1998): Communities and Conservation: Histories and Politics of Community-Based Natural Resource Management (Globalization and the Environment). Lanham: AltaMira Press.

Brown, N. (2003): "Hope against Hype – Accountability in Biopasts, Presents and Futures." In: Science Studies, Vol. 16(2), pp. 3–21.

Brown, M. (2003): Who Owns Native Culture? Cambridge: Harvard University Press.

Brown, M. (2005): "Heritage Trouble: Recent Work on the Protection of Intangible Cultural Property." In: International Journal for Cultural Property, Vol. 12, pp. 40–61.

Brush, S. B. (1994): "A Non-Market Approach to Protecting Biological Resources'." In: T. Greaves (ed.), Intellectual Property Rights for Indigenous Peoples: A Source Book, Oklahoma City, Society for Applied Anthropology.

Brush, S. / Stabinski, D. (1996): Valuing Local Knowledge: Indigenous Peoples and Intellectual Property Rights. Washington D.C.: Island Press.

Brush, S. B. (1995): "Indigenous Knowledge of Biological Resources and Intellectual Property." In: American Anthropologist, Vol. 95(3), pp. 653–671.

Brush, S. B. (1996): "Is Common Heritage Outmoded?" In: S. B. Brush, / D. Stabinski (eds.), Valuing Local Knowledge: Indigenous People and Intellectual Property Rights, Washington, D.C.: Island Press, pp. 143–164.

Brush, S. B. (1999): "Bioprospecting in the Public Domain." In: Cultural Anthropology, 14(4), pp. 535–555.

Bryant, A. T. (1966): Zulu Medicine and Medicine Men, New York: Centaur Press.

Burchell, W. J. (1822): Travels in the Interior of South Africa. Vol. 1, London: Longman, Hurst, Rees, Orme, and Green.

Burchell, W. J. (1824): Travels in the Interior of Southern Africa, Vol. 11, London: Longman, Hurst, Rees, Orne and Green.

Buzelin, H. (2007): "Translation in the Making." In: M. Wolf & A. Fukari (eds.), Constructing a Sociology of Translation, Amsterdam, Philadelphia: John Benjamins Publishing Company.

Buhrmann, V. (1984): Living in Two Worlds. Communication between a White Healer and Her Black Counterpart, Cape Town, Pretoria: Human & Rousseau.

Callon, M. (1986a): "Some Elements of a Sociology of Translation: Domestication of the Scallops and the Fishermen of St. Brieuc Bay." In: J. Law, Law, Power, Action and Belief: A New Sociology of Knowledge? London: Routledge, pp. 196–223.

Callon, M. (1986b): "The Sociology of an Actor-Network: The Case of the Electric Vehicle." In: M. Callon / J. Law / A. Rip (eds.), Mapping the Dynamics of Science and Technology: Sociology of Science in the real World, London: MacMillan Press, pp. 19–34.

Campbell Schuster, S. (1998): Called to Heal, Halfway House: Zebra Press.

Campell, C. (2010): "Southern Africa: Region Failing to Innovate, Says Study" (http://allafrica.com/stories/201008130924.html).

Candea, M. (2010): "Ontology Is Just Another Word for Culture: For the Motion (2)." In: Critique of Anthropology, Vol. 30(2), pp. 152–200.

Carrier, J. G. (1990): "Gifts in a World of Commodities: The Ideology of the Perfect Gift in American Society." In: Social Analysis, Vol. 29, pp. 19–37.

Carrier, J. G. (1992): A Handbook of Economic Anthropology, Cheltenham and Northampton: Edward Elgar.

Carter, C. (2013): "The Brutality of 'Corrective Rape'." New York Times (http://www.nytimes.com/interactive/2013/07/26/opinion/26corrective-rape.html?_r=0).

Chander, A. / Sunder, M. (2004): "The Romance of the Public Domain." In: California Law Review, Vol. 92, pp. 1331–1374.

Cheal, D. (1988): The Gift Economy, New York: Routledge.

Chennels, R. (2010): "Commercial Development of Hoodia" (http://www.kalaharipeoples.net/article.php?i=232&c=22).

Chiseri-Strater, E. (1996): "Turning in upon Ourselves: Positionality, Subjectivity, and Reflexivity in Case Study and Ethnographic Research." In: P. Mortensen & G. E. Kirsch (eds.), Ethics and Representation in Qualitative Studies of Literacy, Urbana: National Council of Teachers.

Chung, J. A. (2009): "Ethnographic Remnants: Range and Limits in the Social Method." In: J. D. Faubion / G. Marcus (eds.), Fieldwork is not What It Used to Be. Learning Anthropology's Method in a Time of Transition, Ithaca, London: Cornell University Press.

Claassen, A. / Cousins, B. (2009): Land, Power & Custom. Controversies Generated by South Africa's Communal Land Rights Act, Cape Town: University of Cape Town Press.

Clark, A. / Fujimura J. H. (1992): The Right Tools for the Job: At Work in the Twentieth-Century Life Sciences, Princeton: Princeton University Press.

Cleveland, D. / Soleri, D. (2002): "Indigenous and Scientific Knowledge of Plant Breeding." In: P. Sillitoe / A. Bicker / J. Pottier (eds.), Participating in Development: Approaches to Indigenous Knowledge, London and New York: Routledge, pp. 206–234.

Cochiaro, G. / Rutert, B. (2013): "Traditional Knowledge Common Pools: The Story of the Kukula Traditional Health Practitioners of Bushbuckridge, Kruger to Canyons (K2C) Biosphere Reserve, South Africa." In: C. Kamu / G. Winter, Common Pools of Genetic Resources: Equity and Innovation in International Biodiversity Law, Abington: Taylor & Francis, pp. 30–38.

Cocchiaro, G. / Lorenzen, J. / Maister, B. / Rutert, B. (2014): "Consideration of a Legal 'Trust' Model for the Kukula Healers' TK Commons in South Africa." In: The Collaborative Dynamics of Innovation and Intellectual Property in Africa, Cape Town: University of Cape Town Press.

Cock, J. / Fig, D. (2000): "From Colonial to Community Based Conservation: Environmental Justice and the National Parks of South Africa." In: Society in Transition, Vol. 31(1), pp. 22–35.

Cocks, M. / Moller, V. (2002): "Use of Indigenous and Indigenised Medicines to Enhance Personal Well-Being: A South African Case Study." In: Social Science and Medicine, Vol. 54, pp. 387–397.

Cohen, J. B. (2009): "Medicine from the Father: Bossiesmedisyne, People, and Landscape in Kannaland." In: Anthropology Southern Africa, Vol. 32 (1&2), pp. 18–26.

Cohen, W. M. / Nelson, R. / Walsh, J. P. (2000): Protecting Their Intellectual Assets: Appropriability: Conditions and Why U.S. Manufacturing Firms Patent (or not), WorkingPaper No. 7552, National Bureau of Economic Research.

Cohn, N. (1970): The Pursuit of the Millennium: Revolutionary Millenarians and Mystical Anarchists of the Middle Ages (revised and expanded), New York: Oxford University Press.

Collins, H. M. (1983): "The Sociology of Scientific Knowledge: Studies of Contemporary Science." In: Annual Review of Sociology, Vol. 2, pp. 265–285.

Collins, H. M. (2010): Tacit and Explicit Knowledge, Chicago: University of Chicago Press.

Collins, H. M. / Yearly, S. (1992): "Epistomological Chicken." In: A. Pickering (ed.), Science as Practice and Culture, Chicago: University of Chicago Press, pp. 301–326.

Comaroff, J. / Comaroff, J. (1991): Of Revelation and Revolution. Christianity, Colonialism and Consciousness in South Africa, Chicago and London: University of Chicago Press.

Comaroff, J. / Comaroff, J. (1993): Modernity and Its Malcontents, Ritual and Power in Postcolonial Africa, Chicago: University of Chicago Press.

Comaroff, J. / Comaroff, J. (1998): "Reflections on the Colonial State, in South Africa and Elsewhere: Fractions, Fragments, Facts and Fictions, Social Identities." In: Journal for the Study of Race, Nation and Culture, Vol. 4(3), pp. 321–362.

Comaroff, J. / Comaroff, J. (1999): "Occult Economies and the Violence of Abstraction: Notes from the South African Postcolony." In: American Anthropologist, Vol. 26(2), pp. 279–303.

Comaroff, J. / Comaroff, J. (2000): "Millenium Capitalism: First Thoughts on a Second Coming." In: Public Culture, Vol. 12(2), pp. 291–343.

Comaroff, J. / Commaroff, J. (2001): Millenium Capitalism and the Culture of Neoliberalism, Durham: Duke University Press.

Comaroff, J. / Comaroff J. (2006): "Law and Disorder in the Postcolony." In: Social Anthropology, Vol. 15(2), pp. 133–152.

Comaroff, J. / Comaroff, J. (2009): Ethnicity, Inc., Scottsville: University of KwaZulu-Natal Press.

Coombe, R. (1995): "The Cultural Life of Things: Anthropological Approaches To Law and Society in Conditions of Globalization." In: American University Journal of International Law and Policy, Vol. 10 (2), pp. 791–836.

Coombe, R. (1998a): The Cultural Life of Intellectual Properties: Authorship, Application, and the Law, Durham, London: Duke University Press.

Coombe, R. (1998b): "Intellectual Property, Human Rights & Sovereignty: New Dilemmas in International Law posed by the Recognition of Indigenous Knowledge and the Conservation of Biodiversity." In: Indiana Journal of Global Legal Studies, Vol. 6(1), Symposium: Sovereignty and the Globalization of Intellectual Property, pp. 59–115.

Coombe, R. (2001): "The Recognition of Indigenous Peoples' and Community Traditional Knowledge in International Law." In: 14 St. Thomas Law Review, pp. 275–285.

Coombe, R. (2003): "Fear, Hope, and Longing for the Future of Authorship and a rivitalized Public Domain in Global regimes of Intellectual Property." In: DePaul Law Review, Vol. 52 (4), pp. 1171–1201.

Coombe, R. (2009): "The Expanding Purview of Cultural Properties and Their Politics." In: Annual Review of Law, Society and Science, Vol. 5, pp. 393–412.

Coombe, R. (2010): "Intellectual Property Issues in Heritage Management Part 2: Legal Dimensions, Ethical Considerations, and Collaborative Research Practices (with George Nicholas, Catherine Bell, John Welch, Brian Noble, Jane Anderson, Kelly Bannister, and Joe Watkins)." In: Journal of Heritage Management, Vol. 3, pp. 117–147.

Coombe, R. (2011): "Cultural Agencies. The Legal Construction of Community Subjects and Their Properties." In: M. Biagiolo / M. Woodmansee / P. Jaszi (eds.), The Making and Unmaking Intellectual Property, Chicago: University of Chicago Press.

Coombe, R. / Alywin, N. (2014): "Marks Indicating Conditions of Origin in Rights-Based Sustainable Development." In: University of California, Davis Law Review, Vol. 47, pp. 75–786.

Cornell, C. / Muvangua, N. (2012): Ubuntu and the Law, New York: Fordham University Press.

Convention of Biological Diversity 1992, United Nations Conference on the Environment and Development (UNCED), Rio de Janeiro, Brazil, February 16, 2016 (https://www.cbd.int/convention).

Crapanzano, V. (2003): "Reflections on Hope as a Category of Social and Psychological Analysis." In: Cultural Anthropology, Vol. 18(1), pp. 3–32.

Crouch, N. / Douwes, E. / Wolfson, M. / Smith Gideon F. / Edwards, T. J. (2008): "South Africa's Bioprospecting, Access and Benefit-Sharing Legislation: Current Realisties, Future Complications, and Proposed Alternatives." In: South African Journal of Science, Vol. 104, pp. 355–366.

Crush, J. / Jeeves, A. (1993): "Transitions in the South African Countryside." In: Canadian Journal of African Studies, Vol. 27(3), pp. 351–360.

Cunningham, A. B. (1988): "Investigation of the Herbal Medicine Trade in Natal-Kwazulu." In: Investigational Report No. 29, Pietermaritzburg: Institute of Natural Resources, University of Natal.

Cullinan, C. (2011): Wild Law. A Manifesto for Earth Justice, Totnes, Devon: Greenbooks.

Cumes, D. (2004): Africa in My Bones. A Surgeon's Odyssey into the Spirit World of African Healing, Cape Town: Spearhead.

Cumes, D. (2013): "South African Indigenous Healing: How It Works." In: Explore: The Journal of Science and Healing, Vol. 9(1), pp. 58–65.

Das Gupta, A. (2011): "Does Indigenous Knowledge Have Anything to do with Sustainable Development?" In: Antrocom Online Journal of Anthropology, Vol. 7(1), pp. 57–64.

Davies, J. / Spencer, D. (2010): Emotions in the Field. The Psychology and Anthropology of Fieldwork Experience, London, Basingstoke: Stanford University Press.

de Beer, J. / Armstrong, C. / Oguamanam, C. / Schonwetter, T. (2014): Innovation & Intellectual Property. Collaborative Dynamics in Africa, Cape Town: University of Cape Town Press.

Decocteau, C. L. (2008): The Bio-Politics of HIV/AIDS in Post-Apartheid South Africa. Dissertation, University of Michigan.

Deleuze, G. (1997): "Desire and Pleasure. Translation of 'Désir et plaisir'." In: Magazine littéraire 325, pp. 59–65 (www.artdes.monash.edu.au/globe/delfou.html).

Deleuze, G. (2006): Two Regimes of Madness: Texts and Interviews 1975–1995, Los Angeles: Semiotext(e).

Deleuze, G. / Guattari, F. (1987): A Thousand Plateaus. Capitalism and Schizophrenia. Continuum, University of Minnesota.

de Maupertuis, P. L. M. (1752): Lettres sur progés des sciences. Dresden.

Department of Science and Technology, Republic of South Africa: Technology for Sustainable Livelihoods (www.dst.gov.za/index.php/chief-directorate-innovation-for-inclusive-development?id=2099).

Devisch, R. (1993): Weaving the Threads of Life. The Gyn-Eco-Logical Healing among the Yaka, Chicago: University of Chicago Press.

Descola, P. (2013): Beyond Nature and Culture, Chicago: University of Chicago Press.

DeWaal, M. (2012): Witch-hunts: The Darkness That Won't Go Away (www.dailymaverick.co.za/article/2012-05-30-witch-hunts-the-darkness-that-wont-go-away/#.Vj4ypaT49ac).

Dilger, H. (2011): "Targeting the Empowered Individual: Transnational Policy-Making, the Global Economy of Aid and the Limitation of 'Biopower' in the Neoliberal Era." In: H. Dilger / A. Kane / S. Langwick (eds.): Mobility, Medicine, and Power in Global Africa: Transnational Health and Healing, Bloomington: Indiana University Press.

Dilger, H. / Kane, A. / Langwick, S. (2012): "Introduction. Transnational Medicine, Mobile Experts." In: Mobility, Medicine, and Power in Global Africa: Transnational Health and Healing, Bloomington: Indiana University Press, pp. 1–31.

Dilger, H. / Hardolt, B. (2010): Medizin im Kontext. Krankheit und Gesundheit in einer vernetzten Welt, Frankfurt a.M.: Peter Lang.

Diob, C. A. (2000): Towards the African Renaissance: Essays in Culture and Development, 1946–1960, Trenton: Red Sea Press.

Douglas, M. (1966): Purity and Danger, London: Routledge.

Downey, G. L. / Dumit, J. (1995): "Locating and Inventing." In: G. Downey / J. Dumit, Cyborgs and Citadels: Anthropological Interventions in Emerging Sciences and Technologies, Santa Fee: School of American Research Press.

Drahos, P. (1996): A Philosophy of Intellectual Property, Dartmouth, Aldershot and Brookfield: Ashgate/Dartmouth Publishing.

Drahos, P. (1999): Intellectual Property, Aldershot: Ashgate/Dartmouth Publishing.

Drahos, P. (2014): Intellectual Property, Indigenous People and Their Knowledge, Cambridge: Cambridge University Press.

Drahos, P. / Braithwaite, J. (2002): Information Feudalism: Who Owns the Knowledge Economy? London: Earthscan Publications.

Drahos, P. / Frankel, S. (2012): Indigenous Peoples' Innovation and Intellectual Property Pathways to Development, Canberra: Australia National University Press.

Dovie, D. B. K. / Witkowski, E.T. F. / Shackleton, C. M. (2005): "Monetary valuation of livelihoods for Understanding the Composition and Complexity of Rural Households." In: Agriculture and Human Values, Vol. 22, pp. 87–103.

Dutfield, G. (2006): Piracy as Terrorism, Copying as Theft: The New Intellectual Property Fundamentalism in International Law and Politics, None, pp. 1361–4169.

Dutfield, G. (2002); Intellectual Property, Biogenetic Resources & Traditional Knowledge, Sterling: Stylus Publishing.

Dutfield, G. (2003): Protecting Traditional Knowledge and Folklore. A review of Progress in Diplomacy and Policy Formulation, UNCTAD-ICTSD (http://www.iprsonline.org/resources/docs/Dutfield%20-%20 Protecting%20TK%20and%20Folklore%20-%20Blue%201.pdf).

Dutfield, G. (2004): Intellectual Property, Biogenetic Resources and Traditional Knowledge, London: Earthscan.

Dutfield, G. (2009): Intellectual Property Rights & the Life Science Industries: Past, Present & Future (2nd ed.), New York: World Scientific.

Du Troit, B. M. (1980): "Religion, Ritual, and Healing among Urban Black South Africans." In: Urban Anthropology, Vol. 91, pp. 21–49.

Egerton, R. B. (1992): Sick Societies: Challenging the Myth of Primitive Harmony, New York: Free Press.

Eisenberg, D. M. / Kessler, Roland C. / Foster, C. / Norlock, F. E. / Calkins, D. R. / Delbanco, T. L. (1993): "Unconventional Medicine in the United States: Prevalence, Costs, and Patterns of Use." In: New England Journal of Medicine, Vol. 328(4), pp. 246–252.

Eisner, T. (1989): "Prospecting for Nature's Chemical Riches." In: Issues in Science and Technology, Vol. 6(2), pp. 31–34.

Eisner, T. (1994): "Chemical Prospecting: A Global Imperative." In: Precedings of the American Philosophical Society, Vol. 138 (3), pp. 385–393.

Ellen, R. / Harris, H. (2000): "Introduction." In: R. Ellen / P. Parks / A. Bicker (eds.), Indigenous Environmental Knowledge Transformations. Critical Anthropological Perspectives, Amsterdam: Taylor & Francis.

Escobar, A. (1995): Encountering Development. The Making and Unmaking of the Third World, Princeton: Princeton University Press.

Escobar, A. (1998): "Whose Knowledge, Whose Nature? Biodiversity, Conservation, and the Political Ecology of Social Movements." In: Journal of Political Ecology, Vol. 5, pp. 53–83.

Escobar, A. (2010): "Postconstructivist Political Ecologies." In: M. R. Redclift / G. Woodgate (eds.), The International Handbook of Environmental Sociology, Cheltenham: Edward Elgar Publishing (2nd ed.), pp. 91–106.

Fassin, D. (2007): "Humanitarianism as a Politics of Life." In: Public Culture, Vol. 19(3), pp. 499–520.

Ferguson, J. (1994): The Anti-Politics Machine: Development, Depoliticization, and Bureaucratic Power in Lesotho, Minneapolis: University of Minnesota Press.

Faubion, J. D. / Marcus, G. (2009): Fieldwork is not What it Used to Be. Learning Anthropology's Method in a Time of Transition, Ithaca and London: Cornell University Press.

Flavier, J. M. (1995): "The Regional Program for the Promotion of Indigenous Knowledge in Asia." In: D. M. Warren / L. J. Slikkerveer / D. Brokensha (eds.), The Cultural Dimension of Development: Indigenous Knowledge Systems, London: Intermediate Technology Publications, pp. 479–487.

Falzon, M.-A. (2009): Introduction: Multi-Sited Ethnography: Theory, Praxis and Locality in Contemporary Research, Farnham and Burlington: Ashgate Publishing.

Faquar, J. (2012): "Knowledge in Translation: Global Science, Local Things." In: L. Green / S. Levine (eds.), Medicine and the Politics of Knowledge, Cape Town: Human Sciences Research Council Press, pp. 153–170.

Fassin, D. (2010): "Humanitarianism as a Politics of Life." In: B. Good / M. Fischer / S. S. Willen / M. DelVecchio Good, et al. (eds.): A Reader in Medical Anthropology. Theoretical Trajectories, Emergent Realities, Oxford: Wiley-Blackwell.

Feris, L. (2009): Protecting and Promoting Traditional Knowledge. In-Course Manual and Resource Book. Training Course in Access and Benefit Sharing from Genetic Resources and Associated Traditional Knowledge, Cape Town.

Felhaber, T. (1997): Traditional Healers' Primary Care Book. Combining Western and Traditional Medicine, Cape Town: Kagiso Publisher: Observatory.

Fischer, M. (2012): "Lively Biotech and Translational Research." In: Sundar Rajan K. (ed.), Lively Capital. Biotechnologies, Ethics, and Governance in Global Markets, Durham: Duke University Press.

Fischer, M. (1997) "Doing Good? The Politics and Antipolitics of NGO Practices." In: Annual Review of Anthropology, Vol. 26, pp. 439–464.

Flint, K. (2008): Healing Traditions. African Medicine, Cultural Exchange, and Competition in South Africa, 1820–1948, Athens: Ohio University Press.

Flint, K. (2012): "Reinventing 'Traditional' Medicine in Postapartheid South Africa." In: D. M. Gordon / S. Krech, S. III (eds.), Indigenous Knowledge and the Environment in Africa and North America, Athens: Ohio University Press.

Forbes, V. S. (ed.) (1986): Carl Peter Thunberg Travels at the Cape of Good Hope 1772–1775, Cape Town: Van Riebeeck Society.

Foucault, M. (2002[1966]): The Order of Things. An Archaeology of the Human Sciences, London: Taylor & Francis.

Foucault, M. (1991): "Governmentality." In: G. Burchell / G. C. Gordon / P. Miller (eds.), The Foucault Effect: Studies in Governmentality, London: Harvester Wheatsheaf, pp. 87–102.

Foucault, M. (2002): "Subject and Power." In: J. Faubion (ed.) / R. Hurley (transl.), Vol. 3. Essential Works of Foucault 1954–1984, London: Penguin.

Foucault, M. (2008): "The Birth of Bio-Politics" – Lecture at the Collège de France 1978–79, Basingstoke: Palgrave Macmillan.

Fourie, T.G. / Swart I. / Snyckers O. (1992): "Folk Medicine: A Viable Starting Point for Pharmaceutical Research." In: South African of Science, Vol. 88, pp. 190–192.

Fowler, A. (2000): The Virtuous Spiral: A Guide to Sustainability Thinking and Practice for Non-Governmental Organisations in International Development, London: Earthscan.

Franklin, S. (2006): "Mapping Biocapital: New Frontiers of Bioprospecting." In: Cultural Geographies, Vol. 13, pp. 301–304.

Franklin, S. / Locke, M. (2003): "Animation and Cessation: The Remaking of Life and Death." In: S. Frankling / S. Lock (eds.), Remaking Life and Death: Toward an Anthropology of the Biosciences, Santa Fee: School of American Research Advanced Seminar Series, pp. 2–22.

Frein, M. / Meier, H. (2008): Die Biopiraten. Milliardengeschäfte der Pharmaindustrie mit dem Bauplan der Natur, Berlin: Ullstein Verlag.

Frost, B. (1998): Struggling to Forgive: Nelson Mandela and South Africa's search for reconciliation, Great Britain: Harper Collins Publishers.

Freemann, M. / Motsei, M. (1992): "Planning Health Care in South Africa – Is There a Role for Traditional Healers?" In: Social Science and Medicine, Vol. 34 (11), pp. 1183–1190.

Friedman, J. (2008): "Anthropological Notes on a Historical Variable." In: H. Minde, Indigenous Peoples: Self-Determination, Knowledge, Indigineity, Delft: Eburon, pp. 29–48.

Galanter, M. (1981): "Justice in Many Rooms. Courts, Private Ordering and Indigenous Law." In: Journal of Legal Pluralism and Unofficial Law, Vol. 19(1), pp. 1–47.

Garforth, L. (2012): "Visibilities of Research: Seeing and Knowing in STS." In: Science, Technology & Human Values, Vol. 37(2), pp. 264–285.

Geertz, C. (1973): "Thick Description: Toward an Interpretive Theory of Culture." In: The Interpretation of Cultures: Selected Essays, New York: Basic Books, pp. 3–30.

Geertz, C. (2005[1972]): "Deep Play. Notes on the Balinese Cockfight." In: Daedalus, Vol. 134(4), pp. 56–86.

Geri, A. (2007): "Knowledge Free and Unfree: Epistemic Tensions and Plant Knowledge at the Cape in the 17th and 18th Centuries." In: International Journal of African Renaissance Studies, Vol. 2(2), pp. 136–182.

Gericke, N. (2001): "Sutherlandia and AIDS Patients. Update 13th March 2001." In: Australian Journal of Medical Herbalism, Vol. 13 (1), pp. 3–17.

Geschiere, P. L. (1997): Modernity and Witchcraft. Politics and the Occult in Postcolonial Africa, Charlottesville and London: University of Virginia Press.

Geschiere, P. L. / van Binsbergen, W. M. J. (2005): Commodificatioon: Things Agency, and Identities, Münster: Lit Verlag.

Geschiere, P. L. / Meyer, B. / Pels, P. (2008): Readings in Modernity in Africa, Indiana: Bloomington.

Gibson, D. (2011): "Ambiguities in the Making of an African Medicine: Clinical Trials of Sutherlandia Trutescens (L.)Br (Lessertia frutescense)." In: African Sociological Review, Vol. 15(1)2011.

Gibson, J. (2005): Intellectual Property, Medicine and Health, Farnham: Ashgate.

Giddens, A. (1991): Modernity and Self-Identity: Self and Society in the Late Modern Age, Cambridge: Polity Press.

Giddens, A. (1994): "Living in a Post-Traditional Society." In: U. Beck / A. Giddens / S. Lash, Reflexive Modernization. Politics, Tradition and the Aestetics in the Modern Social Order, London and Basingstoke: Stanford University Press.

Goldman, M. (1997): "Customs in Common: The Epistemic World of the Commons Scholars." In: Theory and Society, Vol. 26(1), pp. 1–37.

Gluckmann, M. (1965): Politics, Law and Ritual in Tribal Society, Oxford: Basil Blackwell.

Gluckmann, M. (1969): Ideas and Procedures in African Customary Law, Oxford: International African Institute by the University of Oxford Press.

Godbout, J. (in collaboration with Caillé, A.) (1998): The Word of the Gift, Montreal, Kingston, London and Ithaca: McGill-Queen's University Press.

Godelier, M. (1998): The Enigma of the Gift, Chicago: University of Chicago Press.

Goody, J. (1986): The Interface Between the Written and the Oral, Cambridge: Cambridge University Press.

Gordon, C. (ed.) (1980): Knowledge/Power. Selected Writing and Interviews. Foucault, Michel. 1972–1977, New York: Pantheon Books.

Graebner, D. (2001): Towards an Anthropological Theory of Value. The False Coin of Our Own Dreams, New York: Palgrave.

Grebe, S. K. / Singh, R. J. (1999): "LC-MS/MS in the Clinical Laboratory – Where to from Here?" In: Clinical Biochemical Review, Vol. 32 (1), pp. 5–31.

Green, E. (1997): "Purity, Pollution and the Invisible Snake in Southern Africa." In: Medical Anthropology: Cross Cultural Studies in Health and Illness, Vol. 17(1), pp. 83–100.

Green, E. / Jung, A. / Djedje, A. (1994): "The Snake in the Stomach: Child Diarrhea in Central Mozambique." In: Medical Anthropology Quarterly, Vol. 8(1), pp. 4–24.

Green, L. (ed.) (2013): Contested Ecologies. Dialogues in the South on Nature and Knowledge, Cape Town: HSRC Press.

Green, L. (2012): "Beyond South Africa's Indigenous Knowledge – Science Wars." In: South African Journal of Science, Vol. 108 (/78), pp. 1–10.

Green, L. (2008): "Anthropologies of Knowledge and South Africa's Knowledge Systems Policy." In: Anthropology Southern Africa, Vol. 31(1&2), pp. 48–57.

Green, L. (2007): "Cultural Heritage, Archives & Citizenship: Reflections on Using Virtual Reality for Presenting Different Knowledge Traditions in the Public Sphere." In: Critical Arts, Vol. 21(2), pp. 101–122.

Greene, S. (2004): "Indigenous People Incorporated? Culture as Politics, Culture as Property in Pharmaceutical Bioprospecting." In: Current Anthropology, Vol. 45 (2), pp. 211–237.

Gregory, C. (1982): Gifts and Commodities, London: Academic Press.

Griffiths, A. (2013): "Legal Pluralism." In: R. Banakar / M. Travers (eds.), An Introduction to Law and Society, Oxford: Hart Publishing, pp. 269–287.

Grifo, F. / Rosenthal, J. (1997): Biodiversity and Human Health, Washington: Island Press.

Gupta, A. / Ferguson, J. (1997): Anthropological Locations. Boundaries and Grounds of a Field Science, Berkeley, Los Angeles, London: University of California Press.

Gustavson, L. C. / Cytrynbaum, J. D. (2003): "Illuminating Spaces: Relational Spaces, Complicity, and Multi-Sited Ethnography." In: Field Methods, Vol. 15(3), pp. 252–270.

Hacking, I. (2000): The Social Construction of What? Cambridge: Harvard University Press.

Hage, G. (2005): "A not so Multi-Sited Ethnography of a not so Imagined Community". In: Anthropological Theory, Vol. 5(4), pp. 463–475.

Habsbawm, E. J. / Ranger, T. O. (eds.) (1993): The Invention of Tradition, Cambridge: Cambridge University Press.

Hahn, R. (1995): Sickness and Healing: An Anthropological Perspective, New Heaven: Yale University Press.

Hall, J. (1995): Sangoma: My Odyssey into the Spirit World of Africa, New York: Touchstone Books.

Hall, R. / Williams, G. (1991): "Land Reform in South Africa: Problems and Prospects." In: M. Baregu / C. Landsberg (eds.), From Cape to Congo: Southern Africa's Evolving Security Architecture, Boulder Lynne: Rienner, pp. 97–130.

Hammond-Tooke, W. D. (1978): "Do the South-Eastern Bantu Worship Their Ancestors?" In: W. J. Argyle / E. Preston-Whyte (eds.), Social system and tradition in southern Africa: essays in honor of Eileen Krige, Cape Town: Oxford University Press, pp. 134–164.

Hammond-Tooke, W. D. (1985): "Who Worships Whom? Agnates and Ancestors among Nguni." In: African Studies, Vol. 44(1), pp. 47–64.

Hammond-Tooke, W. D. (1989): Rituals and Medicines: Indigenous Healing in South Africa, Johannesburg: A.D. Donker.

Hammond-Tooke, W. D. (1998): "Selective borrowing? The Possibility of San Shamanistic Influence on the Southern Bantu Divination and Healing Practice." In: Southern African Archeological Bulletin, Vol. 53, pp. 9–15.

Hammod-Tooke, W. D. (2002): "The Uniqueness of Nguni Mediumistic Divination in Southern Africa." In: Africa, Vol. 72(2), pp. 277–292.

Handelsman, J. (2005): "How to find new Antibiotics." In: The Scientist, Vol. 19 (19) (www.the-scientist.com/?articles.view/ articleNo/16737/title/How-to-Find-New-Antibiotics).

Hanks, W. F. / Severi, C. (2014): "Translating Worlds: The epistemological space of translation." In: Hau: Journal of Ethnographic Theory, Vol. 4(2), pp. 1–16.

Hann, C. M. (1998) Property Relations: Reviewing the Anthropological Tradition, Cambridge University Press.

Hannerz, U. (2003): "Being There…and There…and There! Reflections on Multi-Sited Ethnography." In: Ethnography, Vol. 4(2), pp. 201–216.

Haraway, D. (1991): "A Cyborg Manifesto. Science, Technology, and Socialist-Feminism in the late Twentieth Century." In: Simians, Cyborgs and Women: The Reinvention of Nature, New York: Routledge.

Haraway, D. (1988): "Situated Knowledges: The Science Question in Feminism and the Privilege of Partial Perspective." In: Feminist Studies, Vol. 14 (3), pp. 575–599.

Hardin, G. (1968): "The Tragedy of the Commons." In: Science, Vol. 162 (3859), pp. 1243–1248.

Harding, S. / Figueroa, R. (2002): Science and Other Cultures: Issues in Philosophies of Science and Technology, London: Routledge.

Harnett, S. M. / Osterhuizen, V. / de Venter, M. (2005): "Anti-HIV Activities of Organic and Aqueous Extracts of Sutherlandia Frutencens and Lobostemon Trigonus." In: Journal of Ethnopharmacology, Vol. 96, pp. 113–119.

Harvey, A. L. (2002): Natural Product Pharmaceuticals: A Diverse Approach to Drug Discovery, Richmond, Surrey: PJB Publications.

Harvey, D. (1993): "The Dialectics of Social and Environmental Change." In: Social Register, Vol. 30, pp. 1–51.

Hastrup, K. (2010): "Emotional Topographies. The Sense of Place in the Far North." In: J. Davis / D. Spencer (eds.), Emotions in the Field: The Psychology and Anthropology of Fieldwork Experience, Palo Alto: Stanford University Press, pp. 191–211.

Hayden, C. (2003): When Nature Goes Public. The Making and Unmaking of Bioprospecting in Mexico, Princeton and Oxford: Princeton University.

Hayden, C. (2007): "Bioscience, Exchange, and the Politics of Benefit-Sharing." In: Social Studies of Science, Vol. 37(5), pp. 729–758.

Hazzelrigg, L. E. (1969): "A Reexamination of Simmel's 'The Secret and the Secret Society': Nine Propositions." In: Social Force, Vol. 47 (3), pp. 323–333.

Heller, M. A. (1998): "Tragedy of the Anticommons: Property in the Transition from Marx to Markets." In: Harvard Law Review, 111(3), pp. 622–688.

Hess, C. / Ostrom, E. (2011): Understanding Knowledge as a Commons. From Theory to Practice, Cambridge and London: MIT Press.

Helmreich, S. (2010): "The Emergence of Multispecies Ethnography." In: Cultural Anthropology, 25(4), pp. 545–575.

Herwitz, D. (2010): Heritage, Culture, and Politics in the Postcolony, New York: Colombia University Press.

Hewart, M. L. (1970): Bantu Folklore (Medical and General), New York: Negro University Press.

Hirokazu, M. (2004): The Method of Hope. Anthropology, Philosophy, and the Fijan Knowledge, London and Basingstoke: Stanford University Press.

Hirokazu, M. (2006): "Economy of Dreams: Hope in Global Capitalism and its Critique." In: Cultural Anthropology, Vol. 21(2), pp. 147–172.

Hirsch, E. / Strathern, M. (2004): Transactions and Creations. Property Debates and the Stimulus of Melanesia, New York and Oxford: Berhahn Books.

Hirst, M. (1998): "A River of Metaphors: Interpreting the Xhosa diviner's myth." In: McAllister (ed.), Culture and the Commonplace: Anthropological Essays in Honor of David Hammond-Tooke, Johannesburg: Witwartersrand University.

Hirst, M. (1993): "The Healer's Art: Cape Nguni Diviners in the Townships of Grahamstown, Eastern Cape, South Africa." In: Curare, Vol. 16 (2), pp. 97–114.

Hirst, M. (1990): The Healer's Art: Cape Nguni Diviners in the Townships of Grahamstown. PhD Thesis, Grahamstown: Rhodes University.

Hitchcock, R. / Vinding, D. (2004): Indigenous Peoples' Rights in Southern Africa, Copenhagen: IWGIA.

Hobart, M. (1993): "Introduction: The Growth of Ignorance?" In: M. Hobart (ed.), An Anthropological Critique of Development. The Growth of Ignorance, London: Routledge, pp. 1–30.

Hobsbawm, E. / Ranger, T. (1992): Invention of Tradition, Cambridge: University of Cambridge Press.

Howes, M. / Chambers, R. (1980): "Indigenous Technical Knowledge: Analysis, Implications and Issues." In: W. D. Brokensha / O. Werner (eds.), Indigenous Knowledge Systems and Development, Lanham, MD: University of America, pp. 329–340.

Hunn, E. (1991): "What is Traditional Ecological Knowledge." In: G. Williams / G. Baines (eds.), Traditional Ecological Knowledge: Wisdom for Sustainable development, Canberra: Centre for Resource and Environmental Studies, ANU.

Hutchings, A. (2007): "Ritual Cleansing, Incense and the Tree of Life – Observations on Some Indigenous Plant Usage in Traditional Zulu and Xhosa Purification and Burial Rites." In: Alternation, 14(2), pp. 189–218.

Hutchings, A. / Haxtin, A. / Lewis, G. / Cunningham, A. (1996): Zulu Medicinal Plants: An Inventory, Durban: University of KwaZulu-Natal.

Hyde, L. (1983): The Gift: Imagination and the Erotic Life of Property, New York: Vintage Books.

Inda, J. X. (2005): "Analytics of the Modern: An Introduction." In: J. X. Inda (ed.), Anthropology of Modernity. Foucault, Governmentality, and Life Politics, Oxford: Blackwell Publishing.

Ingold, T. (2011): Being Alive. Essays on Movement, Knowledge and Description, London and New York: Routledge.

Ingold, T. (2008): "Point, Line and Counterpoint: From Environment to Fluid Space." In: A. Berthoz / Y. Christen (eds.), Neurobiology of 'Umwelt': How Livings Beings Perceive The World. Research and Perspectives in Neurosciences, Heidelberg a.o.: Springer.

Ingold, T. (2007): Lines. A Brief History, New York: Routledge.

Ingold, T. (2002): The Perception of the Environment. Essays on Livelihood, Dwelling and Skills, London and New York: Routledge.

Jackson, M. (1989): Path Towards a Clearing: Radical Empiricism and Ethnographic Inquiry, Bloomington Indiana: University Press.

Jackson, M. (1998): Minima Ethnographica: Intersubjectivity and the Anthropological Project, Chicago: Chicago University Press.

Jackson, M. (2007): "Intersubjective Ambiguities." In: Medische Antropologie, Vol. 19(1), pp. 147–161.

Janzen, J. (1992): Ngoma: Discourses of Healing in Central and Southern Africa, Berkeley: University of California Press.

Jasanoff, S. (ed.) (2004): States of Knowledge: The Co-Production of Science and Social Order, London: Routledge.

James, D. (1999): "Hill of Thorns: Custom, Knowledge and the Reclaiming of a Lost Land in the New South Africa." In: Development and Change, Vol. 31(3), pp. 629–649.

James, D. (2009): "The Tragedy of the Private: Owners, Communities and the State in South Africa's Land Reform Program." In: F. Benda-Beckmann / K. Benda-Beckmann / M. Wiber, Changing Properties of Property, New York and Oxford: Berghahn.

James, W. (1976): Essays in Radical Empiricism, Cambridge: Harvard University Press.

Jebens, H. (ed.) (2004): Cargo, Cult, and Culture Critique, Honolulu: University of Hawaii Press.

Jeffreys, D. (2008): Aspirin: The Remarkable Story of Wonder Drug, London: Bloomsbury Publishing.

Joelving, F. (2011): Would-be-fat-fighter Hoodia Nothing but Side Effects. (https://www.reuters.com/article/us-hoodia/would-be-fat-fighter-hoodia-nothing-but-side-effects-idUSTRE79R6AI20111028).

Juma, C. (1993): Editors of Biodiversity Prospecting: Using Genetic Resources for Sustainable Development, Washington, D.C.: World Resources Institute.

Junod, H. A. (1962): The Life of a South African Tribe, New York: University Books.

Kaplan, M. (1995): Neither Cargo nor Cult: Ritual Politics and the Colonial Imagination in Fiji, Durham: Duke University Press.

Kate, K. T. / Laird, S. A. (1998): The Commercial Use of Biodiversity: Access to Genetic Resources and Benefit Sharing, London: Earthscan.

Katerere, D. R. / Eloff, J. N. (2005): "Antibacterial and Antioxidant Activity of Sutherlandia Frutescens (Fabaceae). A Reputed Anti-HIV/AIDS Phytomedicine." In: Phytotherapy Research, Vol. 19, pp. 779–781.

Keene, L. (2013): "Transmission and Embodiment of History in the Thokoza Sangoma Traditionen." In: The Archival Plattform (http://www.archivalplatform. org/blog/entry/transmission_and_embodiment/).

Kepe, T. (2009): "Shaped by Race: Why 'Race' Still Matters in the Challenges Facing Biodiversity Conservation in Africa." In: Local Environment, Vol. 14(9), pp. 871–878.

King, S. R. / Meza E. / Ayala F. / Forero L. E. / Penna M. et al. (1995): "Croton Lechleri and Sustainable Harvest and Management of Plants in Pharmaceuticals, Phytomedicines and Cosmetic Industries." In: D. S. Wosniak / S. Yuen / M. Garrett / T. M. Shuman, International Symposium on Herbal Medicine, San Diego: International Institute for Human Resources, Health & Human Service, San Diego State University, pp. 305–333.

Knipper, M. (2010): "Traditionelle Medizin als strategische Ressource in Ecuador. Indianische Heilkunde im Kontext." In: H. Dilger / B. Hadolt (eds.), Medizin im Kontext. Krankheit und Gesundheit in einer vernetzten Welt, Frankfurt a. M.: Peter Lang.

Kirkland, T. / Hunter L. M. (2007): "The Bush is No More: Insights on Institutional Change and Natural Resource Availability in Rural South Africa." In: Society and Natural Resources, Vol. 20, pp. 337–350.

Koehn, F. E. / Carter, G. E. (2005): "The Evolving Role of Natural Products in Drug Discovery." In: Nature Reviews Drug Discovery, Vol. 4(3) (http://www.nature. com/nrd/journal/v4/n3/pdf/nrd1657.pdf).

Knorr-Centina, K. (1981): The Manufacture of Knowledge. An Essay on the Constructivist and Contextual Nature of Science, Oxford: Pergamon Press.

Knorr-Centina, K. (1999): Epistemic Cultures: How Sciences Make Knowledge, Cambridge: Harvard University Press.

Knorr-Centina, K. (2001): "Laboratory Studies: The Cultural Approach to the Study of Science." In: J. Sheila / G. E. Markle / J. C. Petersen / T. Pinch (eds.), The Handbook of Science and Technology Studies (2nd ed.), London: Sage, pp. 140–166.

Kohn, E. (2013): How Forests Think? Toward an Anthropology Beyond Human, Los Angeles and London: University of California Press.

Kolb, P. (1979 [1922]): Reise zum Vorgebirge der Guten Hoffnung, Leipzig: Brockhaus.

Kopytoff, I. (1984): "The Cultural Biography of Things." In: Apapdurai, Arjun. The Social Life of Things. Commodities in Cultural Perspective, Cambridge: Cambridge University Press.

Kuper, A. (2003): "Return of the Native." In: Current Anthropology, Vol. 44 (3), pp. 389–402.

Laird, S. (2002): Biodiversity and Traditional Knowledge: Equitable Partnerships in Practice, London: Earthscan.

Laguerre, M. S. (1987): Afro-Caribbean Folk Medicine, South Hadley, MS: Bergin and Garvey.

Langwick, S. (2011): Bodies, Politics, and African Healing. A Matter of Maladies in Tanzania, Bloomington and Indianapolis: Indiana University Press.

Latour, B. (1985): "Give Me a Laboratory and I Will Raise the World." In: K. D. Knorr-Cetina / M. J. Mulkay, Science Observed. Perspectives on the Social Study of Science, London: Sage.

Latour, B. (1987): Science in Action. How to Follow Scientists and Engineers Through Society. Milton Keynes: Open University Press.

Latour, B. (1996): "On Actor-Network Theory. A Few Clarifications Plus More than a Few Complications." In: Soziale Welt, Vol. 47, pp. 369–381.

Latour, B. (1991): We Have Never Been Modern, Cambridge: Harvard University Press.

Latour, B. (1993): The Pasteurization of France, Cambridge: Harvard University Press.

Latour, B. (1999): "On recalling ANT." In: J. Law / J. Hassard (eds.), Actor Network Theory and After, Oxford: Blackwell and the Sociological Review, pp. 15–25.

Latour, B. (2004a): The Politics of Nature. How to Bring the Sciences into Democracy? Cambridge and London: Havard University Press.

Latour, B. (2004b): "On using ANT for Studying Information Systems: A (Somewhat) Socratic Dialogue." In: C. Avgerou / C. Ciborra / F. Land (eds.), The Social Study of Information and Communication. Technology. Innovation, Actors, and Contexts, Oxford and New York: Oxford University Press.

Latour, B. (2005): Reassembling the Social. An Introduction to Actor-Network Theory, Oxford: Oxford University Press.

Latour, B. (2009): The Making of Law – An Ethnography of the Conseil d'Etat, Cambridge: Polity Press.

Latour, B. (2007): "The Recall of Modernity." In: Cultural Studies Review, Vol. 13(1), pp. 11–30.

Latour, B. / Woolgar, S. (1986): Laboratory Life: The Social Construction of Scientific Facts, Princton: Princeton University Press.

Latour, J. (2009): "Actor Network Theory and Material Semiotics." In: B. Turner (ed.), The New Blackwell Companion to Social Theory, Oxford: Blackwell-Willey, pp. 142–158.

Latour, B. / Lépinay, V. A. (2010): The Science of Passionate Interests: An Introduction to Gabriel Tarde's Economic Anthropology, Chicago: Prickly Paradigm Press.

Law, J. (1996): Organizing Modernity, Oxford: Blackwell.

Law, J. (2007): "ANT and Material Semiotics." In: B. Turner (ed.), The New Network to Social Theory (http://www.heterogeneity.net/pub lications/Law2007ANTandMaterialSemiotics.pdf.

Law, J. / Hassard, J. (1999): Actor-Network Theory and After, Oxford: Blackwell.

Law, J. / Mol, A. (2002): Complexities: Social Studies of Knowledge Practices, Durham: Duke University Press.

Laplante, J. (2009): "South African Roots towards Global Knowledge: Music or Molecules?" In: Anthropology of Southern Africa, 32 (1&2), pp. 8–17.

Laplante, J. (2014): "On Knowing and Not Knowing 'Life' in Molecular Biology and Xhosa Healing: Ontologies in the Preclinical Trials of a South African Indigenous Medicine (Muthi)." In: Anthropology of Consciousness, Vol. 25(1), pp. 1–31.

Laplante, J. (2015): "Healing Roots." In: Anthropology in Life and Medicine, Vol. 14, Epistemologies of Healing, New York and Oxford: Berghahn.

Liebig, K. (2001): "Protection of Intellectual Property Rights in the World Trading System: The TRIPS Agreement and Developing Countries." In: German Development Institute briefing paper, January 2001.

Lemanski, C. (2007): "Global Cities in the South: Deepening social and spatial polarization in Cape Town." In: Cities, Vol. 24(6), pp. 448–461.

Levine, S. (2012): Medicine and the Politics of Knowledge, Cape Town: HSRC Press.

Lévi-Strauss, C. (1966): The Savage Mind, Chicago: University of Chicago Press.

Lewis, E. (2010): "If They Return, We'll Braai Them." In: Cape Argues, January 2010 (https://uk.groups.yahoo.com/neo/groups/zimbabwe_news/conver sations/topics/1158).

Lewu, F. B. / Grierson, D. / Afolayan, A. J. (2010): "Influences of Seed Source, Pre-Chilling, Light and Temperature on the Germination of South African Pelargonium Sidoides." In: Journal of Agricultural Science and Technology, Vol. 4, pp. 18–23.

Lowrey, K. (2008): "Incommensurability and New Economic Strategies among Indigenous and Traditional Peoples." In: Journal of Political Ecology, Vol. 15, pp. 61–74.

Luhrman, T. (2010): "What Counts as Data?" In: J. Davies / D. Spencer (eds.), Emotions in the Field, pp. 212–238.

Lund, G. (2003): "Healing the Nation: Medicolonial Discourse and the State of Emergency from Apartheid to Truth and Reconciliation." In: Cultural Critique, Vol. 54, pp. 88–119.

Macilwain, C. (1997): "When Rhetoric Hits Reality in Debate on Bioprospecting." In: Nature, Vol. 392.

Makana, C. (2012): "Healers Slate Muthi Killings." (http://www.sowetanlive.co.za/news/2012/05/09/healers-slate-muthi-killings).

Makhaye, C. (2005): "Muthi, Mops and Murder in Mpophomeni." (http://beta.iol.co.za/news/south-africa/muthi-mobs-and-murder-in-mpophomeni-253139).

Makay, D. (1996): "Agents of Empire: The Banksian Collectors and Evaluation of New Lands." In: D. Miller / P. H. Reill (eds.), Visions of Empire: Voyages, Botany, and Representations of Nature, Cambridge: Cambridge University Press.

Makgoba, W. (1999): African Renaissance. The New Struggle, Cape Town: Mafube – Tafelberg.

Makhubu, L. (1998): "Bioprospecting in an African Context." In: Science, Vol 282(5386), pp. 41–42.

Malinoswski, B. (1922): Argonauts of the Western Pacific, London: Routledge & Kegan Paul.

Mander, M. / Le Breton, G. (2006): "Overview of the Medicinal Plants Industry in South Africa." In: N. Diederichs (ed.), Commercializing Medicinal Plants. A Southern African Guide, Stellenbosch: Sun Press.

Manda, L. D. (2008): "Africa's Healing Wisdom: Spiritual and Ethical Values of Traditional Healthcare Practices." In: R. Nicholson (ed.), Persons in Community. African Ethics in a global Culture, Scottsville: University of KwaZulu-Natal Press.

Mander, M. / Steytler, N. / Diedrichs, N. (2006): "Economics of Medicinal Plant Cultivation." In: N. Diederichs (ed.), Commercialising Medicinal Plants – A Southern African Guide, Stellenbosch: SUN Press, pp. 43–52.

Marcus, G. E. (1995): "Ethnography of/in the World System: The Emergence of Multi-Sited Ethnography." In: Annual Review of Anthropology, Vol. 24, pp. 95–117.

Marcus, G. (1998): Ethnography through Tick and Thin, Princeton: Princeton University Press.

Martin, G. / Vermeylen, S. (2005): "Intellectual Property, Indigenous Knowledge and Biodiversity." In: Capitalism Nature Socialism, Vol. 16, pp. 27–48.

Matsabisa, M. G. / Spotose, T. / Hobo, D. / Javu, M. (2009): "Traditional Health Practitioners' Awareness Training Programme on TB, HIB and AIDS: A Pilot Project for the Kayelitsha Area in Cape Town, South Africa." In: Journal of Medicinal Plants Research, Vol 3(3), pp. 142–147.

Mauss, M. (2011[1954]): The Gift, Mansfield Centre, CT: Martino Publishing.

Mauss, M. (2007): A General Theory of Magic (reprindeted ed.), London: Routledge.

Malinowski, B. (1948): Magic, Science and Religion and Other Essays, Glencoe, Illinois: The Free Press.

Masood, E. (1998): "Social Equity Versus Private Property: Striking the Right Balance." In: Nature, Vol. 392, pp. 537.

Mash, J. L. (2002): Unjust Legality: A Critique of Habermas' Philosophy of Law, Boulder and New York: Rowman and Littlefield.

Mathur, A. (2003): "Who Owns Traditional Knowledge?" In: Economic and Political Weekly, Vol. 38(42), pp. 4471–4481.

Mayeng, B. I. (2009): Traditional Healing and Implications of Policy on the Discipline. UCT Sawyer Seminar Series: Exploring Notions of Body, Health and Illness, Cape Town.

Mbeki, T. (1998): The African Renaissance. Statement of the Deputy President Thabo Mbeki. SABC, Gallagher, August 13.

McElay, C. (2011): The Paradox of Apartheid. Social Segregation and Cultural Collaboration in Medical Discourse. Doctoral Thesis. Georgetown University, USA (https://repository.library.georgetown.edu/bitstream/handle/10822/555508/McElyeathesis.pdf?sequence=2).

Meier zu Biesen, C. (2010): "The Rise to Prominence of Artemisa Annua L. – the Transformation of a Chinese Plant to a Global Pharmaceutical." In: African Sociological Review, Vol. 14(2), pp. 24–46.

Meier zu Biesen, C. (2013): Globale Epidemie – lokale Antworten. Eine Ethnographie der Heilpflanze Artemisia Anua in Tanzania, Frankfurt: Campus.

Meier zu Biesen, C. / Dilger, H. / Nienstedt, T. (2012): Bridging Gaps in Health Care and Healing: Traditional Medicine and the Biomedical Health Care Sector in Zanzibar, Freie Universität Berlin und Südtiroler Ärzte für die Dritte Welt (http://www.polsoz.fu-berlin.de/ethnologie/personenliste/dilger/Meier_zu_Biesen_et_al_Bridg
ing_Gaps_in_Health_Care_and_Healing_FINAL_REPORT_2012.pdf).

Merry, S. A. (1988): "Legal Pluralism." In: Law and Society Review, Vol. 22 (5), pp. 869–96.

Merson, J. (2000): "Bio-Prospecting or Bio-piracy: Intellectual Property Rights and Biodiversity in a Colonial and Postcolonial Context." In: Osiris, Vol. 15, pp. 282–295.

Merz, J. / Magnus, D. / Cho, M. / Caplan, A. L. (2002): "Protecting Subjects Interests' in Genetic Research." In: The American Journal of Human Genetics, Vol. 70 (4), pp. 965–971.

Mgbeotji, I. (2006): Global Biopiracy. Patents, Plants and Indigenous Knowledge. Ithaca, New York: Cornell University Press.

Miller, D. (2005): Materiality, London: Routledge.

Mills, E. / Cooper, C. / Seely, D. / Kanfer, I. (2005): "African Herbal Medicines in the Treatment of HIV: Hypoxiis and Sutherlandia. An Overview of evidence and pharmacology." In: Nutrition Journal, Vol. 4, pp. 19–24.

Mills, E. / Cooper, C. / Kanfer, I. (2005): "Traditional African Medicine in the Treatment of HIV." In: The Lancet Infectious Diseases, Vol. 5, pp. 465–467.

Mills, E. / Foster B. C. / Heeswijk R. V. / Phillips, E. / Wilson K. / Leonard, B. / Kosuge K. / Kanfer, I. (2005): "Impact of African Herbal Medicines on Antiretroviral Metabolism." In: AIDS, Vol. 19(1), pp. 95–97.

Millum, J. (2010): "How Should Benefits of Bioprospecting Be Shared?" In: The Hastings Center Report, Vol. 40(1), pp. 24–33.

Milton, K. (1996): Environmentalism and Cultural Theory: The Role of Anthropology in Environmental Discourse, London and New York: Routledge.

Mitchell, T. (2002): Rule of Experts. Egypt, Techno-Politics, Modernity, Berkeley and Los Angeles: California University Press.

Mofokeng, L. L. (2005): Legal Pluralism in South Africa. Aspects of African Customary, Muslim and Hindu Family Law, Pretoria: Van Schaik Publisher.

Mogobo B. R. (2002): African Philosophy through Ubuntu, Harare: Mond Books, p. 41.

Mol, A. (2000): The Body Multiple: Ontology in Medicinal Practice, Durham: Duke University Press.

Mol, A. (2010): "Koordination und Ordnungsbildung in der Akteur-Netzwerk-Theorie." In: Kölner Zeitschrift für Soziologie und Sozialpsychologie, Vol. 50, pp. 253–269.

Mol, A. (2010): "Actor-Network Theory: Sensitive Terms and Enduring Tensions." In: Kölner Zeitschrift für Soziologie und Sozialpsychologie, Vol. 50(1), pp. 253–269.

Morgan, R. / Wieringa, S. (2005): Tommy Boys, Lesbian Men and Ancestral Wives: Female Same-Sex Practices in Africa, Johannesburg: Jacana Media.

Mofokeng, L. L. (2009): Legal Pluralism in South Africa. Aspects of African Customary, Muslim and Hindu Family Law, Pretoria: Van Schaik Publisher.

Morgera, E. / Buck, M. / Tsioumani, E. (2012): The Nagoya Protocol on Access and Benefit-Sharing in Perspective. Implications for International Law and Implementation Challenges, Leiden: Koninklijke Brill NV.

Morris, A. G. (1997): "The Griqua and the Khoikhoi: Biology, Ethnicity and the Construction of Identity." In: Kronos Journal of Cape History, No. 24, pp. 106–118.

Morris, C. K. (2012): "Pharmaceutical Bioprospecting and the Law: The Case of Umckaloabo in a Former Apartheid Homeland of South Africa." Anthropology News, Vol. 53, p. 6 (www.scicornwall.com/2012/12/pharmaceutical-bioprospecting-and-law.html).

Mossoff, A. (2001): "Rethinking the Development of Patents: An Intellectual History, 1550–1800." In: Hastings Law Journal, Vol. 52(6), pp. 1255–1322.

Mountain, A. (2003): The First People of the Cape: A Look at Their History and the Impact of Colonialism on the Cape's Indigenous People, Claremont and Cape Town: David Philip.

Mulligan, S. / Stoett, P. (2000): "A Global Bio-Prospecting Regime. Partnership or Piracy?" In: Canadian International Journal, Vol. 55(2), pp. 224–246.

Mukinda, J. T. (2005): Acute and Chronic Toxicity of the Flavonoid-Containing Plant Artemisia Afra in Rodents. Dissertation published at the University of Western Cape, Cape Town (http://etd.uwc.ac.za/usrfiles /modules/etd/docs/ etd_init_6157_1176888209.pdf).

Mukinda, J. T. / Syce, J. A. / Fisher, D. / Meyer, M. (2010): "Effect of the Plant Matrix on the Uptake of Luteolin Derivates-Containing Artemisia Afra Aquous-Extract in Caco-2 Cells." In: Journal of Ethnopharmacology, Vol. 130(3), pp. 439–449.

Murray, F. / Stern, S. (2007): "Do Formal Intellectual Property Rights Hinder the Free Flow of Scientific Knowledge? An Emprical Test of the Anti-Commons Hypothesis." In: Journal of Economic Behavior and Organization, Vol. 63(4), pp. 648–687.

Nader, L. (2011): "Ethnography as Theory." In: HAU: Journal of Ethnographic Theory, Vol. 1(1), pp. 211–219.

Nakazora, M. (2015): "Pure Gifts for Future Benefits? Giving Form to the Subject in a Biodiversity Databasing Project in India." In: NatureCulture, Vol. 3(6), pp. 106–121.

Nandy, A. (1984): Science Hegemony and Violence: A Requiem for Modernity, Tokyo: United Nations University. (www.arvindguptatoys.com/ arvindgupta/ hegemony-nandy.pdf). National Recordal System (www.csir.co.za/meraka/National_Recordal_System.html).

Newitt, M. A. (1994): History of Mozambique, London: Hurst & Company.

Ng'etich, K. A. (2005): Indigenous Knowledge, Alternative Medicine and Intellectual property Rights Concerns in Kenya. Conference Paper at the 11th Assembly, Maputo, Mozambique, December 6–11, 2005.

Ngubane, B. (2003): Address by the Minister of Arts, Culture, Science and Technology, at the Signing of a Benefit-Sharing Agreement between the CSIR and the San, March 24, 2003, Molopo Lodge, South Africa (www.polity.org.za/article/ngubane-arts-culture-science-amp-technology-dept-budget-vote-20032004-04042003-2003-04-04).

Ngubane, H. (1976): "Some Notions of Purity and Impurity among the Zulu." In: Journal of the International African Institute, Vol. 46(3), pp. 274–284.

Ngubane, H. (1977): Body and Mind in Zulu Medicine: An Ethnography of Health and Desease in Nyuswa-Zulu Thought and Practice, London and New York: Academic Press.

Ngubane. H. (1981): "Clinical Practice and Organization in Indigenous Healers in South Africa." In: Social Science and Medicine, Vol. 15(3), pp. 361–366.

Niehaus, I. (2012): "Witchcraft and the South African Bantustans: Evidence from Bushbuckridge." In: South African Historical Journal, Vol. 1, pp. 1–18.

Niehaus, I. (2010): "Witchcraft as Subtext: Deep Knowledge and the South African Public Sphere." In: Social Dynamics, Vol. 36 (1), pp. 65–77.

Nigh, R. (2002): "Maya Medicine in the Biological Gaze: Bioprospecting Research as Herbal Fetishism." In: Current Anthropology, Vol. 43(3), pp. 451–477.

Niehaus, I. (2001): Witchcraft, Power, and Politics: Exploring the Occult in the South African Lowfeld, Cape Town: David Philip.

Niehaus, I. (1993): Witch-Hunting and Political Legitimacy: Continuity and Change in Green Valley, Lebowa, 1930–91." In: Africa, Vol. 63(04), pp. 498–530.

Niehaus, I. (2001): "Ethnicity and the Boundaries of Belonging: Reconfiguring Shangaan Identity in the South African Lowfeld." In: African Affairs.,Vol. 101, pp. 557–583.

Niehaus, I. (2005): "Witches and Zombies of the South African Lowfeld: Discourse, Accusations and Subjective Reality." In: Journal of the Royal Institute, Vol. 11(2), pp. 191–210.

Niehaus, I. (2011): Witchcraft and the New Life in South Africa, Cambridge: Cambridge University Press.

Niehaus, I. (with E. Mohlala / K. Shokane) (2001): Witchcraft, Power and Politics: Exploring the Occult in the South African Lowveld, London: Pluto Press.

Nicholas, G. / Bell, C. / Coombe, R. / Welch, J. R. / Noble, B. / Anderson, J. / Bannister, K. / Watkins, J. (2010): "Intellectual Property Issues in Heritage Management." In: Heritage Management, Vol. 3(1), pp. 117–147.

Niezen, R. (2003): The Origin of Indigenism. Human Rights and the Politics of Identity, Berkeley: University of California Press.

Nkabinde, N. Z. (2008): Black Bull, Ancestors and Me. My Life a Lesbian Sangoma, Sunnyside: Janele.

Nkonko Kamwangamalu, M. (1999): "Ubuntu in South Africa: A Sociolinguistic Perspective to a Pan-African Concept." In: Critical Arts: A South-North Journal of Cultural and Media Studies, Vol. 13(2), pp. 25ff.

Nonini, D. (2007): The Global Idea of 'the Commons', New York: Berghahn.

Novas, C. (2006): "The Political Economy of Hope: Patients Organizations, Science and Biovalues." In: BioScience, Vol. 1, pp. 289–305.

Ntutela, S. / Smith, P. / Matika, L. / Mukinda, J. / Arendse, H. / Allie, N. / Estes, M. D. / Mabusela, W. / Folb, P. / Steyn, L. / Johnson, Q. / Folk, W. R. / Syce, J. / Jacobs, M. (2009): "Efficacy of Artemisia Afra Phytotherapy in Experimental Tuberculosis." In: Tuberculosis, Vol. 89 (S1), pp. 33–40.

Oguamanam, C. (2012): Intellectual Property in Global Governance, London and New York: Routledge.

Oloyede, O. (2010): "Epistemological Issues in the Making of an African Medicine: Sutherlandia (Lessertia Frutescens)." In: African Sociological Review, Vol. 13(2), pp. 74–88.

Oloyede, O. (2011): "An Exploration of the Philosophy and Environment of a South African Randomized, Double-Blind, Placebo-Controlled Trial of Lessertia Frutescens Clinical Trials." In: African Sociological Review, Vol. 15(10), pp. 108–123.

Ong, A. / Collier, S. J. (2005): Global Assemblages. Technology, Politics, and Ethics as Anthropological Problems, Maldon, Oxford, Victoria: Blackwell Publishing.

Oomen, B. (2005): Chiefs in South Africa. Law, Culture, and Power in the Post-Apartheid Era, New York: Palgrave.

Osteen, M. (2002): "Gift or Commodity?" In: M. Osteen (ed.), The Question of the Gift. Essays Across the Disciplines, New York: Routledge.

Ostergard, R. / Tubin, M. / Dikirr, P. (2006): "Between the Sacred and the Secular: Indigenous Intellectual Property, International Markets and the Modern African State." In: Journal of Modern African Studies, Vol. 44, pp. 309–333.

Ostrom, E. (1990): Governing the Commons. The Evolution of Institutions for Collective Action, Cambridge: Cambridge University Press.

Parliament of South Africa (1913): Native Land Act (No. 27 of 1913) (also: Bantu Land Act, 1913 and Black Land Act, 1913).

Parry, B. (2002): "Cultures of Knowledge: Investigating Intellectual Property Rights and Relations in the Pacific." In: Antipode, Vol. 34 (4), pp. 670–706.

Parry, J. (1986): "The Gift, the Indian Gift and the 'Indian Gift'." In: Man, Vol. 21(3), pp. 453–473.

Parry, J. / Bloch, M. (eds.) (1989): Money and the Morality of Exchange, Cambridge: Cambridge University Press.

Parry, B. (2004): Trading the Genome. Investigating the Commodification of Bio-Information, New York, Chichster, West Sussex: Columbia University Press.

Pappe, K. W. L. (1847): A List of South African Indigenous Plants Used as Remedies by the Colonists at the Cape of Good Hope, Cape Town: OI Pike.

Pappe, K. W. L. (1850): Florae Carpensis Medicae Prodromis. Cape Town: Robertson.

Phatlane, S. N. (2006): Poverty, Health and Disease in the Era of High Apartheid: South Africa, 1948–1976, Submitted Doctoral Thesis, University of South Africa (Unisa).

Pelgrim, R. (2003): Witchcraft and Policing, Leiden: African Studies Center (https://openaccess.leidenuniv.nl/bitstream/handle/1887/12920/ASC-075287668-076-01.pdf?sequence=2).

Perreau, T. (2003): "Social Capital, Development, and Indigenous Politics in Ecuadorian Amazonia." In: Geographical Review, Vol. 93, pp. 328–348.

Petryna, A. (2003): Life Exposed: Biological Citizens after Chernobyl, Princeton: Princeton University Press.

Peterson, K. (2001): "Bioprospecting for All? Bioprospecting NGOs, Intellectual Property Rights, New Governmentalities." In: PoLAR, Vol. 24(1), pp. 78–91.

Petryna, A. (2009): When Experiments Travel: Clinical Trials and the Global Search for Human Subject, Princeton: Princeton University Press.

Pickering, A. (1992): Science as Practice and Culture, Chicago: University of Chicago Press.

Piennar, A. (2009): The Griqua's Apprentice. Acient Healing Arts of the Karoo, Cape Town: Umuzi.

Pospisil, L. (1971): Anthropology of Law, New York: Harper and Row.

Posey, D. A. / Dutfield, G. (1996): Beyond Intellectual Property: Toward Traditional Resource Rights for Indigenous Peoples and Local Communities, Ottawa: International Development Research Centre.

Posey, D. A. (1999): Cultural and Spiritual Values of Biodiversity, London: United Nations Environmental Program & Intermediate Technology Publications.

Posey, D. A. (2000): "Exploitation of Biodiversity and Indigenous Knowledge." In: C. Cavalcanti (ed.), The Environment, Sustainable Development and Public Policy. Building Sustainability in Brazil, Cheltenham and Northampton: Edward Elgar.

Posey, D. A. (2002a): "Commodification of the Sacred through Intellectual Property Rights." In: Journal of Ethnopharmacology, Vol. 83 (1–2), pp. 3–12.

Posey, D. A. (2002b): "Upsetting the Sacred Balance: Can Study of Indigenous Knowledge Reflect Cosmic Connectedness?" In: P. Silitoe / A. Bicker / J. Pottier, Participating in Development: Approaches to Indigenous Knowledge, London: Routledge, pp. 24–42.

Posey, D. (2004): Indigenous Knowledge and Ethics: A Darrell Posey Reader, New York: Routledge.

Posey, D. / Dutfield, G. (1996): Beyond Intellectual Property: Towards Traditional Resource Rights for Indigenous Peoples and Local Communities, Ottawa: International Development Research Center.

Pratt, M. L. (1992): Imperial Eyes. Travel Writing and Transculturation, New York: Routledge.

Prickett, S. (2009): Modernity and the Reinvention of Tradition. Backing into the Future, Cambridge: Cambridge University Press.

Rabinow, P. (1996): "Artificiality and Enlightenment: From Sociobiology to Biosociality." In: P. Rabinow, Essays on the Anthropology of Reason. Princeton: Princeton University Press.

Rabinow, P. (1999): French DNA. Trouble in Purgatory, Chicago: University of Chicago Press.

Radin, M. J. / Sunder, M. (2004): "Introduction: The Subject and Object of Commodification." In: M. Ertman / J. C. Williams, Rethinking Commodification. Cases and Readings in Law and Culture, New York and London: New York University Press, pp. 8–34.

Ramose, M. B. (2003): "The Philosophy of Ubuntu and Ubuntu as a Philosophy." In: P. H. Coetzee / A. P. J. Roux (eds.), The African Philosophy Reader (2nd ed.), London: Routledge, pp. 230–238.

Reddy, S. (2006): "Making Heritage Legible: Who Owns Traditional Medicinal Knowledge?" In: International Journal of Cultural Property, Vol. 13, pp. 161–168.

Reid, W. V. (1993): Biodiversity Prospecting, Washington: The World Resource Institute.

Reid, W. V. (2002): "Biodiversity Prospecting: Using Genetic Resources for Sustainable Development. A New Release on Life." In: D. Hunter / J. Salzman / D. Zaelke (eds.), International Environmental Law and Policy (2nd ed.), New York: Foundation Press, pp. 942–945.

Reis, R. (1999): "The 'Wounded Healer' as Ideology. The Work of Ngoma in Swaziland." In: R. van Dijk / R. Ries / M. Spierenburg (eds.), The Quest for Fruition Through Ngoma. Political Aspects of Healing in Southern Africa, Athens: Ohio University Press, pp. 61–75.

Reihling, H. (2008): "Bioprospecting the African Renaissance: The new value of muthi in South Africa." In: Journal of Ethnobiology and Ethnomedicine, Vol. 4(9), pp. 4–9.

Reinhold, S. (1994): Local Conflict and Ideology Struggle: Positive Images and Section 28. University of Sussex: unpublished D. Phil. thesis.

Renn, J. (2015): "From the History of Science to the History of Knowledge and Back." In: Centaurus, Vol. 57, pp. 37–53.

Restivo, S. (2010): Bruno Latour. The Once and Future Philosopher. Draft taken from http://salrestivo.org/oldwebsite/LatourFinal.10.pdf on 20.11.2012. Article published in: G. Ritzer / J. Stepnisky, The New Blackwell Companion to Major Social Theorists, Boston: Blackwell, pp. 520–540.

Richter, M. (2003): Traditional Medicines and Traditional Healers in South Africa. Discussion Paper Prepared for the Treatment Action Campaign and AIDS Law Project.

Ritschken, E. (1995): Leadership and Conflict in Bushbuckridge: Struggles to Define Moral Economies within the Context of Rapidly Transforming Political Economies. PhD thesis, University of Witwatersrand.

Roberts, M. (1990): Indigenous Healing Plants. Gauteng: Southern Book Publishers, Halfway House.

Robertson, J. (1999): "Reflexivity Redux: A Pithy Polemic on 'Positonality'." In: Anthropology Quarterly, Vol. 75(4), pp. 785–792.

Robinson, D. (2010): Confronting Biopiracy. Challenges, Cases and International Debates, London and Washinton: Earthscan.

Rouse, J. (1986): Knowledge and Power: Toward a Political Philosophy of Science, Ithaca: Cornell University Press.

Rosaldo, R. (1989): Culture & Truth: The Remaking of Social Analysis, Boston: Beacon Press.

Rose, N. (2007): The Politics of Life Itself. Biomedicine, Power, and Subjectivity in the Twenty-First Century, Princeton: Princeton University Press.

Rose, N. / Novas, C. (2005): "Biological Citizenships." In: A. Ong / S. J. Collier (eds.), Global Assemblages: Technology, Politics, and Ethnics as Anthropological Problems, Oxford: Blackwell Publishing, pp. 43–62.

Rose, N. (2001): "The Politics of Life Itself." In: Theory, Culture and Society, Vol. 18(6), pp. 1–30.

Rose, N. / Valverde M. (1998): "Governed by Law?" In: Social and Legal Studies, Vol. 7, pp. 541–551.

Rosenthal, J. (2006): "Politics, Culture, and Governance in the Development of Prior Informed Consent in Indigenous Communities." In: Cultural Anthropology, Vol. 47(1), pp. 119–142.

Rottenburg, R. (2014): "Experimental Engagements and Metacodes." In: Common Knowledge, Vol. 20(3), pp. 540–548.

Rottenburg, R. (2012): "On Juridico-Political Foundations of Meta. Codes." In: J. Renn (ed.), The Globalization of Knowledge in History. Max Planck Research Library for the History and Development of Knowledge Studies 1, Edition Open Access (www.edition-open-access.de/studies/1/25/index.html).

Rottenburg, R. (2009): Far-Fetched Facts. A Parable of Development Aid, Cambridge and London: MIT Press.

Rottenburg, R. (2014): "Experimental 'Engagments and Metacodes." In: Common Knowledge, Vol. 20(3), pp. 540–548.

Rutert, B. (2012): "Bioprospektion als 'Markt der Möglichkeiten': Hoffnungen, Handlungen und Fakten in Post-Apartheid Südafrika." In: Curare, Vol. 35(3), pp. 229–239.

Rutert, B. / Dilger, H. / Matsabisa, G. M. (2011): Bioprospecting in South Africa: Opportunities and Challenges in a Global Knowledge Economy- a Field in the Becoming. Working Paper Series, 1/11, Center for Area Studies, FU Berlin, CAS.

Sahlins, M. (1976): Culture and Practical Reason, Chicago: University of Chicago Press.

Sampath, P. G. (2004): Regulating Bioprospecting. Institutions for Drug Research, Access and Benefit, Tokio, New York, Paris: United Nations University Press.

Sanders, T. (2003): "Reconsidering Witchcraft: Postcolonial Africa and Analytic (un)Certainties." In: American Anthropologist, Vol. 105(2), pp. 338–352.

Saugestad, S. (2001): "The Inconvenient Indigenous. Remote Area Development in Botswana, Donor Assistance and the First People of the Kalahari." In: Social Anthropology, Vol. 14(2), pp. 290–291.

Schiebinger, L. (2005): Plants and Empire. Colonial Bioprospecting in the Atlantic World, Cambridge and London: Harvard University Press.

Schröder, D. (2009): "Informed Consent: From Medicinal Research to Traditional Knowledge." In: R. Wynberg / D. Schroeder / R. Chennels (eds.), Indigenous Peoples, Consent and Benefit Sharing. Lessons from the San-Hoodia Case, Heidelberg, London, New York: Springer.

Schultze, L. (1928): Zoolgische und Anthropologische Ergebnisse einer Forschungsreise im Westlichen und Zentralen Südafrika, ausgeführt in den Jahren 1903–1905, Vol. 5, part 3, Jena: G. Fischer, pp. 147–227.

Scott, P. (2001): Bioprospecting as a Conservation Tool: History and Background. Crossing Boundaries in Park Management. Proceedings of the 11th Conference on Research and Resource Management in Parks and on Public Lands, edited by David Harmon.

Shore, C. / Wright, S. (eds.) (1997): Anthropology of Policy: Critical Perspectives on Governance and Power, London: Routledge.

Shore, C. / Wright, S. (2011): Policy World. Anthropology and Analysis of Contemporary Power, New York and Oxford: Berghahn Books.

Shreshta, C. H. (2010): "Emotional Apprenticeship: Reflection on the Role of Academic Practice in the Construction of 'the field'." In: J. Davies / D. Spencer (eds.), Emotions in the Field. The Psychology and Anthropology of Fieldwork Experience, Stanford, California: Stanford University Press, pp. 49–73.

Secretariat of the Convention on Biological Diversity (2011): Nagoya Protocol on Access to Genetic Resources and the Fair and Equitable Sharing of Benefits Arising from Their Utilization to the Convention on Biological Diversity (www.cbd.int/abs/doc/protocol/nagoya-protocol-en.pdf).

Sehume, B. (2009): A Phase II Efficacy, Safety, and Tolerability Clinical Study of a Herbal African Traditional Medicines Preparation (PHELA) with Putative Immune modulating Properties. Unpublished Paper. Indigenous Knowledge Health Lead Program. Medical Research Council, South Africa: Cape Town.

Sehume, B. (2010): Pharmaceutical Evaluation of Phela Capsulers Usedin Traditional Medicine. Master Thesis, University of the Western Cape, South Africa.

Seier J.V. / Mdhuli M. / Dhansay M.A. / Loza J. / Laubschner R. / Matsabisa G. (2002): A Toxicity Study of Sutherlandia Leaf Powder (Sutherlandia Microphylla) Consumption. South African Ministry of Health Document.

Shackleton, E. S. / Dzerefos, C. M. / Shackleton, C. M. / Mathabela, E. R. (1996): "Use and Trading of Wild Edible Herbs in the Central Lowfeld Savanna Region South Africa." In: Economic Botany, Vol. 52(3), pp. 251–259.

Shiva, V. (1997): Biopiracy: The Plunder of Nature and Knowledge, Cambridge: South End Press.

Shiva, V. (2007): "Bioprospecting as Sophisticated Biopiracy." In: Journal of Women in Culture and Society, Vol. 32(2), pp. 307–313.

Shiva, V. (2007): "Biodiversity, Intellectual Property Rights, and Globalization." In: B. de Sousa Santos (ed.), Another Knowledge is Possible. Beyond Northern Epistemologies, London and New York: Verso.

Shiva, V. (2002): "Seeds of Suicide. The Ecological and Human Costs of Globalization of Agriculture." In: V. Shiva / G. Bedi (eds.), Sustainable Agriculture and Food Security: The Impact of Globalization, New Delhi: Sage, pp. 169–183.

Simon, C. / Lamla, M. (1991): "Merging Pharmacopoeia: Understanding the Historical Origins of Incorporative Pharmacopoeial Processes among Xhosa Healers in Southern Africa." In: Journal of Ethnopharmacology, Vol. 33(3), pp. 237–242.

Simmel, G. (1906): "The Sociology of Secrecy and of Secret Societies." In: American Journal of Sociology, Vol. 11(4), pp. 441–498.

Simpson, T. / Jackson, V. (1998): "Effective Protection of Indigenous Cultural Knowledge: A Challenge for the Next Millennium." In: Indigenous Affairs, Vol. 3, pp. 44–56.

Sillitoe, P. (2002): "Globalising Indigenous Knowledge." In: P. Sillitoe / A. Bicker / J. Pottier, Participating in Development. Approaches to Indigenous Knowledge, London and New York: Routledge, pp. 108–138.

Smith, A. (1895): A Contribution to the South African Materia Medica. 2nd etn. Lovedale: South Africa.

Smith, C. A. (1966): Common Names of South African Plants. Memoirs of the Botanical Survey of South Africa, No 35, Pretoria: Dep. of Agricultural Technical Services.

Snyder, F. G. (1981): "Colonialism and Legal Form: The Creation of 'Customary Law' in Senegal." In: Journal of Legal Pluralism, Vol. 19, pp. 49.

Soejarto, D. D. / Fon, H. H. S. / Tan, G. T. / Zhang, H. J. / Ma, C. Y. / Franzblau, S. G. / Gyllenhaal, C. / Riley, M. C. / Kadushin, M. R. / Pezzuto, J. M. / Xuan, L. T. / Hiep, N. T. / Hung, N. V. / Vu, B. M. / Loc, P. K. / L. X. Dac / L. T. Binh / N. Q. Chien / N. V. Hai / T. Q. Bich / Cuong, N. M. / Southavong, B. / Sydara, K. / Bouamanivong, S. / Ly, H. M. / Tran van Thuy / Rose, W. C. / Dietzman, G. R. (2005): "Ethnobotany / Ethnopharmacology and Mass Bioprospecting: Issues on Intellectual Property and Benefit-Sharing." In: Journal of Ethnopharmacology, Vol. 100(1–2), pp. 15–22.

Sowman, M. / Wynberg, R. (2012): "Towards Robust Governance for Justice and Environmental Sustainablity: Lessons from Natural Resource Sectors in Sub-Saharan Africa." In: M. Sowman / R. Wynberg (eds.), Governance of Justice and Environmental Sustainability: Lessons Across Natural Resource Sectors in Sub-Saharan Africa. New York and London: Routledge.

Sparrman, A. (2010[1784]): "Reise nach dem Vorgebirge der guten Hoffnung, den südlichen Polarländern und um die Welt, hauptsächlich aber in den Ländern der Hottentotten und Kaffern in den Jahren 1772 bis 1776." Berlin: Haude & Spencer.

Spivak, G. C. (1988): "Can the Subaltern Speak?" In: C. Nelson / L. Grossberg (eds.), Marxism and the Interpretation of Culture, Basingstroke: Macmillan Education, pp. 271–313.

Star, S. L. / Bowker, G. (1999): Sorting Things Out: Classification and Its Consequences, Cambridge, MA: MIT Press.

Star, S. L. (1989): "The Structures of Ill-Structures Solutions: Boundary Objects and Heterogeneous Distributed Problem Solving." In: L. Grasser / N. Huhns (eds.), Distributed Artificial Intelligence, New York: Morgen Publications, pp. 37–54.

Star, S. L. / Griesemer, J. R. (1989): "Institutional Ecology, 'Translation' and Boundary Objects: Amateurs and Professionals in Berkeley's Museum of Vertebrate Zoology, 1907–39." In: Social Studies of Science, Vol. 19(3), pp. 387–420.

Starling, S. (2011): Kalahari Tribe throws Weight at Unilever over Hoodia Rejection (www.nutraingredients.com/Research/Kalahari-tribe-throws-weight-at-Unilever-over-hoodiarejection?utm_source=copyright&utm_medium=On-Site&utm_campaign=copyright).

Starling, S. (2008): Unilever Drops Hoodia (www.nutraingredients).

Steenkamp, P. A. / Harding, N. M. / van Heerden, F. R. / van Wyk, B.-E. (2002): "Idenitfcation of atractyloside by LC-ESI-MS in alleged herbal poisoning." In: Forensic Science International, Vol. 63, pp. 81–92.

Stewart, M. J. / Moar, J. J. / Steenkamp, P. / Kokot, M. (1996): "Findings in Fatal Cases of Poisoning Attributed to Traditonal Remedies in South Africa." In: Forensic Science International, Vol. 101, pp. 177–183.

Strathern, M. (1988): The Gender of the Gift, Oxford: University of California Press.

Strathern, M. (1999a): "Multiple Properties. Multiple Perspectives on Intellectual Property." In: K. Whimp / M. Busse, Protection of Intellectual, Biological and Cultural Property in Papua New Guinea, Canberra: Asia Pacific Press, pp. 47–61.

Strathern, M. (1999b): "What Is Intellectual Property After?" In: The Sociological Review, Vol. 47 (S1), pp. 156–180.

Strathern, M. (1998): "Divisions of Interest and Languages of Ownership." In: C. M. Hann, Property Relations. Renewing the Anthropological Tradition, Cambridge: Cambridge University Press.

Strathern, M. (2000a.): "Multiple Perspectives on Intellectual Property." In: K. Whimp / M. Busse (eds.), Protection of Intellectual, Biological and Cultural Property in Papua New Guinea, pp. 47–61.

Strathern, M. (2000b): "Accountability... and Ethnography." In: M. Strathern (ed.), Audit Cultures: Anthropological Studies in Accountability, Ethics, and the Academy, London and New York: Routledge.

Strathern, M. (2004): Partial Connections, Savage, Maryland: Rowman and Littlefield.

Stengers, I. (2008): "Experimenting with Refrains: Subjectivity and the Challenge of Escaping Modern Dualism." In: Subjectivity, 22, pp. 38–59. (http://dx.doi.org/10.1057/sub.2008.6).

Stoller, P. 2009. The Power of the Between. An Anthropological Odyssey. University of Chicago Press: Chicago.

Stoller, P. / Olkes, C. (1986): In Sorcer's Shadow: A Memoir of Apprenticeship among the Songhay of Niger, Chicago: University of Chicago Press.

Stodulka, T. / Röttger-Rössler, B. (eds.) (2014): Feelings at the Margins – Dealing with Violence, Stigma and Isolation in Indonesia, Frankfurt a. M.: Campus.

Stroeken, K. (2007): Moral Power. The Magic of Witchcraft, New York and Oxford: Berghahn.

Sunder Rajan, K. (2006): Biocapital. The Constitution of Postgenomic Life, London and Durham: Duke University Press.

Sundkler, B. G. M. (1948): Bantu Prophets in South Africa, Cambridge: James Clark & Co.

Summerton, J. V. (2006): "The Organistaion and Infrastructure of the African Traditional Healing System: Reflections from a Sub-District of South Africa." In: African Studies, Vol. 65 (2), pp. 297–319.

Suzman, J. (2002): Minorities in Independent Namibia, London: Minority Rights Group International.

Takeshita, C. (2001): "Bioprospecting and Its Discontents: Indigenous Resistance as Letigimate Politics." In: Alternatives, Vol. 26, pp. 259–282.

Taussig, M. (1980): The Devil and Commodity Fetishism in South America, Chapel Hill: University of North Carolina Press.

Tedlock, B. (2006): "Indigenous Heritage and Biopiracy in the Age of Intellectual Property Rights." In: Explore, Vol. 2(3), pp. 256–259.

Tedlock, B. (1991): "From Participant Observation to the Observation of Participation: The Emergence of Narrative Ethnography." In: Journal of Anthropological Research, Vol. 47(1), pp. 69–94.

Tedlock, B. (2000): "Ethnography and Ethnographic Representation." In: N. K. Denzin / Y. S. Lincoln (eds.), Handbook of Qualitative Research (2nd ed.), Thousand Oaks: Sage.

The Bellagio Declaration of 1993 (http://college.cengage.com/English /amore/demo/ch5_r2.html).

The Crucible Group (1994): People, Plants, and Patents. The Impact of Intellectual Property on Trade, Plant Diversity, and Rural Society. (www.etcgroup.org/content/people-plants-and-patents).

The International Labor Organization (1989): Convention 169 of 1989 (www.ilo.org/dyn/normlex/en/f?p=NORMLEXPUB:12100:0::NO::P12100_INSTRUMENT_ID:312314).

The Republic of South Africa (2004): Communal Land Rights Act (Act No. 11 of 2004) (www.ruraldevelopment.gov.za/phocadownload/Acts/ commu-nal%20land%20rights%20act%2011%200f%202004.pdf).

The Republic of South Africa (2004): Indigenous Knowledge Systems (IKS) Policy.

The Republic of South Africa (2004): National Environmental Management Biodi-versity Act (NEMBA) (No. 10 of 2004).

The Republic of South Africa (2004): Traditional Health Practitioner (THP) Act (No. 35 of 2004).

The Republic of South Africa: Trust Property Control (Act 57 of 1988). Witchcraft Suppression Act (No. 3 of 1957). To Provide for the Suppression of the Practice of Witchcraft and Similar Practices.

The Republic of South Africa (2008): The Bioprospecting, Access and Benefit Sharing Regulatory Framework. A guideline for Users and Providers (https:// www.environment.gov.za/sites/default/files/legislations/bioprospecting_ regulatory_framework_guideline.pdf).

Thornton, R. (2002): "Environment and Land in Bushbuckridge, South Africa." In: L. Zarsky (ed.), Human Right and the Environment: Conflicts and Norms in a Globalizing World, Oxon and New York: Earth Scan.

Thornton, R. (2009): "The Transmission of Knowledge in South African Traditional Healing." In: Africa: The Journal of the International African Institute, Vol. 79(1), pp. 17–34.

Ticktin, M. (2014): "Humanitarianism as Planetary Politics." In: S. Perera / S. Razack (eds), At the Limits of Justice: Women of Color on Terror, University of Toronto Press, pp. 406–420.

Taubes, G. (1995): "Scientists Attacked for 'Patenting' Pacific Tribe." In: Science, Vol. 270, pp. 1112.

Truter, I. (2007): "African Traditional Healers. Cultural and Religious Beliefs In-tertwined in a Holistic Way." In: South African Pharmacological Journal, pp. 56–60.

Tsing, A. (2013): "Sorting out Commodities. How Capitalist Value Is Made through Gifts." In: HAU: Journal of Ethnographic Theory, Vol. 3(1), pp. 21–43.

Tsing, A. (2015): The Mushroom at the End of the World: On the Possibility of Life in Capitalist Ruins, Princeton: Princeton University Press.

Turner, V. (1967): The Forest of Symbols, Ithaca, New York: Cornell University Press.

Turnbull, D. (2003): Masons, Tricksters and Cartographers, London: Routledge.

United Nations Permanent Forum of Indigenous Issues (2007): Declaration of Indigenous Peoples' Rights to Genetic Resources and Indigenous Knowledge (www.ipcb.org/resolutions/htmls/Decl_GR&IK.html).

United Nations Educational, Scientific and Cultural Organization (2002): Draft Glossary (www.unesco.org/culture/ich/doc/src/00272-EN.doc).

United Nations (2007): Declaration of the Rights of Indigenous Peoples (www.un. org/esa/socdev/unpfii/documents/DRIPS_en.pdf).

Unschuld, P. (1975): "Medico-Cultural Conflicts in Asian Settings: An Exploratory Theory." In: Social Science and Medicine, Vol. 9, pp. 303–312.

van der Geest, S. / Reynold White, S. / Hardon, A. (1995): "An Anthropology of Pharmaceuticals. A biographical Approach." In: Annual Review of Anthropology, Vol. 25, pp. 153–175.

van der Geest, S. / Reynold White, S. / Hardon, A. (2006): The Social Lives of Medicine, Cambridge: Cambridge University Press.

van Wyk, B.-E. / van Oudtshoorn, B. / Gericke, N. (2009): Medicinal Plants of South Africa, Pretoria: Briza Publication.

van Gennep, A. (1960): The Rites of Passage. London: Routledge Library Editions.

van Dijk, R. / Spielenberg, M. (2000): The Quest of Fruition through Ngoma. Ohio: Ohio University.

van Sitter, L. (2012): "Nation-Building Knowledge. Dutch Indigenous Knowledge and the Invention of White South Africanism, 1890–1909." In: D. M. Gordon / S. III Krech (eds.), Indigenous Knowledge and the Environment in Africa and North America, Athens: Ohio University Press.

van Wyk, B.-E. (2011): "The Potential of South African Plants in the Development of New Medicinal Products." In: South African Journal of Botany, 77(4), pp. 812–829.

van Wyk, B.-E. (2008): "A Broad Review of Commercially Important Southern African Medicinal Plants." In: Journal of Ethnopharmacology, Vol. 119, pp. 342–355.

van Wyk, B.-E. / Dugmore, H. (2004): Muthi and Myths from the African Bush, Pretoria: Marula Books.

van Wyk, B.-E. / Gericke, N. (2000): People's Plants: A Guide to Useful Plants of Southern Africa, Pretoria: Briza Publishers.

van Wyk, B.-E. / Albrecht, C. (2008): "A Review of the Taxonomy, Ethnobotany, Chemistry and Pharmacology of Sutherlandia Frutescens (Fabaceae)." In: Journal of Ethnopharmacology, Vol. 119(3), pp. 620–629.

van Wyk, B.-E. / van Outshoorn, B. / Gericke, N. (2009) Medicinal Plants of South Africa, Pretoria: Brisa.

van Wyk, B.-E. / Wink, M. (2014): Phytomedicines, Herbal Drugs, and Poisons, Chicago: University of Chicago Press.

van Binsbergen, W. (1991): "Becoming a Sangoma: Religious Anthropological Field-Work in Francistown, Botswana." In: Journal of Religion in Africa, pp. 309–344.

van Binsbergen, W. (2002): The Translation of Southern Africa Sangoma Divination towards a Global Format, and the Validity of the Knowledge It Produces. Paper presented at the symposium "Worldviews, Science and Us", Brussels, Centre Leo Apostel, Free University Brussel, Belgium, 10th June 2003.

van Gennep, A. (1960): The Rites of Passage, London: Routledge.

van Genugten, W. / Meijknecht, A. (2011): Harnessing Intellectual Property Rights for Development Objectives, Nijmegen: Legal Publishers.

Verran, H. (2001): Science and an African Logic, Chicago and London: University of Chicago Press.

Verdery, K. / Humphrey, C. (2004): Property in Question. Value Transformation in the Global Economy, Oxford and New York: Berg.

Vermeylen, S. (2013): "Nagoya Protocol and Customary Law. The Paradox of Narratives in the Law." In: Law Environment and Development (LEAD) Journal, Vol. 9(2), pp. 180–201.

Vermeylen, S. / Martin, G. / Clift, R. (2008): Intellectual Property Rights Systems and the Assemblage of Local Knowledge Systems." In: International Journal of Cultural Property, Vol. 15 (2), pp. 201–221.

Vermeylen, S. (2007): Between Law and Lore. PHD thesis, Guildford: University of Surrey at Guildford.

Viveros de Castro, E. (1998): "Cosmological Deixies and Amerindian Perspectvism." In: Journal of the Royal Anthropological Institute, Vol. 4, pp. 469–488.

von Benda Beckman, K. (1981): "Forum Shopping and Shopping Forums. Dispute Settlement in Minangkabau Village in West Sumatra." In: Journal of Legal Pluralism, Vol. 19, pp. 117–159.

von Benda-Beckmann, K. (2001): "Legal Pluralism." In: Tai Culture, Vol. VI (1&2), pp. 18–40.

von Benda-Beckmann, F. (2002): Who's Afraid of Legal Pluralism?" In: Journal of Legal Pluralism, Vol. 47, pp. 37–82.

von Benda-Beckmann, F. / von Benda-Beckmann, K. / Wiber, M. (2007): Changing Properties of Property. New York / Oxford: Berghahn Books.

von Linné, C. / Agnethler, G. (2015): Systema Naturae, New York: The Scholar's Choice.

Waldby, C. (2002): "Stem Cells, Tissue Cultures and the Production of Biovalue." In: Health: An Interdisciplinary Journal for Social Study of Health, Illness and Medicine, Vol. 6(3), pp. 305–323.

Waldram, James B. (1998): "The Efficacy of Traditional Medicine: Current Theoretical and Methodological Issues." In: Medical Anthropology Quarterly, Vol. 14(4), pp. 603–625.

Watson, P. (2005): Idea. A History of Thought and Invention. From Fire to Freud, New York: Harper Collins Books.

Watson-Verran, H. & Turnball, D. (1995): "Science and Other Indigenous Knowledge Systems." In: S. Jasnoff / G. Markie / J. Peterson / T. Pinch, Handbook of Science and Technology Studies, Thousand Oaks: Sage, pp. 114–140.

Watts, M. (1999): "Contested Communities, Malignant Markets, and Gilded Governance: Justcie Resource Extraction, and Conservation in the Tropics." In: C.

Zerner (ed.), People, Plants and Justice: The Politics of Nature Conservation, New York: Columbia University Press, pp. 21–51.

White, S. / van der Geest, S. / Hadon, A. (2002): Social Lives of Medicines, Cambridge: Cambridge University Press.

Williams, V. L. / Balkwill, E. / Witkoski, K. T. F. (2000): "Unraveling the Commercial Market for Medicinal Plants and Plant Parts on the Witwatersrand. South Africa." In: Economic Botany, Vol. 54(3), pp. 310–327.

Waldby, C. (2002): "Stem Cells, Tissue Cultures and the Production of Biovalue." In: Health: An Interdisciplinary Journal for Social Study of health, Illness and Medicine, Vol. 6(3), pp. 305–323.

Weiner, A. (1985): "Inalienable Wealth." In: American Anthropologist, Vol. 12(2), pp. 210–227.

Weiner, A. (1992): Inalienable Possessions: The Paradox of Keeping While Giving, Berkeley: University of California Press.

Wessinger, C. (1996): Millennialism, Persecution, and Violence: Historical Cases, New York: Syracuse University Press.

West, P. (2005): "Translation, Value, and Space: Theorizing an Ethnographic and Engaged Environmental Anthropology." In: American Anthropologist, Vol. 107 (4), pp. 632–642.

WHO (2000): General Guidelines for the Methodologies on Research and Evaluation of Traditional Medicine. World Health Organization, Geneva, Janury 24, 2019 (http://apps.who.int/medicinedocs/pdf/whozip42e/ whozip42e.pdf).

WHO (2004): Guidelines on Good Agricultural and Collection Practices (GACP) for Medicinal Plants, Geneva: World Health Organization (http://apps.who.int/ medicinedocs/en/d/Js4928e/).

Wilson, W. / Goggin, K. / Williams, K. / Gerkovich, M. / Gqaleni, N. / Syce, J. / Bartman, P. / Johnson, Q. / Folk, W. (2012): Safety of Sutherlandia Fructescens in HIV-Seropositive South African Adults: An Adaptive Double-Blind Randomize Placebo Controlled Trial (https://sahivsoc.org/Files/Douglas%20Wilson%20-%20Safety%20 of%20Sutherlandia%20fructescens%20%2827%20Nov,%2013h30%29.pdf).

WIPO Documentation Toolkit, January 24, 2019 (http://www. wipo.int/export/sites/www/tk/en/resources/pdf/tk_toolkit_draft.pdf).

Wolf, M. (1999): "The Emergence of a Sociology of Translation." In: M. Wolf / A. Fukari (eds.), Constructing a Sociology of Translation, Amsterdam: John Benjamins Publishing.

Wreford, J. (2009): The Pragmatics of Knowledge Transfer: An HIV/AIDS Intervention with Traditional Health Practitioners in South Africa, Centre for Social Science Research (CSSR), University of Cape Town, No. 260.

Wreford, J. T. (2008): Working with Spirit. Experiencing Izangoma Healing in Contemporary South Africa, New York and Oxford: Berghahn Books.

Wreford, J. / Esser, M. / Hippler, S. (2007): Involving Traditional Health Practitioner in HIV/AIDS Interventions: Lessons from the Western Cape, Centre for Social Science Research (CSSR), University of Cape Town, No. 210.

Wynberg, R. / Schroeder, D. / Chennels, R. (eds.) (2009): Indigenous Peoples, Consent and Benefit Sgaring. Lessons from the San-Hoodia Case, Heidelberg, London and New York: Springer.

Wynberg, R. (2005): "Rhetoric, Realism and Benefit-SharinUse of Traditional Knowledge of Hoodia Species in the Development of an Appetite Suppressant." In: The Journal of World Intellectual Property, Vol. 7(6), pp. 851–876.

Wynberg, R. / Laird, S. (2009): "Bioprospecting, Access and Benefit Sharing: Revisiting the Grand Bargain." In: R. Wynberg / D. Schroeder / R. Chennels, Indigenous Peoples, Consent and Benefit Sharing, Dortrecht, London, Heidelberg and New York: Springer.

Yudice, G. (2003): The Expediency of Culture, Durham: Duke University Press.

Zenkler, J. (2010): "Traditionelle Medizin und Afrikanische Renaissance in Südafrika." In: Dilger & Hadolt: Medizin im Kontext.

Zenker, J. (2011): The Modernisation of Traditional Healing in South Africa: Healers, Biomedicine and the State, Halle/Saale: Dissertationsschrift: Philsophische Fakultät.

Zenker, O. (2011): "Autochthony, Ethnicity, Indigeneity and Nationalism: Time-Honouring and State-Oriented Modes of Rooting Individual-Territory-Group-Triads in a Globalizing World." In: Critique of Anthropology, Vol. 31(1), pp. 63–81.

Zenker, O. (2012): "The Juridication of Political Protest and the Politicisation of Legalism in South African Land Restitution." In: J. Eckert / B. Donahoe / C. Strümpell / Z. Ö. Biner (eds.), Law against the State: Ethnographic Forays into Law's Transformations, Cambridge: Cambridge University Press.

Zenker, O. (2014): "New Law against an Old State: Land Restitution as a Transition to Justice in Post-Apartheid South Africa." In: Development and Change. Special Issue: Transition and Justice: Negotiating the Terms of New Beginnings in Africa, Vol. 45(3), pp. 502–523.

Ziervogel, D. (1954): The Eastern Sotho, Pretoria: Van Schaik.

Additional Websites

ABS Capacity Development Initiative (www.abs-initiative.info).

African Centre for Biosafety (2016): Major breakthrough in the fight against biopiracy: Pelargonium patents (www.evb.ch/fileadmin/files/documents / Biodiversitaet/Paper_knowledge_not_for_sale.pdf).

Afrinatural Holdings (www.afrinatural.com).

Cape Nature (www.capenature.co.za).

Gaiaresearch (www.gaiaresearch.co.za).

Medical Research Council Innovation Centre (www.innovation.mrc. ac.za/malaria.pdf).

South African Department of Science and Technology (www.dst.gov.za).

South African San Institute's website (www.san.org.za).

Sutherlandia.org (www.sutherlandia.org).

Traditional Healers Organization, Johannesburg (www.traditional health.org.za/t/documents/biodiversity_and_intellectual_property_rights_02.html).

Zizamele Herbs (www.zizamele.com/about_us/about_zizameleherbs.html).

Social and Cultural Studies

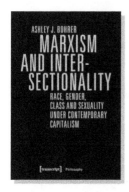

Ashley J. Bohrer
Marxism and Intersectionality
Race, Gender, Class and Sexuality
under Contemporary Capitalism

2019, 280 p., pb.
29,99 € (DE), 978-3-8376-4160-8
E-Book: 26,99 € (DE), ISBN 978-3-8394-4160-2

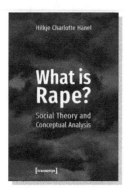

Hilkje Charlotte Hänel
What is Rape?
Social Theory and Conceptual Analysis

2018, 282 p., hardcover
99,99 € (DE), 978-3-8376-4434-0
E-Book: 99,99 € (DE), ISBN 978-3-8394-4434-4

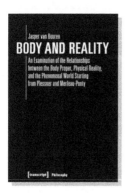

Jasper van Buuren
Body and Reality
An Examination of the Relationships
between the Body Proper, Physical Reality,
and the Phenomenal World Starting from Plessner
and Merleau-Ponty

2018, 312 p., pb., ill.
39,99 € (DE), 978-3-8376-4163-9
E-Book: 39,99 € (DE), ISBN 978-3-8394-4163-3

**All print, e-book and open access versions of the titles in our list
are available in our online shop www.transcript-verlag.de/en!**

Social and Cultural Studies

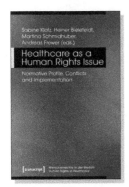

Sabine Klotz, Heiner Bielefeldt,
Martina Schmidhuber, Andreas Frewer (eds.)
Healthcare as a Human Rights Issue
Normative Profile, Conflicts and Implementation

2017, 426 p., pb., ill.
39,99 € (DE), 978-3-8376-4054-0
E-Book: available as free open access publication
E-Book: ISBN 978-3-8394-4054-4

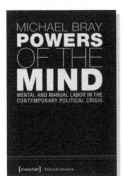

Michael Bray
Powers of the Mind
Mental and Manual Labor
in the Contemporary Political Crisis

2019, 208 p., hardcover
99,99 € (DE), 978-3-8376-4147-9
E-Book: 99,99 € (DE), ISBN 978-3-8394-4147-3

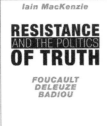

Iain MacKenzie
Resistance and the Politics of Truth
Foucault, Deleuze, Badiou

2018, 148 p., pb.
29,99 € (DE), 978-3-8376-3907-0
E-Book: 26,99 € (DE), ISBN 978-3-8394-3907-4
EPUB: 26,99 € (DE), ISBN 978-3-7328-3907-0

**All print, e-book and open access versions of the titles in our list
are available in our online shop www.transcript-verlag.de/en!**

CPSIA information can be obtained
at www.ICGtesting.com
Printed in the USA
JSHW021307240420
5281JS00001B/2

9 783837 647945